Teen Health

Course 1

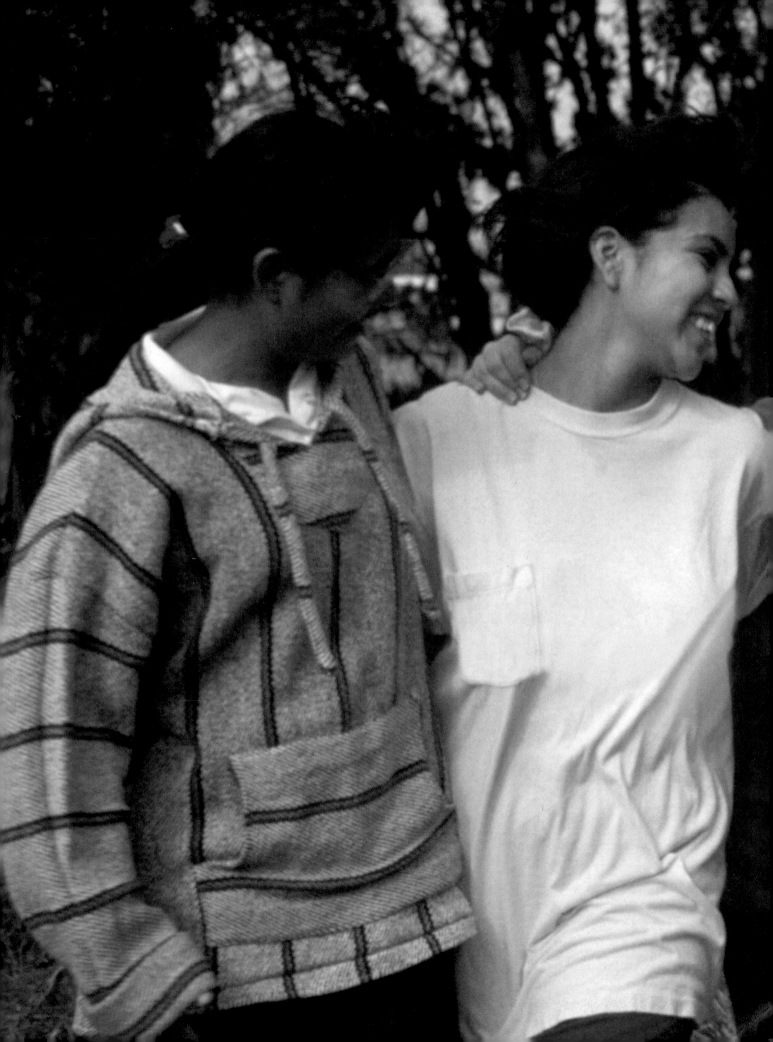

Teen Health
Course 1

Mary Bronson Merki, Ph.D.

Michael J. Cleary, Ed.D.

Betty M. Hubbard, Ed.D., C.H.E.S.

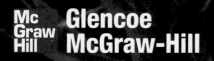

Glencoe
McGraw-Hill

New York, New York   Columbus, Ohio   Chicago, Illinois   Peoria, Illinois   Woodland Hills, California

Meet the Authors

Mary Bronson Merki, Ph.D., has taught health education in grades K–12. As Health Education Specialist for the Dallas School District, Dr. Merki developed and implemented a district-wide health education program, *Skills for Living,* which was used as a model by the state education agency. She also helped develop and implement the district's Human Growth, Development, and Sexuality program, which won the National PTA's Excellence in Education Award. In 1992 and 1998, she was selected as Teacher of the Year by her peers. In 1996 and again in 2000, she was recognized in *Who's Who Among American Teachers.* Dr. Merki recently retired after 30 years of teaching in Texas public schools.

Michael J. Cleary, Ed.D., is Professor and School Health Education Coordinator at Slippery Rock University. Dr. Cleary taught at Evanston Township High School in Evanston, Illinois, and later became the Lead Teacher Specialist at the McMillen Center for Health Education in Fort Wayne, Indiana. Dr. Cleary has published and presented widely on curriculum development and portfolio assessment in K–12 health education. Dr. Cleary is the coauthor of *Managing Your Health: Assessment for Action.* He is a Certified Health Education Specialist.

Betty M. Hubbard, Ed.D., C.H.E.S., has taught health education in grades K–12 as well as health education methods classes at the undergraduate and graduate levels. She is a professor at the University of Central Arkansas, teaching classes in curriculum development, mental health, and human sexuality. Dr. Hubbard supervises student teachers and conducts in-service training for health education teachers in school districts throughout Arkansas. Her publications, grants, and presentations focus on research-based, comprehensive health instruction.

Glencoe/McGraw-Hill

A Division of The McGraw·Hill Companies

Printed in the United States of America.

Send all inquiries to:
Glencoe/McGraw-Hill
21600 Oxnard Street, Suite 500
Woodland Hills, California 91367

ISBN 0-07-823935-4 (Course 1 Student Text)
ISBN 0-07-823936-2 (Course 1 Teacher Wraparound Edition)

5 6 7 8 9   004   07 06 05 04

Health Consultants

UNIT 1
A Healthy Foundation

Stephanie S. Allen
Senior Lecturer
Baylor University, Louise
Herrington School of
Nursing
Dallas, Texas

Victoria Bisorca, C.H.E.S.
Lecturer
California State University,
Long Beach
Long Beach, California

Howard S. Shapiro, M.D.
Associate Professor
University of Southern
California School of
Medicine
Los Angeles, California

Linda Stevenson, Ph.D., R.N.
Assistant Professor
Baylor University, Louise
Herrington School of
Nursing
Dallas, Texas

UNIT 2
Promoting Physical Health

Roberta Larson Duyff, R.D.
Food and Nutrition
Consultant/President
Duyff Associates
St. Louis, Missouri

Mark Giese, Ed.D.
Chair, Department of Health,
Science, and Kinesiology
Northeastern State University
Tahlequah, Oklahoma

Jan King
Teacher
Neshaminy School District
Langhorne, Pennsylvania

Tinker D. Murray, Ph.D.
Professor and Coordinator of
the Exercise and Sports
Science Program
Southwest Texas State
University
San Marcos, Texas

Alice Pappas, Ph.D., R.N.
Associate Professor/Associate
Dean
Baylor University, Louise
Herrington School of
Nursing
Dallas, Texas

Don Rainey
Instructor, Coordinator of the
Physical Fitness and
Wellness Program
Southwest Texas State
University
San Marcos, Texas

**Sherman Sowby, Ph.D.,
C.H.E.S.**
Professor of Health Science
California State University,
Fresno
Fresno, California

Catherine Strain, R.D.
Associate Professor
Marian College
Indianapolis, Indiana

UNIT 3
Protecting Your Health

Sally Champlin, C.H.E.S.
Faculty
California State University,
Long Beach
Long Beach, California

Jill English, Ph.D., C.H.E.S.
Assistant Professor
California State University,
Fullerton
Fullerton, California

Sharon Gonzales, R.N.
Nurse
Thomas Grover Middle School
Princeton Junction, New Jersey

David Sleet, Ph.D.
Associate Director for Science
Division of Unintentional
Injury Prevention
Centers for Disease Control
and Prevention (CDC)
Atlanta, Georgia

Reviewers

Beverly J. Berkin, C.H.E.S.
Health Education Consultant
Bedford Corners, New York

Donna Breitenstein, Ed.D.
Professor & Coordinator of Health Education
Director of North Carolina School Health
    Training Center
Appalachian State University
Boone, North Carolina

Julie Campbell-Fouch
Health Teacher, Department Chair
Stanford Middle School
Long Beach, California

Pamela R. Connolly
Subject Area Coordinator for Health and
    Physical Education, Diocese of Pittsburgh
Curriculum Coordinator for Health and Physical
    Education, North Catholic High School
Pittsburgh, Pennsylvania

Pat Freedman
Instructional Coordinator for Student Wellness
Humble Independent School District
Humble, Texas

Ginger Lawless, C.H.E.S.
Dyslexia and School Health Education Specialist
Fort Bend Independent School District
Sugar Land, Texas

James Robinson III, Ed.D.
Professor, Assistant Dean for Student Affairs
The Texas A&M University System
Health Science Center
School of Rural Public Health
College Station, Texas

Michael Rulon
Health/Physical Education Teacher
Johnson Junior High School
Adjunct Faculty, Laramie County
    Community College
Cheyenne, Wyoming

Jeanne Title
Coordinator, Prevention Education
Napa County Office of Education and Napa
    Valley Unified School District
Napa, California

Brief Contents

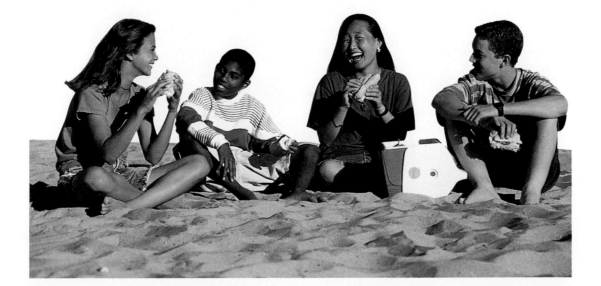

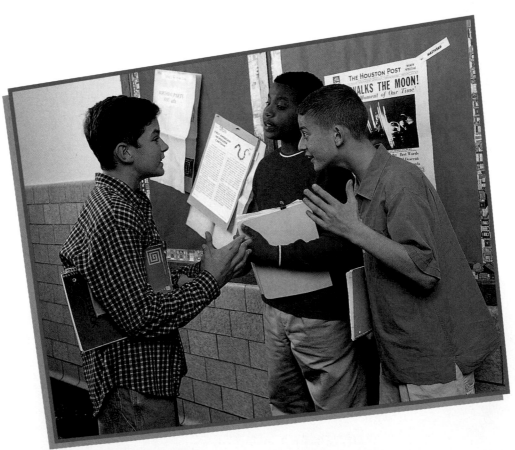

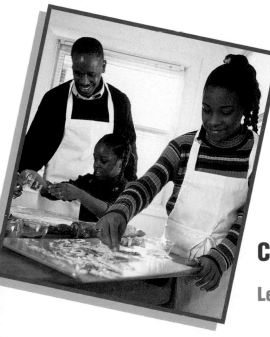

x

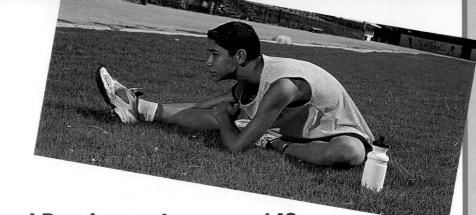

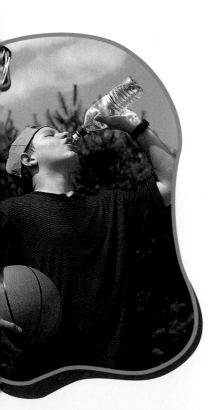

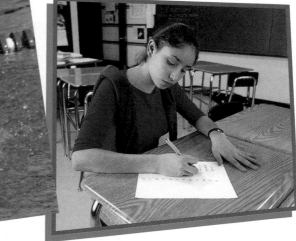

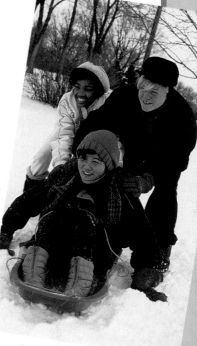

Features

Hands-On Health

HEALTH SKILLS ACTIVITIES

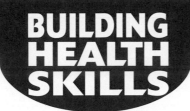
BUILDING HEALTH SKILLS

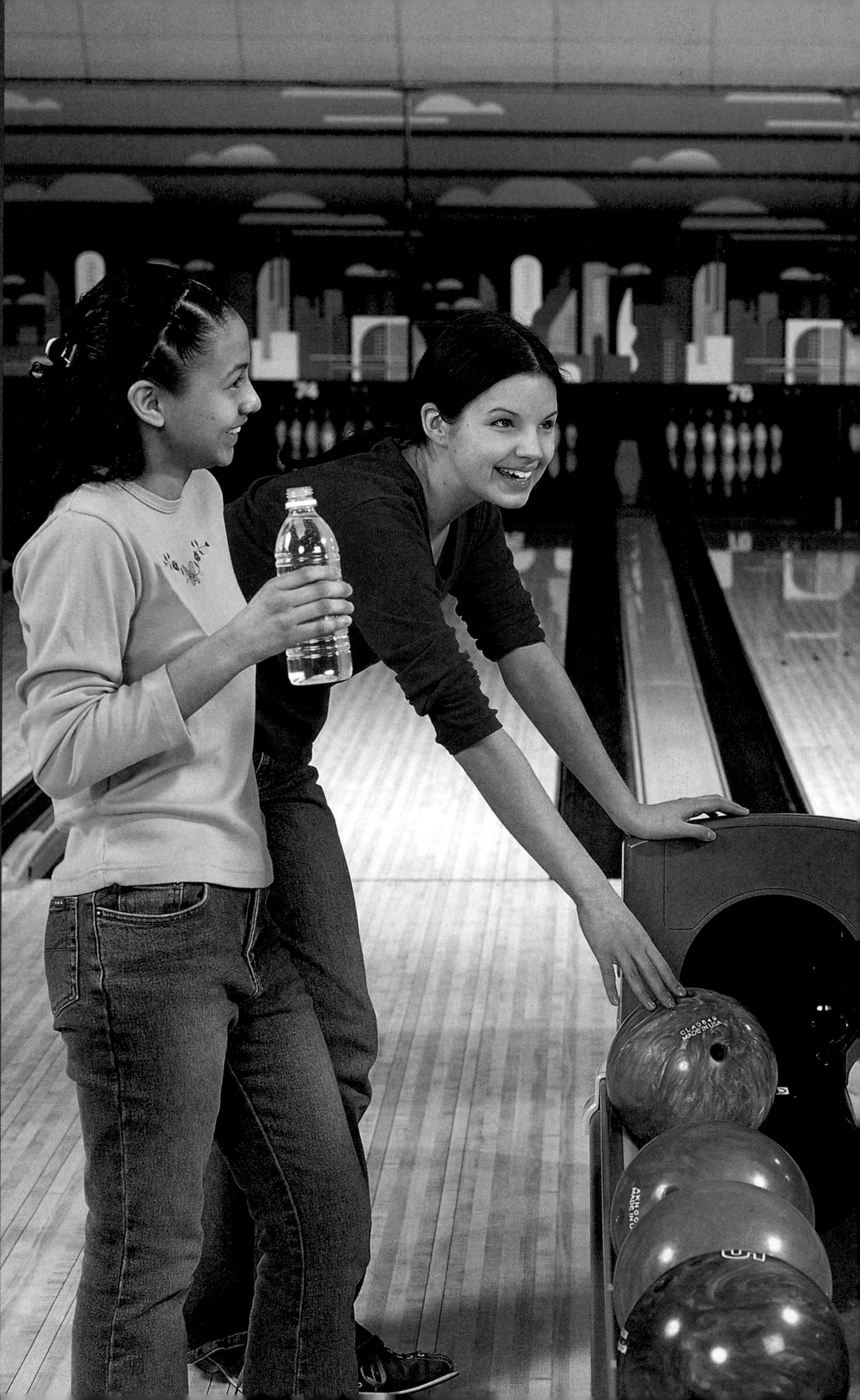

A Healthy Foundation

Technology Project

Word Processing Project
Share what you know about important health decisions in a report or a letter to your family.
- Log on to health.glencoe.com.
- Click on Technology Projects and find the "Practice with Word Processing" activity.
- Use Save, Edit, and Format functions to personalize your report.

In Your Home and Community

Goal Setting
Make a plan to spend a few hours a week with your family in an activity other than watching television. Eat dinner together, play a board game, do volunteer work in your community, read a book out loud, or sit and talk about an issue that is important to one of you. See if you can plan an outing based on one of your discussions. Set a goal to have these family evenings on a regular basis.

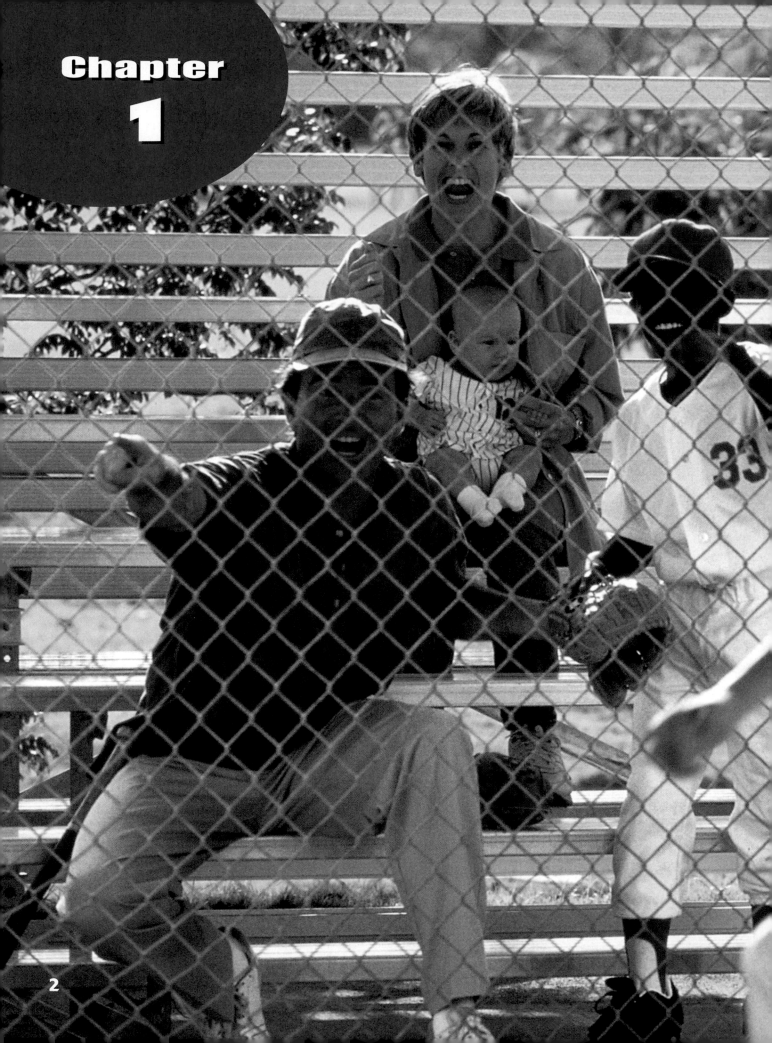

Living a Healthy Life

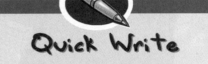

Your Health and Wellness

Quick Write

Describe in a sentence or two what you think it means to lead a healthy life.

LEARN ABOUT...

- the relationship between health and wellness.
- keeping your physical, mental/emotional, and social health in balance.

VOCABULARY

- health
- wellness
- habit

Taking Charge of Your Health

You may have heard the saying, "Today is the first day of the rest of your life." Think about the meaning of this statement. What you do today affects you throughout your life. This is especially true where your health is concerned.

Health is *a combination of physical, mental, emotional, and social well-being.* It might help you to think of health as a triangle—see **Figure 1.1**. One part of the triangle is your physical health—the condition of your body. Another part is your mental and emotional health—your thoughts and feelings. The third part of the triangle is your social health—the way you relate to other people.

What other parts of the health triangle are these teens working on?

Playing soccer is one way to improve your physical health.

Maintaining Your Health Balance

Being healthy means keeping your health triangle in balance. Here are some ways to work on all three sides of your health triangle:

- **Physical.** Get regular physical activity, eat nutritious foods, and get enough rest.
- **Mental/emotional.** Take time to study, to think, and to express your feelings in healthy ways.
- **Social.** Spend time with both family and friends.

Remember that changes you make to one side of your health triangle will also affect the other two sides. For example, if you spend more time playing sports, your physical health will improve. This will also help you feel better about yourself, improving your mental health.

FIGURE 1.1

The Health Triangle

Keeping your health triangle in balance is one of the keys to lifelong health.

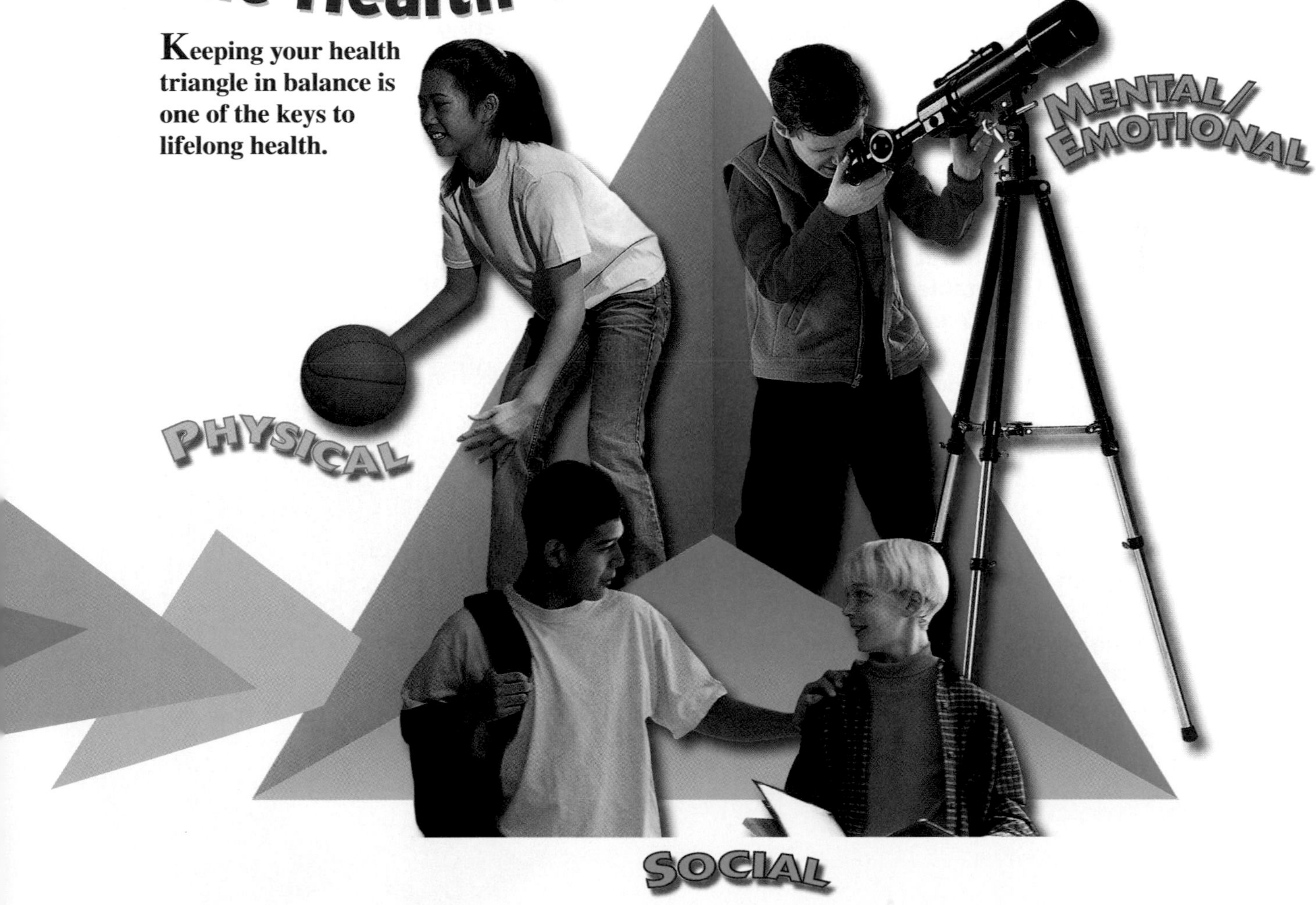

MENTAL/EMOTIONAL

PHYSICAL

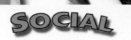

SOCIAL

Keep in mind that all three sides of your health triangle will not develop at the same rate. This is normal. It's also normal to find your health triangle temporarily out of balance. The important thing is to notice when one side is out of balance and take steps to change. This balance is the key to lifelong health and wellness.

Hands-On Health

YOUR PERSONAL HEALTH

Do you have a clear and accurate view of your own health triangle? Take this personal health inventory to find out.

WHAT YOU WILL NEED
- pencil or pen
- paper

WHAT YOU WILL DO
Number the paper 1–6 for each health area. Think about each of the following statements and respond with *yes* or *no*.

Physical Health
1. I eat at least three well-balanced meals each day.
2. I snack on healthful foods such as fruits and vegetables.
3. I get at least 60 minutes of physical activity daily.
4. I sleep at least eight hours a night.
5. I avoid the use of tobacco, alcohol, and other drugs.
6. I have good personal hygiene habits.

Mental/Emotional Health
1. I accept myself and feel good about who I am.
2. I can name several things that I can do well.
3. I generally keep a positive attitude.
4. I ask for help when I need it.
5. I am able to handle stress.
6. I try to improve myself.

Social Health
1. I relate well to family, friends, and classmates.
2. I try to work out any differences I have with others.
3. I express my feelings in positive ways.
4. I treat others with respect.
5. I can say no to risky behaviors.
6. I communicate well with others.

IN CONCLUSION
Give yourself 1 point for each *yes*. A score of 5–6 in any area reflects good health. If you score 0–2 in any area, try to improve that part of your health triangle.

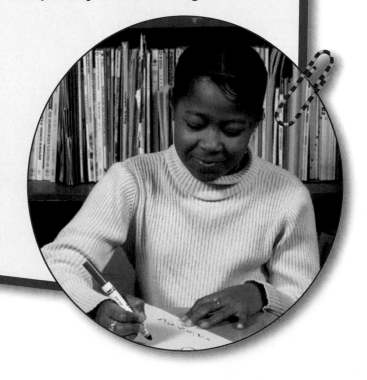

Wellness

Wellness is *a state of well-being, or balanced health.* To maintain wellness, take care of health problems as they come up. You should also try to protect and improve your health.

You can achieve wellness through good health habits. A **habit** is *a pattern of behavior that you follow almost without thinking.* One good habit is washing your hands before you eat. It's much easier to develop good habits now than to change bad habits later.

✓ Reading Check

Each part in a compound word is a word by itself, as in *notebook.* Find at least three compound words in Lesson 1.

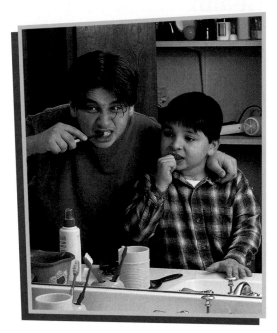

Good health habits help you maintain a high level of wellness. *Explain how this teen's habits protect his and his brother's health.*

Lesson 1 Review

Using complete sentences, answer the following questions on a sheet of paper.

Reviewing Terms and Facts

1. **Vocabulary** Define *health* and *wellness.*
2. **List** What are the three parts of the health triangle?
3. **Describe** Give an example of good social health.

Thinking Critically

4. **Analyze** Explain how a change to one side of the health triangle can affect the other two sides.

5. **Hypothesize** Why do you think it is easier to develop good health habits than to break bad ones?

Applying Health Skills

6. **Analyzing Influences** Think of one good health habit that you have. Write a paragraph explaining how you first developed the habit. Then describe how the habit contributes to your health and wellness.

Building Health Skills

Quick Write

List three things you do to maintain your health. Preview this lesson and identify the health skills that you are practicing when you do each of these activities.

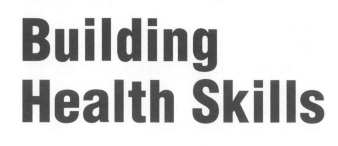

LEARN ABOUT...

- what skills help you stay healthy.
- how you can promote your health and the health of others.

VOCABULARY

- prevention

Skills for Good Health

One of the keys to wellness is the prevention of illness. **Prevention** is *keeping something from happening.* You can prevent illness and injury in many ways. For example:

- **Physical Health.** Get regular medical and dental checkups. Wear protective gear when you play sports. Always wear safety belts.
- **Mental and Emotional Health.** Talk to your parents or guardians about health-related concerns. Learn to manage stress. Think positively.
- **Social Health.** Try to get along with family and friends. Avoid gossiping or spreading rumors. Choose friends who avoid tobacco, alcohol, and other drugs.

All the examples listed above demonstrate health skills. These are skills that help you become healthy and stay healthy. The health skills that you develop now will have a positive effect throughout your life. **Figure 1.2** shows ten important health skills.

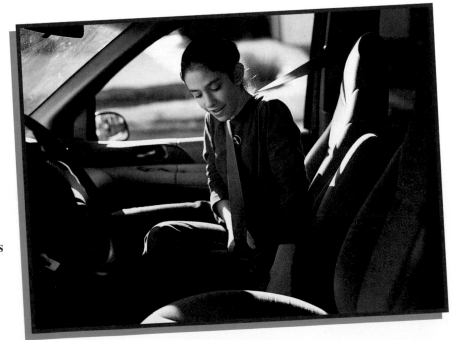

Wearing a safety belt is one way to prevent injury. *What other ways can you think of?*

FIGURE 1.2

THE HEALTH SKILLS

These ten skills affect your physical, mental/emotional, and social health. These skills can help you, not just during your teen years, but throughout your entire life.

Health Skill	What It Means to You
Accessing Information	You know how to find reliable health information and health-promoting products and services.
Practicing Healthful Behaviors	You take action to reduce risks and protect yourself against illness and injury.
Stress Management	You find healthy ways to manage and reduce the stress in your life.
Analyzing Influences	You recognize the many factors that influence your health, including culture, media, and technology.
Communication Skills	You express your ideas and feelings and listen when others express theirs.
Refusal Skills	You can say no to risky behaviors.
Conflict Resolution	You work out problems with others in healthy ways.
Decision Making	You think through problems and find healthy solutions.
Goal Setting	You plan for the future and work to make your plans come true.
Advocacy	You take a stand and make a difference in your home, school, and community.

Accessing Information

Knowing how to access, or obtain, reliable health information is an important skill. Sources of information include:

- **Knowledgeable Adults:** parents and guardians, health professionals, teachers, religious leaders, and others.
- **Library Resources:** encyclopedias and nonfiction books on medicine, science, nutrition, and fitness.
- **Mass Media:** news reports and articles by health professionals, scientists, and others.
- **The Internet:** up-to-the-minute information provided by government agencies and qualified health professionals.
- **Community Resources:** government agencies, hospitals, clinics, colleges, and health organizations like the American Red Cross.

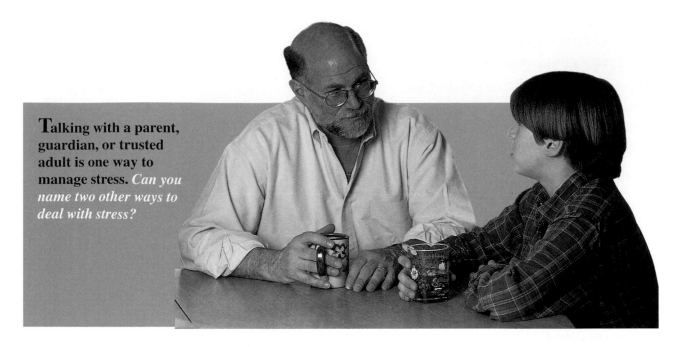

Talking with a parent, guardian, or trusted adult is one way to manage stress. *Can you name two other ways to deal with stress?*

Taking Care of Yourself

The next two health skills involve self-management, or taking care of yourself.

- **Practicing Healthful Behaviors.** You can take care of yourself by practicing healthful behaviors, or actions that help maintain good health. These include eating nutritious foods, staying active, getting enough sleep, and taking time to relax when you feel tired.
- **Stress Management.** You can also take care of yourself by learning to cope with stress. Stress is part of life. Sometimes you may not be able to control the amount of stress in your life. However, you can control how you react to it. Managing stress means finding a way to deal with it rather than letting it control you.

Analyzing Influences

Why do you do the things you do? Many factors influence your behavior. These factors can be internal or external.

- *Internal* influences come from inside you. For example, your personal likes and desires influence the foods you eat, the activities you choose, and the friends you spend time with.
- *External* influences come from outside sources. People can influence you, including parents, teachers, and friends. Television shows, books, advertisements, and movies can also influence your behavior. Finally, you are influenced by your culture, your environment, and the laws of your community.

Communicating with Others

The next group of skills involves the way you communicate with other people. Communication is the clear exchange of ideas and information. That means telling others how you feel and listening to and understanding how they feel.

- **Refusal Skills.** Sometimes you have to say no to others. For example, people you know may try to pressure you into doing something that you think is wrong. Refusal skills help you say no in an effective way, without feeling uncomfortable.

- **Conflict Resolution.** When you have conflicts, or disagreements, with others, it's best to settle them in a way that satisfies everyone. Conflict resolution usually requires talking matters over calmly and reasonably. Both people must work together to find a solution to the problem.

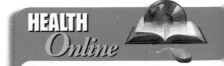

HEALTH *Online*

Building health skills helps you take charge of your life. Find out more in Web Links at **health.glencoe.com.**

HEALTH SKILLS ACTIVITY

COMMUNICATION SKILLS

When Friends Change

Tia and Carlos have been friends since second grade. Lately, though, Tia has noticed a change in Carlos. The two friends used to meet at their lockers after school and talk about what happened that day. Twice in the last week, Carlos told Tia he would be there, but then he didn't show up. The last time it happened, Tia had something important to tell Carlos. The next day she heard from another friend that Carlos had told people that Tia was boring. What should Tia do?

What Would You Do?

Write a dialogue between Tia and Carlos. Have Tia tell Carlos how she feels about his behavior. Then have Carlos explain why he is acting that way. Use the speaking skills shown below.

- Use "I" messages.
- Use clear, simple statements.
- State your thoughts and feelings honestly.
- Make eye contact and use appropriate body language.

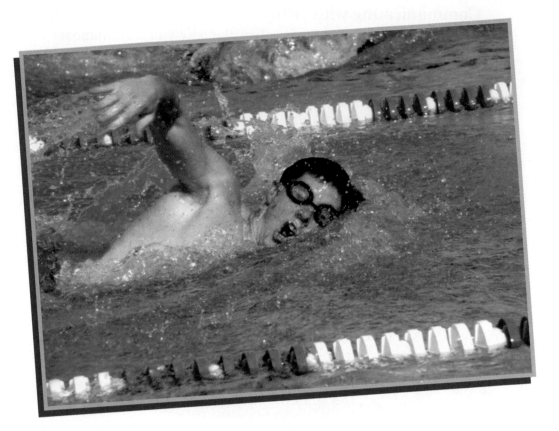

Martin wants to spend more time on his favorite hobby, swimming. *What specific goals might he set for himself?*

Decision Making and Goal Setting

Decision making and goal setting are related skills. For example, suppose you hear about tryouts for the track team. First, you might make a decision to try out. Then you could set a goal to start running every day for practice. That goal would help you improve your speed so you would be more likely to make the team.

Making decisions and setting goals are step-by-step processes that require careful thought. They are important skills that help you shape your life in a positive way.

Advocacy

Most health skills help you keep yourself healthy. However, advocacy has more to do with the health of others. To advocate something means to support it or speak out in favor of it. When you advocate for health, you encourage other people to live healthy lives. You can practice advocacy by showing that you feel strongly about healthful behaviors. You can also provide people in your home, school, or community with the information they need to make healthful choices.

Health Skills and Wellness

Throughout your teen years, you will learn and practice many different skills. For example, you build your skills in reading and math, music and art, and perhaps sports. Like any skill, the ten health skills must be learned and then practiced regularly. Then, as you develop your health skills, you can apply them to everyday activities. Doing so will help you lead a healthy life. Your health skills will also help you keep your health triangle in balance.

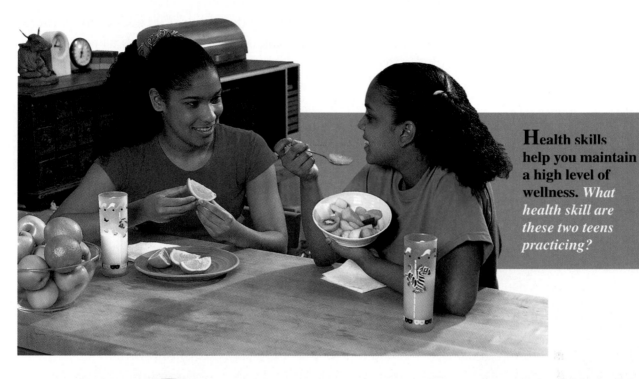

Health skills help you maintain a high level of wellness. *What health skill are these two teens practicing?*

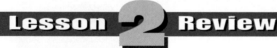

Lesson 2 Review

Using complete sentences, answer the following questions on a sheet of paper.

Reviewing Terms and Facts

1. **Vocabulary** Define the word *prevention*. Use it in an original sentence.
2. **Recall** How do internal influences differ from external influences? Give two examples of each.
3. **Give Examples** Give an example of a situation in which you might need to practice refusal skills.

Thinking Critically

4. **Apply** Think of a decision you made recently about your health. Then name one or more goals you might set as a result of that decision.
5. **Analyze** Why is advocacy considered a health skill?

Applying Health Skills

6. **Accessing Information** Make a poster showing possible sources of information that someone might use to find answers to health-related questions.

Decisions and Your Character

Quick Write

List three health-related decisions that you had to make during the past week. Which one was the hardest to make? Why?

LEARN ABOUT...

- how your decisions reflect your character.
- how you can make responsible decisions.
- how your decisions affect your health.

VOCABULARY

- decision
- consequence
- risk
- cumulative risk
- values
- character

Types of Decisions

Every day you face many decisions. **Decisions** are *choices that you make.* Some decisions are minor, such as picking out clothes to wear. Other decisions can have serious **consequences**, or *results.* During your teen years, you'll have many important decisions to make.

When making decisions, it is important to consider the risk involved. **Risk** is *the chance of harm or loss.* Any decision that involves a risk to your health is an important one and requires careful thought. Here are some examples of decisions that affect your health:

- **Physical Health.** What kinds of foods will I eat? How much physical activity will I get?
- **Mental/Emotional Health.** How much time will I spend studying? Which people can I talk to about my problems?
- **Social Health.** Who will my friends be? What activities will I do in my free time?

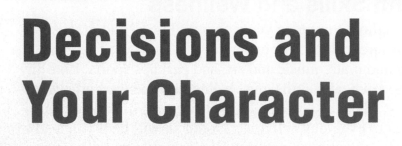

Choosing to wear a bike helmet is an important decision for your health. *What other decisions affect your health?*

How to Make Healthy Decisions

For important decisions, you need to take a thoughtful, step-by-step approach. An important decision can seem overwhelming—like a huge mountain you have to climb. You may worry that you'll make the wrong choice. You may even do nothing and hope that you won't have to make any choice at all.

However, making a decision doesn't have to be scary. The "secret" is to view decision making as a *process*—that is, a series of steps. **Figure 1.3** shows several steps you can follow.

FIGURE 1.3

The Decision-Making Process

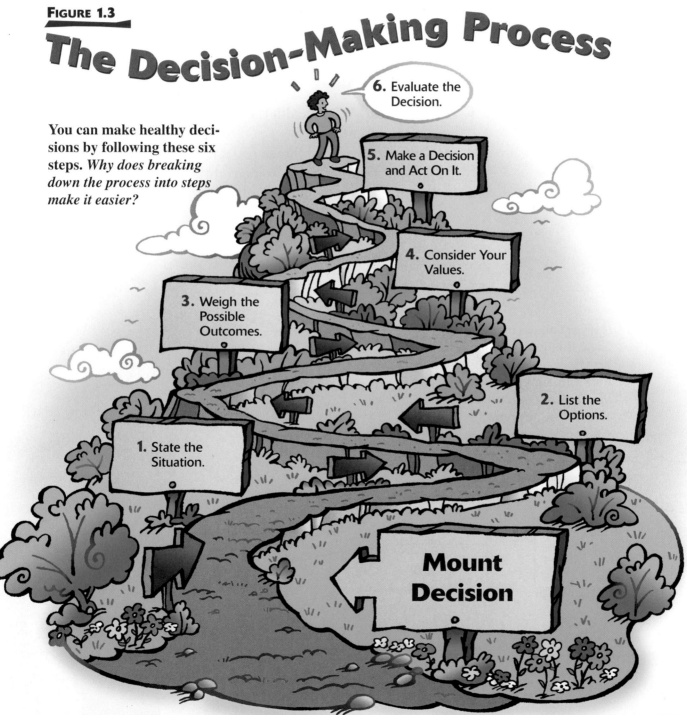

You can make healthy decisions by following these six steps. *Why does breaking down the process into steps make it easier?*

6. Evaluate the Decision.

5. Make a Decision and Act On It.

4. Consider Your Values.

3. Weigh the Possible Outcomes.

2. List the Options.

1. State the Situation.

Mount Decision

Reading Check

Make up a memory device similar to H.E.L.P. to remember the good character traits listed on page 17.

Step 1: State the Situation

To make a healthy decision, first understand the situation. This isn't always simple. You need to consider all the facts and who else is involved.

Step 2: List the Options

Once you have a clear view of the situation, think of your options. Don't limit yourself to just one or two choices. Try to think of all the possibilities. If you can, you may want to ask other people for suggestions, too. A family member, teacher, or friend will often come up with ideas you hadn't thought of.

Step 3: Weigh the Possible Outcomes

Consider your options carefully. Use the word *help* to guide your choice.

- **H (Healthful)** What health risks, if any, will this option present?
- **E (Ethical)** Does this choice reflect what you and your family believe to be right?
- **L (Legal)** Does this option violate any local, state, or federal laws?
- **P (Parent Approval)** Would your parents approve of this choice?

Joey set a goal to learn the trumpet. Even though it will be difficult at first, his efforts will make him happier in the long run. *Can you think of a decision that is hard in the short term but desirable in the long term?*

For some decisions, you'll also need to consider **cumulative risk**. Cumulative (KOO·myuh·luh·tiv) risk is *the addition of one risk factor to another, increasing the chance of harm or loss.* For example, riding your bike without a helmet is one risk factor. Riding in traffic is another. Riding at night is a third. Each of these risk factors is serious. When combined, they greatly increase your chances of severe injury.

Step 4: Consider Your Values

Values are *beliefs you feel strongly about that help guide the way you live.* Your values are based on what's important to you and your family. They're also based on what you believe is right or wrong. If your values are strong, any decision you make should be in agreement with them. If it isn't, you probably won't feel comfortable with the decision.

Values are part of your **character**, or *the way you think, feel, and act.* Examples of good character include:

- **Trustworthiness.** Trustworthy people are reliable and honest. You can count on them to keep their promises.
- **Respect.** Displaying respect means showing regard for other people and for authority.
- **Responsibility.** You show responsibility by being willing to accept the credit or the blame for what you do.
- **Fairness.** Being fair means treating everyone equally and honestly.
- **Caring.** You can show others you care for them by treating them with understanding and consideration. Caring people are kind and try to help others when they can.
- **Citizenship.** Good citizens obey rules and laws. They do what they can to help their school, community, and country.

These character traits influence your decisions in many ways. For example, suppose you saw a friend stealing. As a caring friend, you might want to keep silent to protect your friend. However, your sense of fairness might prompt you to speak out.

Developing Good Character

Decisions and Character

You know that your character affects the decisions you make. You can also use your decisions to help build good character. When you are faced with a decision, ask yourself: *What would a trustworthy person do? A responsible person? A caring person?*

Step 5: Make a Decision and Act on It

You've thought about and compared the options. You've considered the risks and consequences. Now you're ready to make a decision and act on it. Choose the course of action that seems best and is consistent with your values. You should feel comfortable with your choice, even if it isn't a "perfect" solution. If none of your choices satisfy you, go back to Step 2 and look for new options.

Step 6: Evaluate the Decision

After carrying out your decision, evaluate the results. What were the positive results? Were there negative results? Were there any unexpected outcomes? Was there anything you could have done differently? If the action you took was not as successful as you'd hoped, try again. Use the decision-making process to find another way to deal with the situation.

HEALTH SKILLS ACTIVITY

DECISION MAKING

Leaving the Party

Kim and her best friend Bethany are attending a party at a friend's home. After about an hour, Kim notices that several teens have taken beer from the refrigerator and are drinking it. She tells Bethany that she feels uncomfortable and wants to call her dad to take them home. However, Bethany says she wants to stay and might even try a few sips herself. Kim has to decide what to do.

What Would You Do?

Apply the six steps of the decision-making process to Kim's problem. What decision would you make if you were Kim? Write an explanation of your decision.

1. STATE THE SITUATION.
2. LIST THE OPTIONS.
3. WEIGH THE POSSIBLE OUTCOMES.
4. CONSIDER YOUR VALUES.
5. MAKE A DECISION AND ACT ON IT.
6. EVALUATE THE DECISION.

Good Character, Responsible Decisions

When you think your decisions out carefully, you are more likely to make healthy choices. These decisions can improve your physical, mental/emotional, and social health. They help you steer your life the way you want it to go.

Having good character helps you make healthy decisions. For example, if you are a responsible person, you recognize the consequences of your actions. You think carefully about decisions that affect your health. You are more likely to avoid health risks.

At the same time, responsible decisions build good character. When you are able to make your own decisions, you become more responsible. You take action and accept the consequences. Healthy decisions also encourage respect between you and your friends and family members.

Jenny has made a decision to volunteer at her local library. *How does this decision show good character? How does it help reinforce good character?*

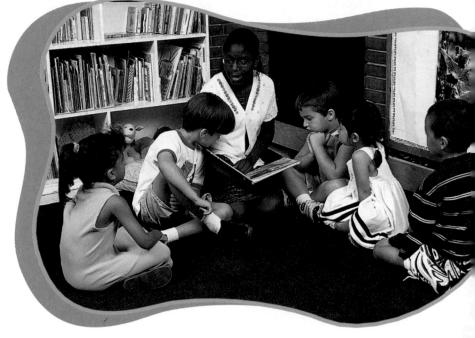

Lesson 3 Review

Using complete sentences, answer the following questions on a sheet of paper.

Reviewing Terms and Facts

1. **Vocabulary** Define the terms *decision* and *consequences*. Write a sentence explaining how the terms are related.
2. **Explain** What should you consider when making decisions?
3. **List** What are the six steps of the decision-making process?
4. **Recall** Why is it important to consider your values when you make a decision?

Thinking Critically

5. **Analyze** How are responsible decisions related to good character?
6. **Select** Choose one of the six steps in the decision-making process and describe its importance to the process.

Applying Health Skills

7. **Advocacy** Make a colorful poster or create a puppet show that could help younger children work through the decision-making process. Remember to keep it simple so they can understand and apply the process. Share your work with your class.

Setting Health Goals

Quick Write

List three things that you would like to accomplish in the next year. Which of the three is most important to you? Why?

LEARN ABOUT...

- why it is important to have goals.
- how to set goals.
- how to reach your goals.

VOCABULARY

- goal
- short-term goal
- long-term goal

Kinds of Goals

A **goal** is *something that you hope to accomplish*. Some goals are broad, such as wanting to be happy or successful. Others are more specific, such as getting a part in a school play or earning enough money to buy new sports equipment.

Your goals may be short-term or long-term. A **short-term goal** is *one that you plan to accomplish in a short time*. A **long-term goal** is *one that you hope to achieve within a period of months or years*. Short-term goals often lead to long-term goals. For example, you may hope to become a doctor someday. To reach this long-term goal, you may have short-term goals such as doing well in science classes. By setting goals, you take charge of your life. See **Figure 1.4**.

Setting a goal for yourself gives you something to work toward. *What goals have you set for yourself?*

FIGURE 1.4 Why Set Goals?

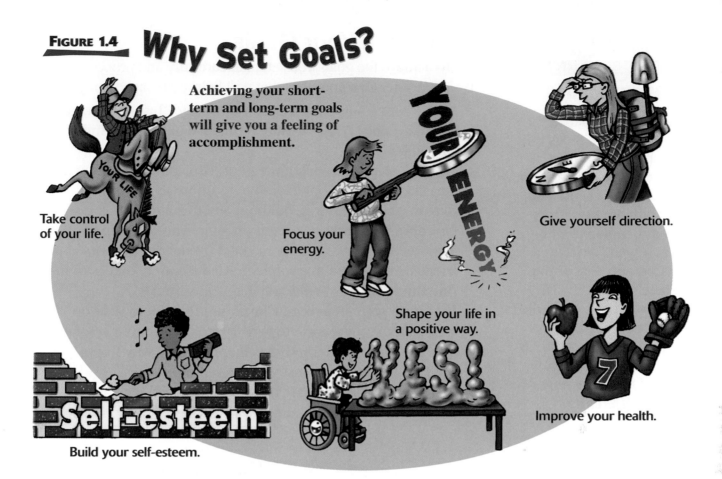

Take control of your life.

Achieving your short-term and long-term goals will give you a feeling of accomplishment.

Focus your energy.

Your Life

Your Energy

Give yourself direction.

Build your self-esteem.

Self-esteem

Shape your life in a positive way.

YES!

Improve your health.

Choosing Your Goals

When you set goals, it's important to consider several factors. First, what are your needs? Everyone has certain basic needs. You need food, clothing, love, and companionship. Second, what are your values? Just as values help you make decisions, they also help you set goals. For example, if your education is important to you, one of your goals may be to get good grades.

Next, think about your interests. The things that interest you the most are the ones you'll probably want to include in your goals. Then consider your skills, abilities, and knowledge. What do you do well? What abilities and knowledge do you need to gain? If you hope to excel as a writer, one of your goals might be to develop your vocabulary.

Keep in mind that your goals should be realistic. If you dream of becoming a great violinist, don't expect to reach your goal in six weeks. Sometimes you'll need more information in order to set a realistic goal. In that case, talk with a parent, teacher, coach, or other trusted adult.

✓ Reading Check

Which term best describes how the information in the Choosing Your Goals section is organized: *sequence, comparison,* or *cause-and-effect*?

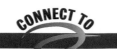

CONNECT TO
Language Arts

GOALS IN LITERATURE
Many stories focus on characters who set specific goals and work to achieve them. Read a book or short story about someone who set a goal. Write a paragraph describing the character's goal and what she or he did to reach it. *Was the character successful? If so, why? If not, what could he or she have done differently?*

Achieving Your Goals

To achieve the goals you set, plan carefully and proceed step by step. Here are some steps that will help you reach your goals:

- **Make your goals specific.** Don't just say, "I want to become a better runner." Say, "I want to run an eight-minute mile by November 1."
- **List the steps to reach your goal.** Break big goals down into smaller tasks. For example, to improve at baseball, plan to practice hitting, fielding, and throwing.
- **Get help from others.** Identify people who can help you achieve your goals. Family members, teachers, coaches, and friends are good sources of help. Also identify sources of information, such as books and magazine articles.
- **Evaluate your progress.** Check periodically to see how well you're progressing toward your goal. Should you be doing anything differently? Is there a better way to proceed? If necessary, adjust your plan or seek help.
- **Reward yourself.** Treat yourself in a special way and celebrate your accomplishments.

HEALTH SKILLS ACTIVITY

GOAL SETTING

Achieving Health Goals

In Lesson 1, you completed a personal health inventory. Review your responses to the inventory. Were some areas of your health weaker than you would like them to be? You can set a goal to improve your physical, mental/emotional, or social health. Remember the guidelines you have learned.

- Consider your needs, values, and interests.
- Consider your skills, abilities, and knowledge.
- Set realistic goals.
- Make your goals specific.
- List the steps to reach your goals.
- Get help from others.
- Evaluate your progress.
- Reward yourself.

ON YOUR OWN
Set two or three short-term health goals based on items for which you answered *no* on the health inventory on page 6. Make a plan for achieving your goals.

Changing Your Goals

To achieve your goals, it helps to stay motivated. Being motivated means that you are eager to reach your goal. Remind yourself why you set the goal in the first place. If your needs, values, interests, and abilities have not changed, then you will probably realize that the goal is still important to you.

However, some of your needs, values, interests, and abilities probably will change during your teen years. You will be having new experiences and meeting new people. You'll grow and develop as a person. As a result, you may revise or abandon old goals and add new ones. That's fine. Setting and achieving goals should always be a flexible process.

Goal setting is a skill you will use throughout your life. Don't be afraid to adjust your short-term or long-term goals as you go along. Just remember to follow the guidelines you've learned for choosing and achieving your goals.

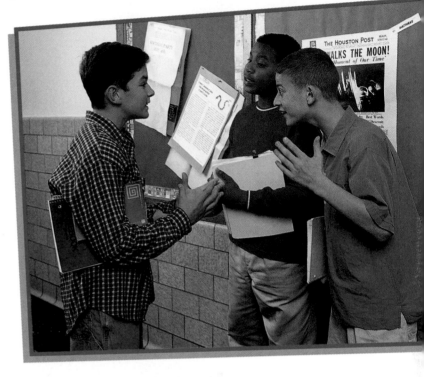

This teen set a goal to express his feelings in a healthy way and to disagree without getting angry. *What are your goals?*

Lesson 4 Review

Using complete sentences, answer the following questions on a sheet of paper.

Reviewing Terms and Facts

1. **Vocabulary** Define *short-term goal* and *long-term goal*. Use the two terms in an original sentence.
2. **Explain** Why is it important to set short-term and long-term goals?
3. **Recall** What factors should you consider when choosing your goals?
4. **Identify** Describe five steps that can help you achieve your goals.

Thinking Critically

5. **Analyze** Explain the meaning of this statement: "Setting and achieving goals should always be a flexible process."
6. **Apply** Give an example of a goal you have now that may change in the future. Explain why.

Applying Health Skills

7. **Goal Setting** Write down one of your long-term goals. List at least two short-term goals that can help you achieve your long-term goal. Then outline the steps you will take to reach each short-term goal.

EXPLORING INFLUENCES ON YOUR HEALTH

Model

In this chapter you learned how to make decisions that protect your health. Many internal and external factors influence your decisions. When you understand these influences, you can better understand the health choices you make. Thomas, shown below, is trying to choose an after-school snack. Read about what influences his decision.

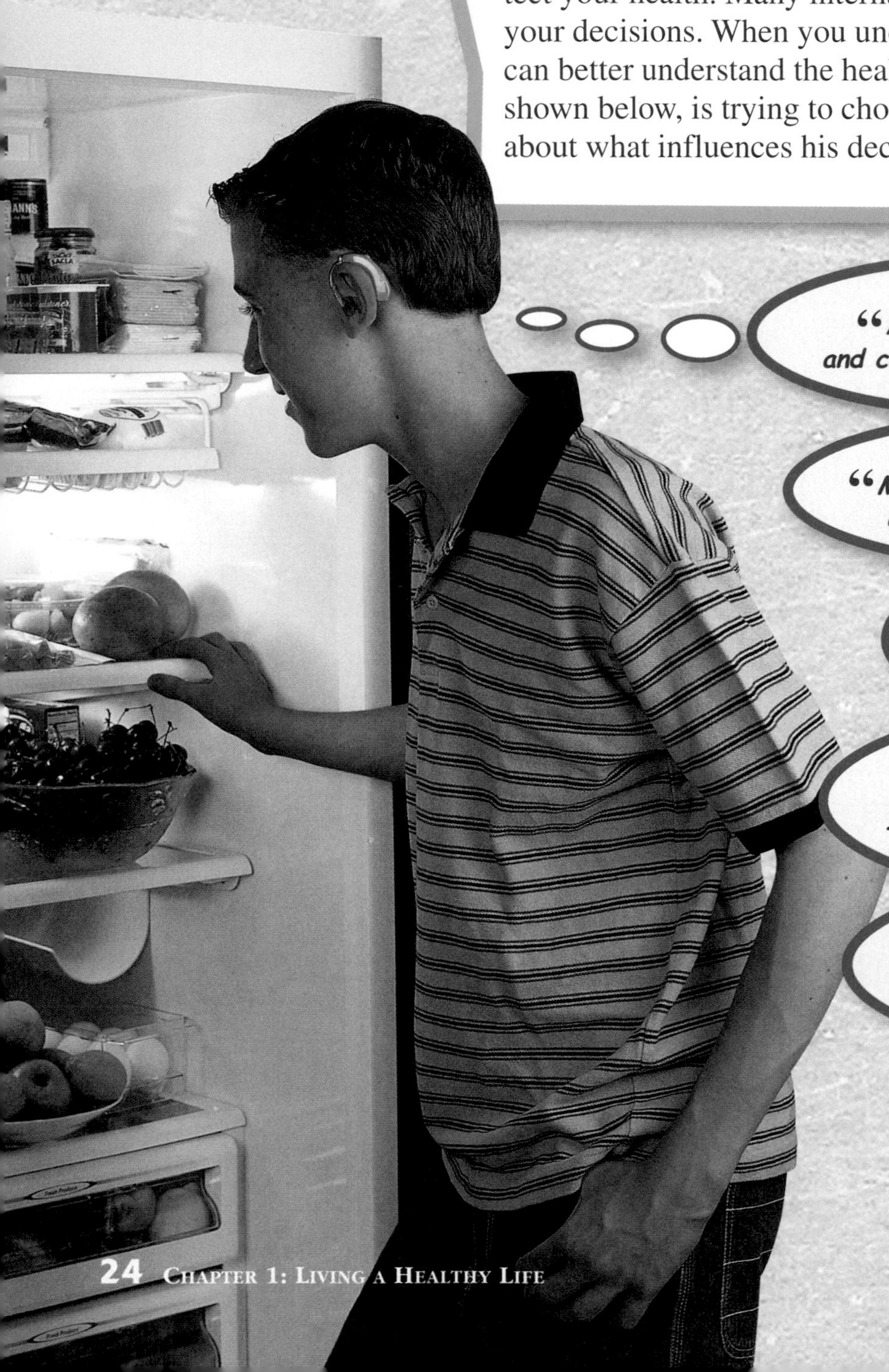

FRIENDS
"Ari always has milk and cookies after school."

FAMILY
"Mom is always telling me to eat more vegetables."

MEDIA
"I could try that cereal I saw advertised on TV."

CURIOSITY
"Here are some mangoes— I've never tried those before."

LIKES AND DISLIKES
"I've really got a craving for some crackers and cheese."

Practice

The chart on this page shows several choices that affect your health. The left side of the chart lists factors that can influence those choices. Copy the chart onto your own paper and fill it in. For example, if your family influences your choices about the food you eat, put an "X" next to "Family" in the column labeled "Food Choices." You may mark more than one box in each row and in each column. After you have completed the chart, answer these questions:

1. What factors influence you the most? The least?
2. Do internal or external influences affect you more?
3. Why is it important to understand what influences you?

Apply/Assess

In small groups, go over the results of your charts. Make a larger copy of the chart on butcher paper using colored markers. On this chart, record the number of students who checked each influence for each health choice. As a group, present an oral or written report of your findings to the class. In the summary, describe which influences affect your group the most and the least. Identify the influences as internal or external. Then explain why teens should understand the influences on their health.

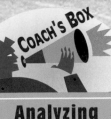

COACH'S BOX

Analyzing Influences

Both internal and external influences affect your choices. These influences may include:

Internal
- interests
- likes/dislikes
- fears
- curiosity

External
- family
- friends
- media
- culture

Self-√Check
- Did we describe which influences affect our group the most? The least?
- Did we identify whether internal or external factors most affect teens in our group?

Choices						
Influences	**Food Choices**	**Physical Activity**	**Tobacco and Alcohol**	**Stress**	**Friendships**	**Activities**
Interests						
Likes and Dislikes						
Fears						
Curiosity						
Total for internal influences						
Family						
Friends						
Media						
Culture						
Total for external influences						

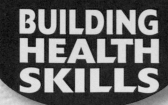

DECISION MAKING

CHOOSING HEALTHY BEHAVIORS

Model

Hannah has an important decision to make. Her family is moving to another state this spring. Hannah is upset because she has a big part in a dance recital this June. Hannah's parents have offered to let her stay with her aunt until the end of the school year. Let's see how Hannah uses the six steps of decision making to make a choice.

STEP 1: STATE THE SITUATION.
"I don't want to miss my recital, but I've never been away from my family before."

STEP 2: LIST THE OPTIONS.
"I could move with my family or stay with Aunt Susan."

STEP 3: WEIGH THE POSSIBLE OUTCOMES.
"If I move in the spring, I will be with my family. I will get to choose my bedroom, and I will get a chance to make friends at my new school. If I stay with Aunt Susan, I will get to dance in the recital, and I will have more time with my old friends."

STEP 4: CONSIDER YOUR VALUES.
"Dancing is very important to me, and this recital will give me valuable experience. I also value my relationship with my family."

STEP 5: MAKE A DECISION AND ACT.
"I will stay with Aunt Susan so I can dance in the recital. The time away from my family should go quickly because I will be busy and because I enjoy being with Aunt Susan."

STEP 6: EVALUATE THE DECISION.
"I feel good about this decision. The rewards were worth the drawbacks."

Practice

Read the following scenario. Then apply the six-step decision-making process to Anthony's situation. Outline the steps of the decision-making process on your own paper.

Anthony and Matthew have been best friends since they were very young. A month ago, Anthony became friends with William, a new student. Matthew does not get along with William. He never wants to spend time with Anthony when William is there. Now William has invited Anthony to go to a professional basketball game with him and his parents. However, the game is on the same day as Matthew's birthday party. What should Anthony do?

Apply/Assess

Describe a situation in which a person must make a decision about his or her health. Write your situation on a sheet of paper and put your name at the top. After your teacher reviews your situation, apply the first five decision-making steps to the scenario. Consider your two best options. Explain how this decision would improve the person's health.

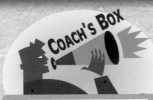

COACH'S BOX

Decision Making

1. State the situation.
2. List the options.
3. Weigh the possible outcomes.
4. Consider your values.
5. Make a decision and act.
6. Evaluate the decision.

Self-✓Check

- Did I use the first five steps of the decision-making process?
- Did I consider two options?

SUMMARY

LESSON·1 Health is the combination of physical, mental/emotional, and social well-being. To achieve a high level of wellness, you need to pay equal attention to all three sides of your health triangle.

LESSON·2 The ten health skills help you maintain lifelong health and prevent illness and injury.

LESSON·3 Decisions you make about your health require thought and planning. The six-step decision-making process helps you make good choices. Your character influences your decisions.

LESSON·4 Setting goals can help you gain control of your life and give your life a positive direction.

Reviewing Vocabulary and Concepts

On a sheet of paper, write the numbers 1–10. After each number, write the term from the list that best completes each sentence.

- advocacy
- communication
- habit
- health
- internal
- mental
- physical
- prevention
- refusal skills
- wellness

Lesson 1

1. The combination of physical, mental/emotional, and social well-being is _____.
2. Eating nutritious foods is an example of good _____ health.
3. _____ health relates to the way you feel about yourself.
4. A(n) _____ is a pattern of behavior that you follow almost without thinking.
5. The achievement of a high level of overall health is _____.

Lesson 2

6. _____ means keeping something from happening.
7. _____ influences are factors that affect your actions and decisions that come from within you.
8. The clear exchange of ideas and information is called _____.
9. _____ help you say no in an effective way, without feeling uncomfortable.
10. You can encourage other people to live healthy lives by practicing _____.

On a sheet of paper, write the numbers 11–20. Write *True* or *False* for each statement below. If the statement is false, change the underlined word or phrase to make it true.

Lesson 3

11. The chance of harm or loss is <u>consequence</u>.
12. <u>Decisions</u> are choices that you make.
13. <u>Values</u> are beliefs you feel strongly about that help guide the way you live.
14. The way a person thinks, feels, and acts is called <u>risk</u>.
15. The addition of one risk factor to another, increasing the chance of harm or loss, is <u>cumulative risk</u>.

Lesson 4

16. A <u>goal</u> is something you hope to accomplish.
17. Graduating from high school and going on to college is an example of a <u>short-term goal</u>.
18. When choosing your goals, you should consider your needs, values, and <u>abilities</u>.
19. Making your goals <u>general</u> will help you achieve them.
20. Your goals are <u>unlikely</u> to change during your teen years.

Thinking Critically

Using complete sentences, answer the following questions on a sheet of paper.

21. **Explain** Why do you think some teens take unnecessary risks with their health?
22. **Synthesize** Write a plan that breaks down the long-term goal of achieving physical fitness into several short-term goals that can be reached one at a time.
23. **Interpret** How do external influences affect your decisions?
24. **Compare and Contrast** Explain the similarities and differences between a short-term goal and a long-term goal.
25. **Analyze** What does it mean to be a responsible person?

Career Corner

Health Teacher

Do you like learning about health? Do you think you have a gift for helping others learn? A career as a health teacher might be for you. This career requires excellent communication skills and the ability to motivate others. You'll also need a four-year teaching degree with courses in health education. One way to prepare for this career is by tutoring others. For more information, visit Career Corner at health.glencoe.com.

Chapter 2

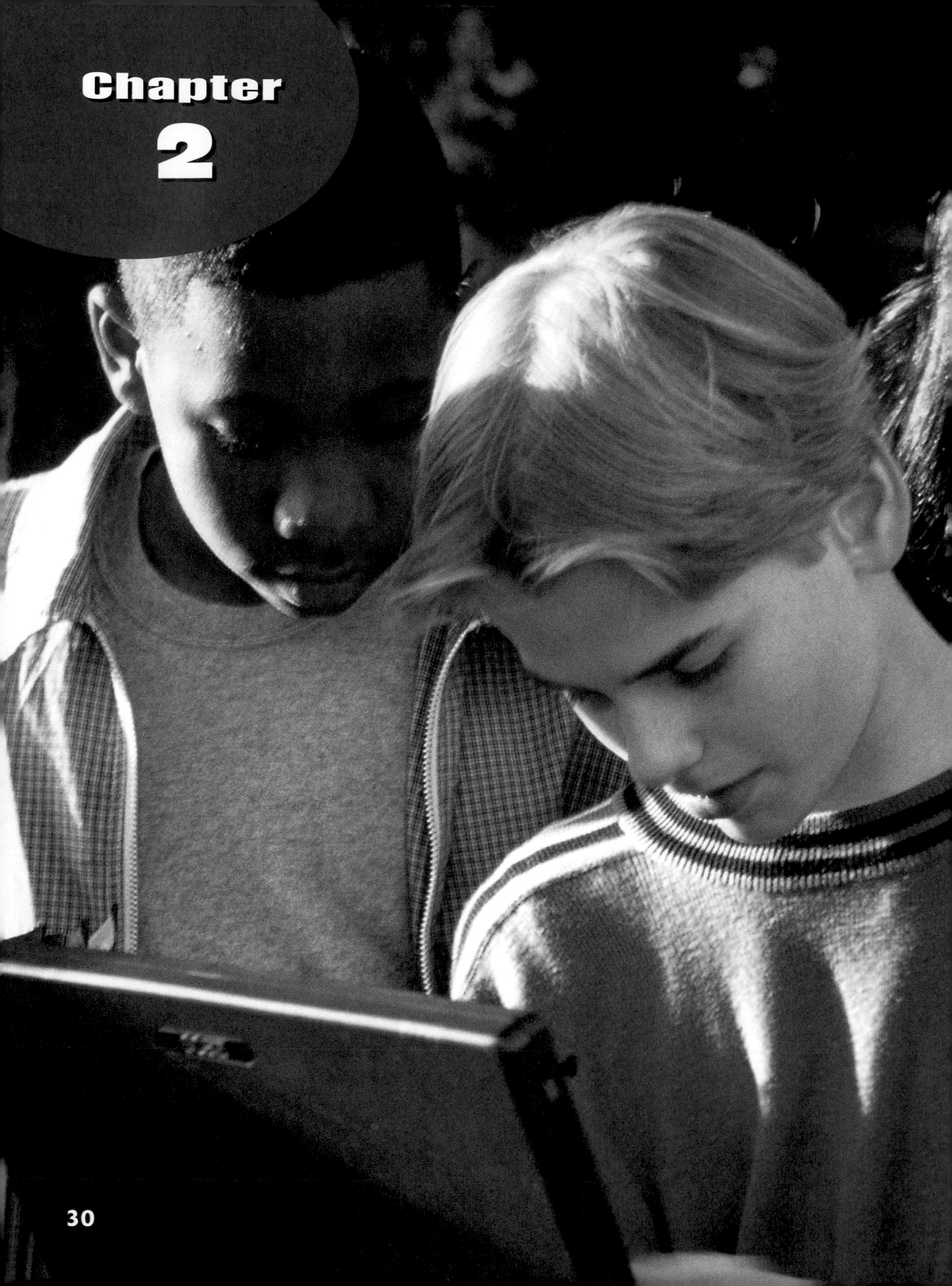

Mental and Emotional Health

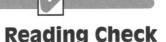

Quick Write

Write a brief description of the way you view yourself. In general, do you tend to see yourself in a positive way? How do you think your view of yourself affects your health and your behavior?

Before you begin Chapter 2, rate your mental and emotional health. Take the Health Inventory at health.glencoe.com.

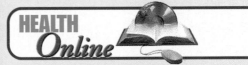

Reading Check

Read the chapter and lesson titles. Then write at least one question you would like to explore for each lesson. As you read, jot down the answers to your questions.

Feeling Good About Yourself

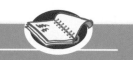

Quick Write

Make a list of five words or phrases you would use to describe yourself. Briefly explain how each word or phrase fits you.

LEARN ABOUT...

- what your self-concept is.
- what influences your self-concept.
- how you can build a positive self-concept.

VOCABULARY

- self-concept
- reinforce
- self-esteem

Self-Concept and Your Health

The person you see in a mirror is only one part of who you are. There are many other important parts of the total you. Discovering these parts is one of your tasks in growing up. It's an exciting time! You are learning

- about your opinions.
- what matters most to you.
- what you like and don't like.
- whom you like to be with.
- what you do well.
- what you'd like to improve.

Each discovery gives you a clearer picture of who you are. How you think others see you adds still more to the picture. Altogether, your **self-concept** is *the view you have of yourself.* It is also called your self-image.

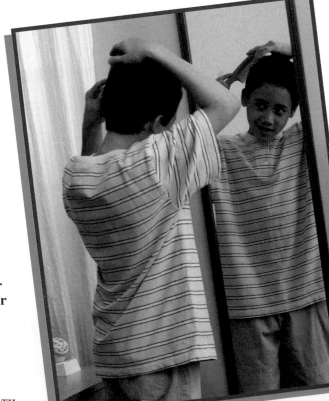

Getting to know yourself is an important task during your teen years. *What are some questions you have about yourself?*

Who Influences Your Self-Concept?

Many people influence your self-concept. Your parents or guardians are the first and greatest influence. Messages they send you have a lasting effect. Grandparents, sisters, brothers, and other relatives have an effect, too. At school, friends and teachers are yet another influence on your self-concept.

People around you send messages by what they say to you or how they treat you. The messages can be positive or negative. Messages such as "Nice job" will **reinforce**, or *support,* your self-concept. Sending positive messages is a two-way street. You are more likely to support those who have supported you in the past. Notice how positive messages support Jim's self-concept in **Figure 2.1**.

☑️ **Reading Check**
Use context clues. Locate unfamiliar words on these pages. Reread the sentences around them to find their meanings.

FIGURE 2.1

Building a Positive Self-Concept

Positive messages help reinforce a person's self-concept. *How can you send positive messages to others?*

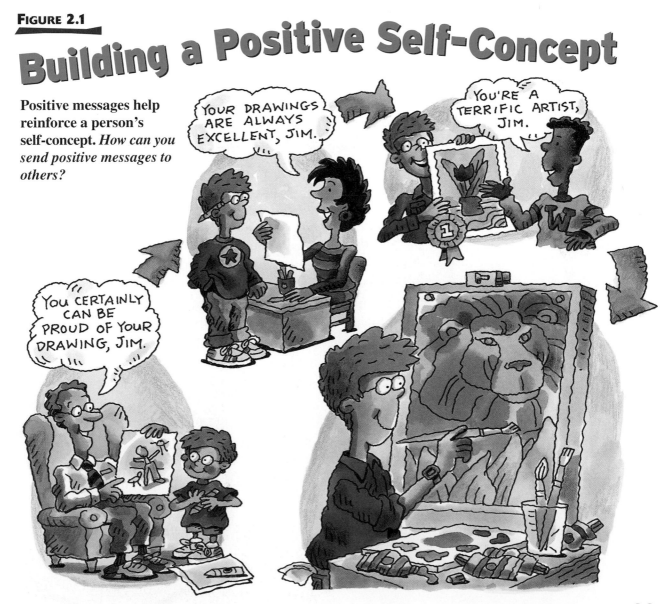

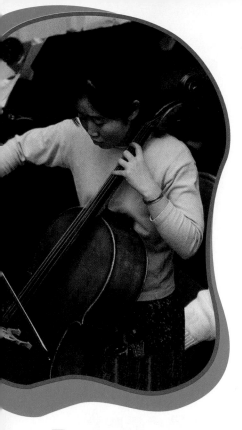

Focusing on what you do well helps you develop a positive self-concept. **What is another way to develop a positive self-concept?**

Developing a Positive Self-Concept

There are several ways to develop a positive self-concept. First of all, concentrate on what you do well. That gives you the confidence to try new things. Having the courage to try something new also reinforces your self-concept. Some other ways to develop a positive self-concept include:

- Think positive thoughts about yourself and others.
- Say positive things to friends and family members.
- Learn more about yourself and the person you want to be.
- Don't dwell on hurtful remarks you get from others.
- Accept encouragement from others and use it to discover your strengths.
- Develop realistic expectations—no one is perfect.

Practicing self-reflection is another way to build up your self-concept. Take time to think about who you want to be. Look at yourself honestly. Make a list of things you want to improve, and reward yourself for your successes.

HEALTH SKILLS ACTIVITY

COMMUNICATION SKILLS

Reinforcing a Friend's Self-Concept

You have learned about how to develop a positive self-concept. Did you know that you can use many of the same tools to reinforce your friends' self-concepts? You can:

- Tell your friends how much you like them and why.
- Help your friends learn about themselves. Explore different interests and ideas with them.
- Let your friends know that you believe in them. Encourage them to work toward their goals.
- If friends have trouble reaching their goals, help them to set more realistic expectations. Remind them of their strengths. Help them avoid dwelling on failures.

WITH A GROUP

Role-play a scene involving two friends. One friend is upset about not getting a part in the school play. Use the skills taught in this chapter to help rebuild this teen's self-concept.

Benefits of a Positive Self-Concept

Having a positive self-concept helps you build healthy self-esteem. Your **self-esteem** is *the ability to like and respect yourself.* Self-esteem enables you to:

- Have confidence in yourself.
- Feel appreciated, loved, and secure.
- Care about yourself and want to look after your health.
- Care about others and want to get along with them.
- Bounce back after a disappointment.

A positive self-concept helps you appreciate and improve your good points. You will make confident decisions and stand up for what's important to you.

A positive self-concept and high self-esteem will help you achieve what you set out to do. *How does a positive self-concept contribute to success?*

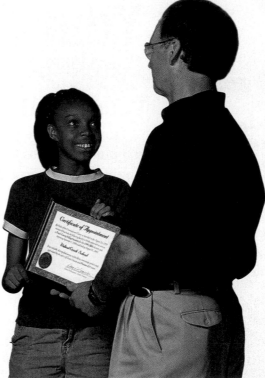

Lesson 1 Review

Using complete sentences, answer the following questions on a sheet of paper.

Reviewing Terms and Facts

1. **Vocabulary** Define the terms *self-concept* and *self-esteem*. Write a sentence that includes both terms.
2. **Identify** Name three people who have had a positive influence on your self-concept.
3. **Give Examples** Name three ways you can develop a positive self-concept.

Thinking Critically

4. **Explain** Why is having a positive self-concept important to your overall health?
5. **Describe** Write a paragraph starting with the phrase "I feel good about myself because . . ."

Applying Health Skills

6. **Goal Setting** Make a list of your three best qualities. Write a journal entry describing how you plan to make the most of these strengths over the next few weeks. Follow your plan carefully for a week. Then write another entry describing the results.

Understanding Your Emotions

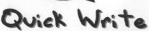

Quick Write

Make a list of five ways you show that you are happy. Now list five ways you show that you are angry. Do you find one feeling easier to express than the other? What does that mean to you?

LEARN ABOUT...

- the kinds of emotions you experience.
- how you can express strong feelings in healthful ways.
- where you can get help in dealing with your emotions.

VOCABULARY

- emotion
- hormones
- abstinence

Your Emotions

How do you feel right now? Are you happy, sad, or angry? Happiness, sadness, and anger are emotions, or *feelings*. In a single day, you probably experience many different emotions.

Types of Emotions

You may be more comfortable with some emotions than others. Most people like to feel happy, well-liked, and appreciated. When you're feeling this way, you enjoy life more. You feel more confident and you respond well to others.

However, emotions such as anger, fear, and sadness are also normal. It's how you express them that makes a difference. For example, being nervous about Friday's math test may drive you to study hard and do well.

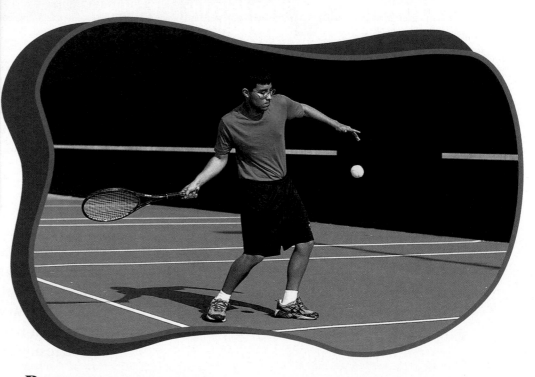

Physical activity is one healthy way to release your emotions. *How do you feel after you have been active?*

Emotional Changes During Adolescence

Things that happen around you can affect your emotions. Your emotions also have a lot to do with what's happening inside you. This is especially true during your teen years. Teens often experience sudden changes of emotion. Your hormones (HOR·mohnz) are partly responsible for these shifts. **Hormones** are *powerful chemicals, produced by glands, that regulate many body functions.*

During your teen years, hormones cause rapid changes in your body. They can cause emotional changes, too. The results can be confusing. One minute you feel on top of the world. The next minute you're down in the dumps. In short, you're having mood swings—like the teen in **Figure 2.2**.

CONNECT TO

Science

FEELINGS—INSIDE AND OUTSIDE
Emotions can cause physical changes in the body. You may feel lots of energy. Your heart may beat faster, and your muscles may become tense. *How does your body respond to emotions such as anger, nervousness, or excitement?*

FIGURE 2.2

Adolescent Mood Swings

Emotional shifts, sometimes called mood swings, are common for teens. Both ends of the swing are normal.

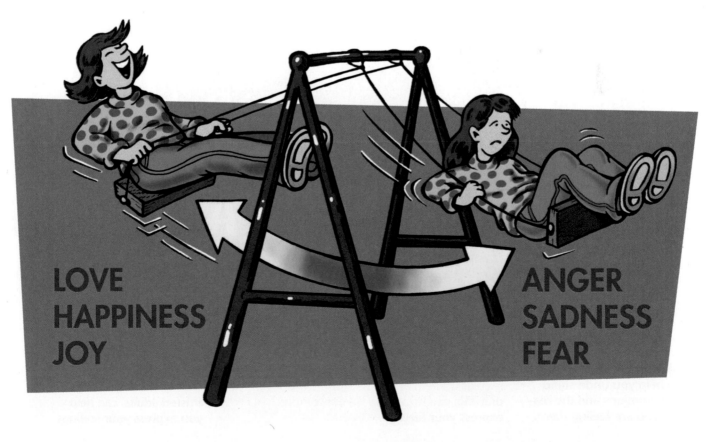

LOVE
HAPPINESS
JOY

ANGER
SADNESS
FEAR

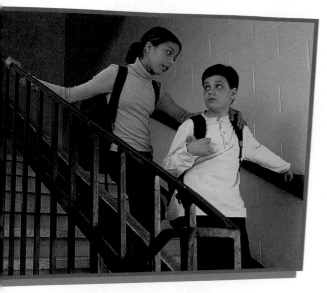

Expressing Your Emotions

As you've learned, emotions are neither good nor bad. It's the way you express, or release, them that counts. Holding emotions inside you can be damaging to all sides of your health triangle. These include:

- **Physical health**—trouble sleeping, sleeping too much, stomachaches, headaches.
- **Mental/emotional health**—tension, trouble concentrating, anger, being disorganized.
- **Social health**—arguments with friends or family members, violent behavior, withdrawing from others, sulking.

The good news is that you can learn to express emotions in healthful ways. **Figure 2.3** shows some positive ways of dealing with emotions.

When you offer support and encouragement, you help a friend express emotions in a healthy way. *What are some other ways to show you care?*

FIGURE 2.3

Dealing with Your Emotions

Here are four healthy ways to express strong emotions.

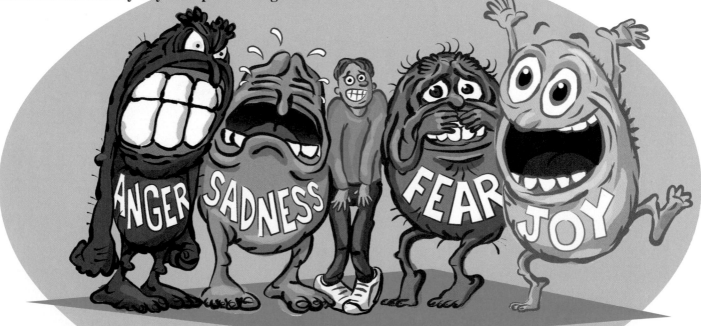

Thinking it out can help you understand your emotions and the reasons you are feeling them.

Creating something such as a poem or a drawing, can help you express your feelings.

Physical activity can help you work out your feelings.

Talking to others such as friends, siblings, or trusted adults, can help you express your feelings.

Practicing Abstinence

Everyone has some basic emotional needs, such as the need to be loved and accepted. Unfortunately, some teens try to fill their emotional needs by engaging in risky behavior. These teens may join gangs. Some may use tobacco, alcohol, or illegal drugs. Others may become sexually active. These behaviors, however, do not really meet emotional needs. Dealing with emotions in healthy ways includes resisting these kinds of unhealthy behaviors.

Abstinence (AB·sti·nuhns) is *refusing to participate in health-risk behaviors.* When you practice abstinence, you avoid situations that are dangerous. This protects your health and the health of others.

HEALTH SKILLS ACTIVITY

ACCESSING INFORMATION

People Who Can Help

Do your emotions get the best of you sometimes? Have you tried several strategies and found that you are still troubled or confused? There are lots of people who can help.

- **TRUSTED ADULTS.** Talking to your parents, guardians, and other relatives can help you understand your emotions. People such as ministers and youth leaders can also help.
- **TEACHERS, SCHOOL NURSES, AND COUNSELORS.** The people who work at your school are ready to help when you experience troubling emotions or need help with a problem.
- **HEALTH CARE PROVIDERS.** Doctors, nurses, and professional counselors can provide valuable help.

ON YOUR OWN
Think about a time when your emotions troubled you. What did you do? Where did you go for help? What will you do the next time you feel troubled?

Sometimes, your peers may pressure you to take part in dangerous or unhealthy behaviors. Times like these really test your emotions. You want to maintain your friendships, but you also want to make healthful decisions. It may help to remember that friends who do dangerous things could get into trouble. Being around them may get you into trouble, too. It could also cost you the respect of parents and other people you care about. You could even lose respect for yourself.

Dealing with this pressure will be easier if you practice refusal skills. Refusal skills let you say no and help you stay in emotional control. Chapter 3 tells you more about refusal skills. It also teaches you how to use communication skills. These skills involve strategies for speaking and listening. Both are important as you learn to deal with your emotions.

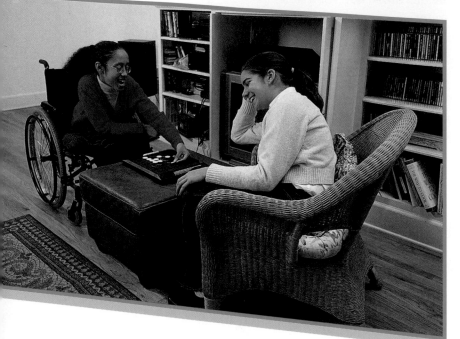

Caring friends will not pressure you to engage in risky behaviors. *Name some healthy activities you and your friends enjoy doing together.*

Lesson 2 Review

Using complete sentences, answer the following questions on a sheet of paper.

Reviewing Terms and Facts
1. **Vocabulary** Define the word *emotion* and use it in a sentence.
2. **Explain** Why are mood swings common among teens?
3. **List** Name three healthy ways to express strong emotions.

Thinking Critically
4. **Describe** Write a paragraph starting with the phrase "I will express my emotions in a healthy way by . . ."

5. **Apply** You are angry because your brother or sister has borrowed your headphones without asking and you want to use them. How will you deal with your emotions and work out the problem with your sibling?

Applying Health Skills
6. **Advocacy** Make a list of five ways that you could encourage other teens to practice abstinence from risky behaviors.

Managing Stress

Stress: A Natural Part of Life

Zach is going to be the quarterback this afternoon, but he has only played this position once. His mouth feels dry and his stomach feels like butterflies are fluttering inside it. Kendall has just found out that she won the part she wanted in the school play. Her heart is pounding. What's going on?

Zach and Kendall feel **stress**. Stress is *your body's response to changes around you.* Ordinary events like forgetting a locker combination or taking a test can cause stress. Big changes like starting a new school, parents divorcing, or a friend moving away also create stress. No matter what the situation, try to remember that stress is a natural part of life.

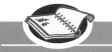

Quick **W**rite

List some situations in which you felt nervous or anxious. Tell what you did to relieve those troubling feelings.

LEARN ABOUT...

- what stress is.
- how your body responds to stress.
- how you can manage stress.

VOCABULARY

- stress
- eustress
- distress
- stressor
- adrenaline
- fatigue

Jerry is feeling stress as he rushes to finish his test. *What kinds of situations are stressful for you?*

☑

Reading Check
Identify some of the causes of stress. Then name some of the negative and positive effects of stress.

Types of Stress

Stress can be positive or negative. *Positive stress* is called **eustress** (YOO·stres) and can help you accomplish tasks, reach goals, and escape danger. It motivates athletes to work hard during practice. As a result, they perform well in competition. Can you think of a positive stress?

Distress, or *negative stress,* gets in your way and holds you back. Personal problems at home or at school produce negative stress. So do natural disasters like storms or floods. Too much negative stress can be unhealthy.

Your Body's Response to Stress

What makes your hands sweat when you worry or your heart jump when you're really happy? It's your body's way of responding to **stressors**, which are *objects, people, places, and events that trigger stress.* A stressor sets off a chain of events called the "fight-or-flight response," shown in **Figure 2.4**.

FIGURE 2.4

THE FIGHT-OR-FLIGHT RESPONSE

This illustration shows some of the physical changes stress can cause.

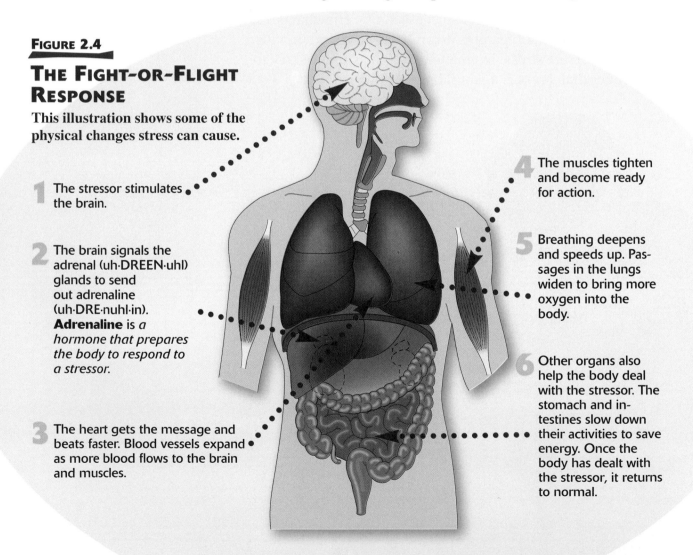

1 The stressor stimulates the brain.

2 The brain signals the adrenal (uh·DREEN·uhl) glands to send out adrenaline (uh·DRE·nuhl·in). **Adrenaline** is *a hormone that prepares the body to respond to a stressor.*

3 The heart gets the message and beats faster. Blood vessels expand as more blood flows to the brain and muscles.

4 The muscles tighten and become ready for action.

5 Breathing deepens and speeds up. Passages in the lungs widen to bring more oxygen into the body.

6 Other organs also help the body deal with the stressor. The stomach and intestines slow down their activities to save energy. Once the body has dealt with the stressor, it returns to normal.

Stress and Fatigue

Dealing with too much stress can cause fatigue (fuh·TEEG), or *extreme tiredness*. There are two types of fatigue. Physical fatigue affects your body. Vigorous physical activity can cause physical fatigue. Rest is the best remedy. Emotional fatigue can come from feelings of worry, sadness, or boredom. You can deal with it by removing the source of stress, increasing your activity level, or learning ways to manage the stress.

Ways to Manage Stress

How do you keep negative stress from damaging your health? Sometimes you can avoid a stressor. If a bully harasses you on your way home from school, you can walk home a different way. Some stressors, however, are simply part of life. You need to learn to manage them. These tips can help.

- **Recognize stress.** A funny feeling in your stomach, fast breathing, and a pounding heart—all of these can be signals that you are feeling stress.
- **Manage your time.** Set aside regular times to do homework and chores. That way you won't have to rush to get them done at the last minute.

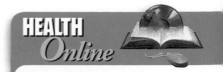

HEALTH *Online*

Visit Web Links at health.glencoe.com and learn more about dealing with stress in your life.

Positive stress can help you accomplish tasks and reach goals. *How can positive stress affect your schoolwork?*

- **Set your priorities.** Make a list of things you want to accomplish. Decide how important each task is. Focus on one thing at a time. Too many activities—such as practices, club meetings, or after-school work—can lead to stress.
- **Redirect your energy.** Stress increases your energy. Use that energy to do something positive. You could enjoy a hobby or offer to help a family member with a project.

Hands-On Health

HEAD-TO-TOE STRESS RELIEF

Removing stressors is the best way to relieve your stress. Sometimes, however, it can help just to reduce your body tension. This activity will guide you through a series of steps that can help you relax.

WHAT YOU WILL NEED
- a sock
- two tennis balls

WHAT YOU WILL DO
1. Begin by relaxing your face. Find the place where your upper jaw connects to your lower jaw. Place two fingers over this spot on either side of your face. Gently rub your fingertips in a circular motion. This eases tension in your jaw.
2. The next step will relax your neck. Place the two tennis balls inside the sock. Drape the sock across the back of your neck. Adjust the sock so that one tennis ball falls on either side of your neck.

    Place one hand over each of the tennis balls. Use your hands to roll the balls slowly back and forth against your neck muscles. You can try rolling the balls in circles, too.

3. For the next step, stand with your feet shoulder width apart. Bend your knees slightly. Place your hands on your knees.

    Slowly bend over at the hips. Try to keep your neck and back in a straight line. When you are leaning all the way forward, slowly arch your back upward, like a cat stretching. Then gradually release the stretch until your back is straight again.

IN CONCLUSION
How did these exercises affect your body tension? Do you feel tenser than you did before? Less tense? About the same? Would you recommend these exercises as a way to relax?

As a class, brainstorm some other ways to relax your body. You can include other types of activities besides exercises.

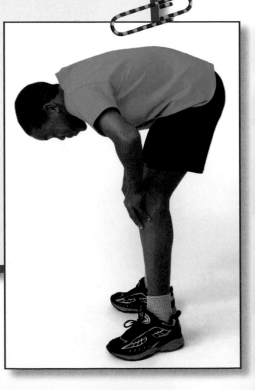

- **Talk to someone.** Talking about stress can relieve the pressure. A parent, friend, or school counselor may give you some good advice.
- **Relax.** Take a deep breath, and exhale slowly. Do it again. Try to calm yourself when you feel stress. Take time to be alone and fill your mind with positive thoughts. You could also relax by reading or listening to soothing music.
- **Put things in perspective.** Remember that you are not alone; everyone has stress and problems. Do not make your problems seem bigger than they really are.
- **Increase your activity.** Becoming more active releases the physical energy that builds up when you feel stress. Physical activity naturally calms the body.

Redirecting your energy by being physically active is a good way to manage stress. *What other strategies for managing stress work for you?*

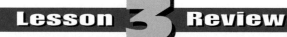

Lesson 3 Review

Using complete sentences, answer the following questions on a sheet of paper.

Reviewing Terms and Facts

1. **Vocabulary** Define the terms *stress, eustress,* and *distress.* Use each word in an original sentence.
2. **Give Examples** Name one type of positive stress and one type of negative stress in your life.
3. **List** Name two ways your body responds to stress.
4. **Identify** What are the two types of fatigue?

Thinking Critically

5. **Synthesize** Why do you think adrenaline is sometimes called "the emergency hormone"?
6. **Analyze** Explain how stress can affect your physical, mental/emotional, and social health.

Applying Health Skills

7. **Stress Management** Harley feels very stressed because he has a lot of homework. How would you suggest Harley deal with his stress?

HANDLING STRONG EMOTIONS

Model

As a teen, you experience many different emotions. Part of growing up is learning to respond to your emotions in a healthy way. Read about Brittany, a thoughtful and active middle school student. Brittany finds a note that her friend Sonya wrote. In the note, Sonya said that Brittany was "full of herself." When Brittany reads the note, she feels like yelling at Sonya. Instead, she sits down and writes out the steps for handling strong emotions.

DETERMINE THE EMOTION.
I feel sad and betrayed.

EVALUATE THE CAUSE.
Sonya is talking about me behind my back. She wrote something that was unkind and untrue.

ASK FOR HELP (IF NEEDED).
I can handle these emotions myself, but I may want to talk to my sister about my feelings after school.

LEARN TO RESPOND.
I'm going to call Sonya tonight. I'll tell her I found her note and ask her to explain what she wrote.

Practice

Read the following scenario about a teen experiencing strong emotions.

Jason was riding home from school on his new bike. As he coasted down a hill, he ran over a broken bottle and flattened his tire. Jason had to push his bike the rest of the way home. It was hot and humid—a bad ending to a difficult day at school.

1. What emotion is Jason experiencing?
2. What caused this emotion?
3. Do you think Jason needs help to handle this emotion? If so, where could he go for help?
4. What would be a healthy response to this emotion?

Apply/Assess

Think of a situation that created a strong or a long-lasting emotion in you. Show what you know about feelings by illustrating the steps for handling emotions.

Divide butcher paper or poster board into four sections. In the first section, draw a picture that shows how you felt. In the second section, list the causes. In the third section, list people who could help you handle your emotions. Draw a healthy response to this emotion in the last section. Explain your drawing to other students, and tell why your response is healthy.

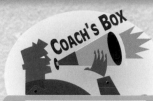

Practicing Healthful Behaviors

You can deal with strong emotions by following these steps:
- Determine the emotion.
- Evaluate the cause.
- Ask for help if needed.
- Learn to respond in a way that does not hurt anyone.

Self-√Check

- Did I illustrate an emotion?
- Did I show a healthy response?
- Can I explain why it is a healthy response?

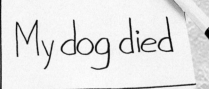

MANAGING YOUR TIME

Model

Some teens feel like there are never enough hours in the day for all they want to do. As a result, they often feel stress. One way to handle this stress is to learn how to use time wisely. Read about a teen named Grady facing a stressful situation.

Grady tells his parents that he will make the Honor Roll this semester. To accomplish that goal, Grady takes home his textbooks regularly. He sets aside time every evening for homework. When exams come, he knows his subjects well. He only needs a short review to get a good grade. He makes the Honor Roll. Grady feels stress-free and proud of his accomplishment.

Practice

Write a story about a teen who is having a stressful day. In the story, show how a shortage of time contributes to the teen's stress. Then, at the end, suggest ways the teen could better manage his or her time. Explain how those changes would help reduce the teen's stress.

Apply/Assess

The first step in learning how to use your time wisely is to see how you currently spend your time. On a sheet of notebook paper, draw a day planner like the one shown below. Fill in each of the sections with a short phrase describing how you usually spend that hour of the day. Include items like school, sleep, meals, TV, social activities, homework, family activities, chores, and personal hobbies.

On the back of your page, draw a day planner for Saturday or Sunday. Fill it in with short phrases that show how you spend your time on a typical day during the weekend.

Look at your day planner. Are you surprised by anything you see? Now think about some of the sources of stress in your life. Could managing your time help you avoid these stressors? At the bottom of the page, list two or three ways you could manage your time more effectively. Then briefly explain how managing your time could help you reduce stress and improve your health.

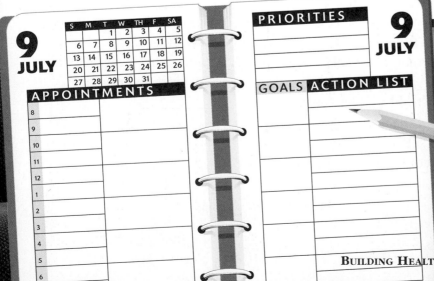

SUMMARY

LESSON•1 Your self-concept is the way you see yourself. Messages from others influence your self-concept. Developing a positive self-concept helps you improve your mental and emotional health. Understanding and appreciating yourself helps you build a positive self-concept.

LESSON•2 All emotions are normal. The way you express your emotions, however, may be healthy or unhealthy.

Expressing emotions in healthy ways is important to good mental and emotional health.

LESSON•3 Stress is your body's internal response to changes around you. Stress may be positive or negative. Too much stress can harm your health. There are many strategies you can use to manage stress.

Reviewing Vocabulary and Concepts

On a sheet of paper, write the numbers 1–12. After each number, write the term from the list that best completes each statement.

- abstinence
- decisions
- emotional shifts
- emotions
- express
- hormone
- parents/ guardians
- realistic
- refusal skills
- reinforce
- self-concept
- self-esteem

Lesson 1

1. The view you have of yourself is your _____.
2. The first and greatest influence on your self-concept when you are young is your _____.
3. Positive messages will _____ your self-concept.
4. One way to help yourself develop a positive self-concept is to have _____ expectations.
5. The ability to like and respect yourself is called _____.
6. A positive self-concept helps you make confident _____.

Lesson 2

7. Happiness, sadness, and anger are examples of _____.
8. A _____ is a powerful chemical, produced by glands, that regulates many body functions.
9. Mood swings, or _____, are common for young people.
10. Talking to others, physical activity, and creating something are all ways to _____ your emotions.
11. _____ means refusing to participate in health-risk behaviors.
12. Dealing with peer pressure is easier if you practice _____.

Lesson 3

On a sheet of paper, write the numbers 13–17. Write *True* or *False* for each statement below. If the statement is false, change the underlined word or phrase to make it true.

13. Your body's response to changes around you is <u>stress</u>.
14. Negative stress, the kind that gets in your way and holds you back, is called <u>stressor</u>.
15. A <u>distress</u> is an object, person, place or event that triggers stress.
16. The hormone that prepares the body to respond to a stressor is called <u>adrenaline</u>.
17. <u>Fatigue</u> is extreme tiredness.

Using complete sentences, answer the following questions on a sheet of paper.

18. **Interpret** Explain how messages from parents and friends affects your self-concept.
19. **Suggest** Identify three ways to improve your self-concept.
20. **Analyze** Describe some healthy ways of expressing emotions that you have found to be effective.
21. **Explain** List three objects, people, places, or events that act as stressors for you. Explain why you find them stressful.
22. **Compare and Contrast** Compare and contrast the causes of physical fatigue with the causes of emotional fatigue.

Career Corner

School Counselor

Do you like to help others solve problems? Would you like to help young people discover their talents and plan their futures? If so, consider a career as a school counselor. These professionals work in a school setting. They help students with school, family, or personal problems. They also work with students in informal groups to develop career goals.

School counselors need a four-year college degree and two years graduate training in counseling. Read more about this and other health careers by visiting Career Corner at **health.glencoe.com.**

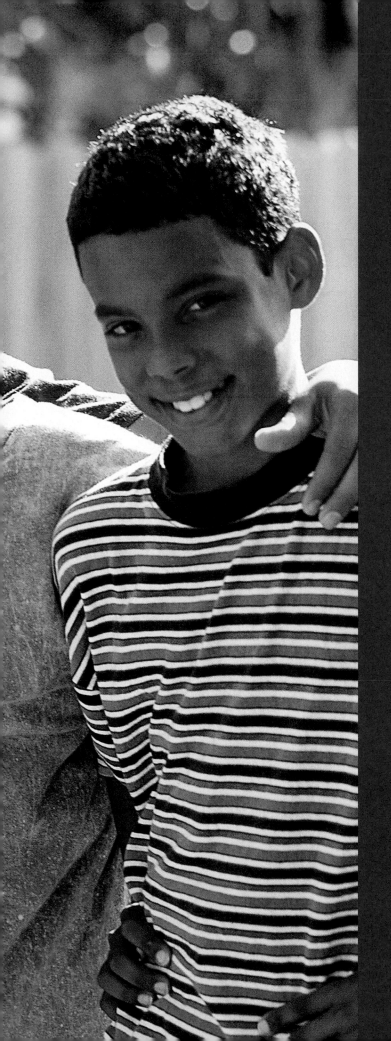

Social Health

Quick Write

List all the questions you have about how to get along with others. For example, you might like to know how you can communicate better or how to resolve problems in your family. After reading this chapter, see how many of your questions have been answered.

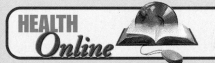

Rate your ability to communicate effectively. Take the Health Inventory for Chapter 3 at health.glencoe.com.

✓ Reading Check

Make predictions. What information do you think this chapter will include? On what are you basing your response? Read the chapter and see if your predictions were correct.

Your Family

Quick Write

Write a short letter to a new pen pal describing some activities you do regularly with your family. Explain how these activities bring you closer together as a family.

LEARN ABOUT...

- how family members care for each other.
- different kinds of families.
- your role within your family.
- ways to handle problems in families.

VOCABULARY

- family
- nurture
- abuse
- sexual abuse
- neglect

Belonging to a Family

Ever since you were a baby, you have been connecting and bonding with your parents and other members of your family. The **family** is *the basic unit of society*. As a group, it provides for the needs of its members. **Figure 3.1** shows some basic ways people in families care for each other.

FIGURE 3.1

HOW FAMILIES CARE FOR THEIR MEMBERS

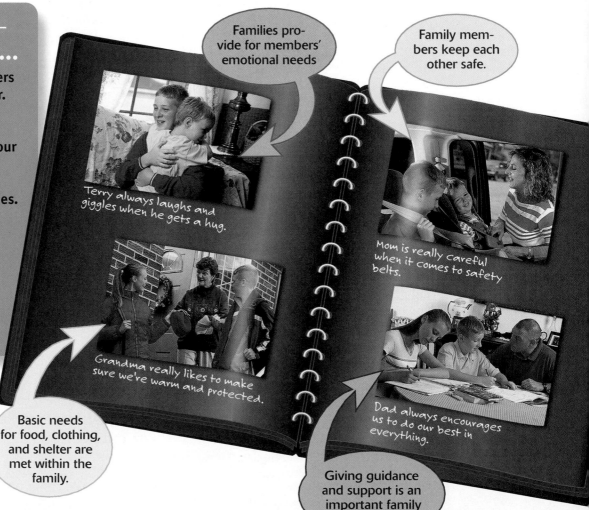

Families provide for members' emotional needs

Family members keep each other safe.

Terry always laughs and giggles when he gets a hug.

Mom is really careful when it comes to safety belts.

Grandma really likes to make sure we're warm and protected.

Dad always encourages us to do our best in everything.

Basic needs for food, clothing, and shelter are met within the family.

Giving guidance and support is an important family function.

FIGURE 3.2

Building Strong Families

Love, caring for one another, and respecting each other's needs make up the foundation of a healthy family. *What can you do to keep this foundation strong?*

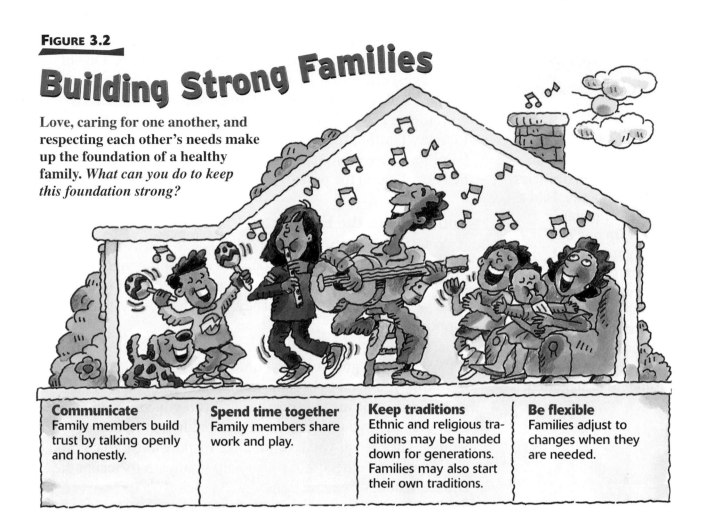

Communicate	**Spend time together**	**Keep traditions**	**Be flexible**
Family members build trust by talking openly and honestly.	Family members share work and play.	Ethnic and religious traditions may be handed down for generations. Families may also start their own traditions.	Families adjust to changes when they are needed.

Types of Families

There are many kinds of family structures. A nuclear family is made up of two parents and one or more children. An extended family is a nuclear family plus other relatives, such as grandparents. Couples are families with no children. A child or children living with only one parent make up a single-parent family.

Blended families are formed when two people who marry each other bring children from earlier marriages into their new family. Children living with grandparents make up yet another type of family. Sometimes, a child who has lost his or her parents is raised by another person or couple, who are known as foster parents.

Recognizing Healthy Families

All healthy families share the same goal. They seek to **nurture**, or *provide for the physical, emotional, mental, and social needs* of their members. **Figure 3.2** shows some ways to help build healthy families.

Developing Good Character

Responsibility

As a teen, you may be ready to take on more responsibilities in your family. Fold a sheet of paper in half. On one side list your current responsibilities. On the other side, list some new, perhaps more interesting, responsibilities you believe you are capable of handling.

While the goal of the family remains the same, the family unit has changed a lot over the past 50 to 100 years. One of the biggest changes is that families are smaller. In the past, couples had more children, and other relatives often lived with them. The roles of family members have also changed. In many families today, both parents work outside the home. Families move more often. There are more single-parent families now than in the past.

Your Role in the Family

Your family helps you in many ways. When you were a baby, your family provided you with everything you needed, including food, clothing, and a place to live. Your family also gave you love and attention. They were the first system of support in your life.

Now, as you grow older, your family is helping you develop the skills you need to become an independent adult. Within your family, you are starting to learn who you are. Your family members help you develop your personality, attitudes, and values. They teach you how to make responsible choices and get along with others. They also help you learn to accept the consequences of your actions.

During your teen years, you will begin developing your own set of values and beliefs. Sometimes, you will not agree with your parents. When this happens, talk with them calmly. Even if you feel frustrated, remain respectful.

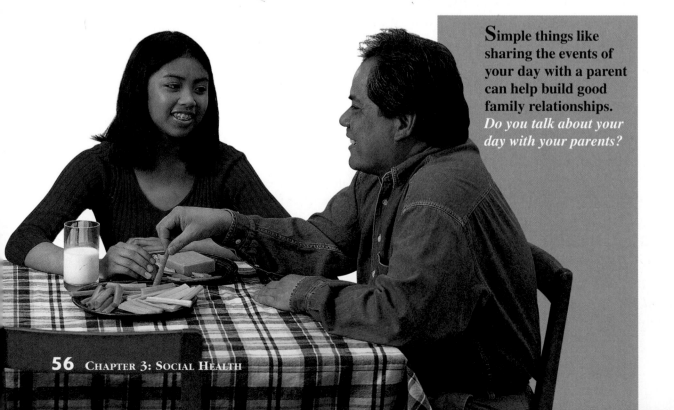

Simple things like sharing the events of your day with a parent can help build good family relationships. *Do you talk about your day with your parents?*

Dealing with Changes

Every family can expect to go through changes. Some changes, like the birth of a new baby or the marriage of grown children, are generally happy events. They also require family members to take on new roles and responsibilities. Other family changes, like moving, can be difficult. Family members can plan ways to help each other adjust.

Separation and divorce can bring on negative stress or feelings of anger, sadness, or guilt. Sharing your feelings with your parents or another trusted adult may help. Let both parents know that you care for them and that seeing them unhappy is painful. Try to help younger brothers and sisters understand and cope.

One of the most difficult changes of all is a death in the family. When this happens, people may feel many emotions, including sadness, fear, or even anger. It is important to express these feelings in healthful ways.

☑ Reading Check

Identifying synonyms will help you build a larger vocabulary. List synonyms for these words: *help, calmly, generally, unhappy.*

HEALTH SKILLS ACTIVITY

DECISION MAKING

Juggling Responsibilities

Hunter is a busy teen. He studies hard and gets good grades. This month, he tried out for the school play and got a small part. Now he has rehearsals about once a week.

Last night Hunter's older sister called him on the phone. She explained that she had to go to the dentist one afternoon this week. She wanted to know if Hunter could baby-sit for her son while she was at the dentist.

Hunter was about to say yes, but then he remembered that he had a rehearsal that day after school. Now he is unsure what to do. He wants to help his sister, but he doesn't want to miss his rehearsal. How can Hunter solve this problem?

WHAT WOULD YOU DO?

Apply the six steps of the decision-making process to Hunter's situation. Compare your responses with those of another classmate. Finally, take a class vote on the best solution for Hunter.

1. STATE THE SITUATION.
2. LIST THE OPTIONS.
3. WEIGH THE POSSIBLE OUTCOMES.
4. CONSIDER YOUR VALUES.
5. MAKE A DECISION AND ACT ON IT.
6. EVALUATE THE DECISION.

Dealing with Family Problems

All families have problems. You have learned about some ways families can deal with changes on their own. However, some problems are far too serious to solve by sharing feelings and helping each other. In these situations the family should seek outside help. Many types of counseling are available.

One of the most serious family problems is **abuse** (uh·BYOOS), or *a pattern of mistreatment of another person.* An adult or a child might be a target of abuse. A family with an abuse problem is not a healthy family. Mistreatment can occur in a number of different forms.

- **Physical abuse.** This form involves excessive use of force. The abused person often shows signs of physical abuse, such as bruises, burns, bite marks, or broken bones.

  - **Emotional abuse.** This form can be harder to spot. It often involves yelling and putting down another family member. Although there may not be physical marks, the emotional scars run deep. The abused person often feels worthless and ashamed.

  - **Sexual abuse.** Examples of **sexual abuse** involve *an adult displaying sexual material to a child, touching a child's private body parts, or engaging in any kind of sexual activity with a child or teen.* It is often difficult to see that a child is being sexually abused.

  - **Neglect.** *The failure of parents to provide basic physical and emotional care for their children* is called **neglect.** Physical neglect occurs when parents do not provide food, clothing, shelter, or medical care for their child. Emotional neglect involves not giving love, affection, and other forms of emotional support.

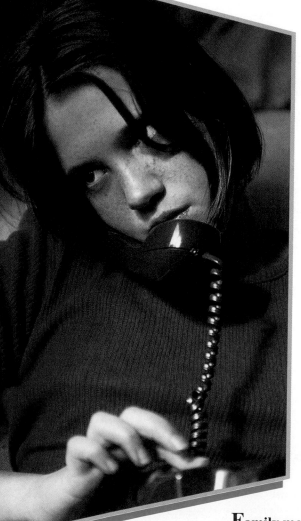

Family members dealing with problems of abuse need to get outside help right away. *What resources are available in your school and community for people dealing with abuse?*

Where Families Can Find Help

A person who is being abused needs outside help right away. The first step in getting help is for the abused person to tell a trusted adult. The abused person may need to be in a safe place. A teacher or school counselor can be a good first person to talk with. Whenever there is immediate danger, the police should be called. The abuser also needs help. Professionals can help the abuser understand the reason for the behavior and why it must change. It is never acceptable to abuse others.

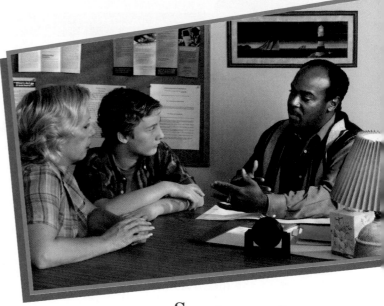

Troubled families can find help from a number of sources. Religious leaders, social service agencies, and hospital social workers provide professional counseling. Crisis center volunteers are also available. You can call them through the numbers listed under "crisis intervention" in your telephone book. School counselors and doctors' offices can suggest support and self-help groups. Some support groups are for the targets of abuse. Others are for the abusers. Both types try to help the people involved.

Sometimes people may need to see a professional family counselor about their problems. *What are some situations in which counseling could be helpful?*

Lesson 1 Review

Using complete sentences, answer the following questions on a sheet of paper.

Reviewing Terms and Facts

1. **Recall** What are the four ways in which families care for their members?
2. **Explain** Describe four ways to keep healthy families strong.
3. **List** Name three different family structures and describe them.
4. **Vocabulary** Define *abuse* and *neglect*. How are they related?

Thinking Critically

5. **Apply** Suppose you and your parents are having a disagreement over what time your curfew should be. Name two pointers that will help you as you work out the conflict with them.
6. **Synthesize** Write two statements you might make to help a friend who is dealing with divorce in the family.

Applying Health Skills

7. **Accessing Information** Use the Yellow Pages and lists of local government offices to find names of private and public organizations where families dealing with abuse can get help. Make a wallet card showing how to contact these places.

Your Friends and Peers

Why We Need Other People

Imagine that you are having a party with a large guest list. You would probably invite relatives, close friends, and people in your neighborhood. You also might invite classmates, teammates, and others in the community. You would invite these people because you have a relationship (ri·LAY·shuhn·ship) with them. **Relationships** are *the connections you have with other people.*

The relationships you have with family members are some of your most important. You also have relationships with friends, teachers, coaches, and people from clubs you belong to. All of these relationships help meet your need to feel loved and wanted, safe and secure. Your relationships give you a sense of belonging and support.

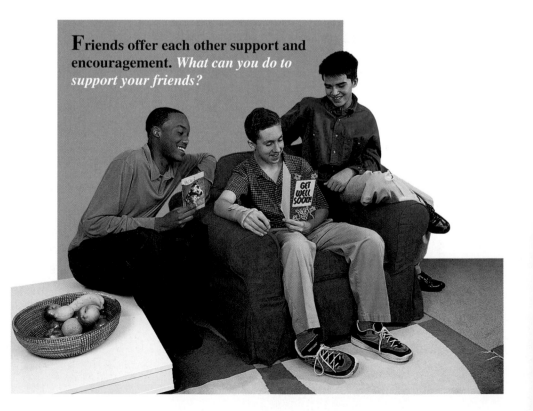

Friends offer each other support and encouragement. *What can you do to support your friends?*

The Value of Friends

Forming ties with friends is one of the most important things you do during your teens. A **friendship** is *a special type of relationship between people who enjoy being together.* Right now, most of your friends are probably the same age and gender as you. However, some of your friends might be the same age as your parents or grandparents.

You form friendships for many reasons. Jenna, for example, likes Sandra because Sandra makes her laugh. Jenna is friendly with Claire because they are in the same karate class. Jenna can have fun with Sandra and still be Claire's friend. **Figure 3.3** shows other kinds of friendships.

Reading Check

Find compound words on pages 60 and 61. Which two words form each of these compound words?

FIGURE 3.3

DIFFERENT FRIENDS FOR DIFFERENT REASONS

You make and keep friends for different reasons. *Which of these reasons apply to you and your friends?*

You have similar interests. Teens become friends because they enjoy the same hobbies, sports, and other activities.

You have similar values. Teens choose people as friends because their beliefs and standards of behavior are similar.

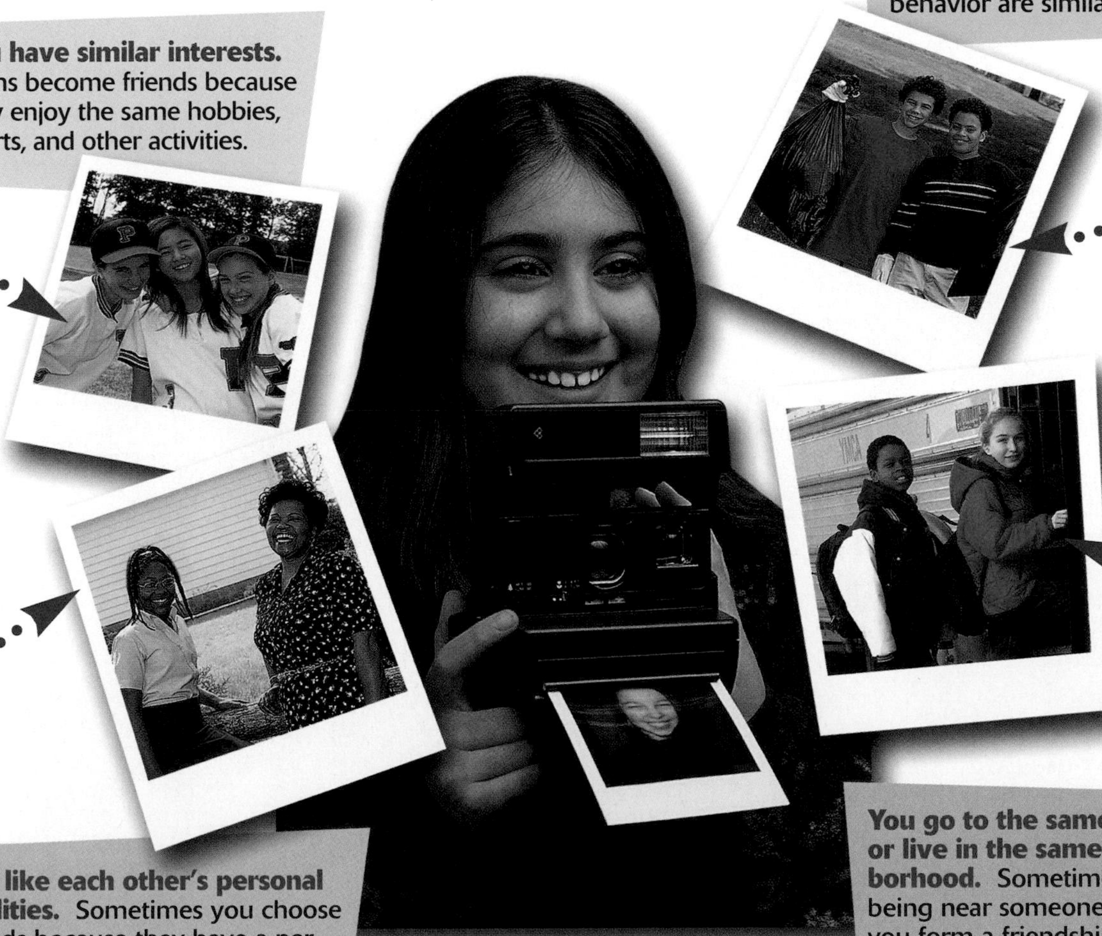

You like each other's personal qualities. Sometimes you choose friends because they have a personal quality that you like, such as a good sense of humor.

You go to the same school or live in the same neighborhood. Sometimes just being near someone helps you form a friendship.

What Makes a Good Friend?

Good friends share a number of special qualities. You and your friends expect these qualities in each other. For example, good friends are loyal and faithful. They will not allow others to say untrue or mean things about you. You also expect them to be **reliable**, or *dependable*. You can count on them to do what they say.

Good friends understand how you feel if you are sad or disappointed. In short, they display **empathy**, or *the ability to identify and share another person's feelings*. They are caring and always want the best for you. They may even care enough to risk a friendship by trying to stop you from doing something that is harmful to you or others.

Some of your friendships are more casual. You may sit with schoolmates in the cafeteria or cheer with them at a football game, but that may be the only time you spend with them. Some of your relationships may be somewhere between casual and close friendships. All your different friendships are an important part of your life.

Your hobbies or interests become even more enjoyable when you share them with a friend. *What hobbies or interests do you have in common with your friends?*

What Is Peer Pressure?

If you named all the people you know who are your age, you'd end up with a very long list. All of *your friends and other people in your age group* are your **peers**. They support you and give you confidence as you move from depending on your family to being on your own. Your peers also have expectations of you. They may pressure you to act and think like everyone else in a group. **Peer pressure** is *the influence you feel to go along with the behavior and beliefs of your peer group.*

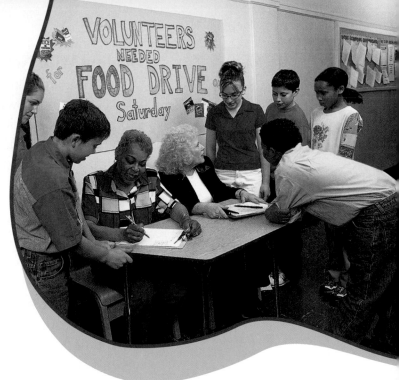

Types of Peer Pressure

Peer pressure can be either positive or negative, subtle or obvious. Positive peer pressure can be a good influence. It can inspire you to improve yourself or do something worthwhile. Peers can be a positive influence, for example, when they

- challenge you to perform well as a member of a team.
- expect you to behave responsibly.
- inspire you to improve your health and your appearance.
- encourage you to do your best in school.
- get you to work with others to improve your school and community.
- expect you to be fair and caring.

When others see you trying to help people, it might motivate them to do the same. *How do your friends motivate you?*

You feel negative peer pressure when others want you to do something that is harmful or goes against your beliefs and values. Your peers put negative pressure on you when they

- urge you to use tobacco, alcohol, or other drugs.
- dare you to do something dangerous or unsafe.
- talk you into being unkind to someone who is different from you and your friends.
- persuade you to do something that goes against your values or something illegal such as shoplifting.
- encourage you to be disrespectful to parents or other adults.
- urge you to fight or get involved with conflicts.

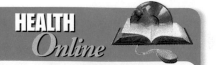

HEALTH *Online*

Make informed decisions when dealing with peer pressure. Use the information you'll find in Web Links at health.glencoe.com.

Dealing With Negative Peer Pressure

Standing up to negative peer pressure can be difficult. You worry about what will happen if you don't go along with the group. Will your friends still like you? Will they leave you out in the future? No matter how difficult, it is important that you develop your own identity, apart from the crowd. It's part of growing up.

Refusal skills, or *methods for saying no,* help you resist negative peer pressure. **Figure 3.4** shows how to handle negative peer pressure using the handy S.T.O.P. formula. Remember that you can always get help from a trusted adult. A parent, older brother or sister, or a counselor will listen to your problem and can help you decide what is the best thing for you to do. They may suggest some options that you haven't considered.

HEALTH SKILLS ACTIVITY

REFUSAL SKILLS

S.T.O.P. the Pressure

You will be more successful at resisting negative peer pressure if you are well prepared. Think of reasons for refusing. Practice what you would say and do. As you practice keep these points in mind. The S.T.O.P. formula makes it easy to remember.

SAY NO IN A FIRM VOICE.
TELL WHY NOT.
OFFER OTHER IDEAS.
PROMPTLY LEAVE.

WITH A GROUP

With three or four classmates, role-play a situation of negative peer pressure. One group member will be the teen facing negative peer pressure. The others will apply the pressure. After each role-play, review the responses of the teen under pressure. Discuss other ways for a teen to refuse in that situation.

FIGURE 3.4

Ways to Resist Negative Peer Pressure

If your peers put negative pressure on you, you could use these methods to say no. *Which approach do you think would work best with the people you know?*

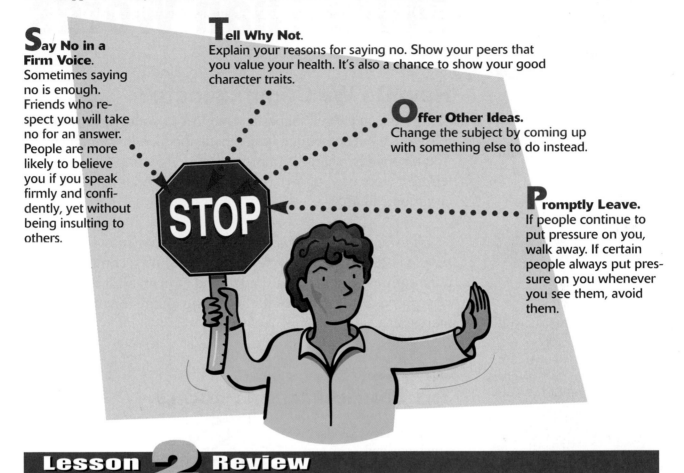

Say No in a Firm Voice. Sometimes saying no is enough. Friends who respect you will take no for an answer. People are more likely to believe you if you speak firmly and confidently, yet without being insulting to others.

Tell Why Not. Explain your reasons for saying no. Show your peers that you value your health. It's also a chance to show your good character traits.

Offer Other Ideas. Change the subject by coming up with something else to do instead.

Promptly Leave. If people continue to put pressure on you, walk away. If certain people always put pressure on you whenever you see them, avoid them.

Lesson 2 Review

Using complete sentences, answer the following questions on a sheet of paper.

Reviewing Terms and Facts

1. **Vocabulary** Define the terms *relationship* and *friendship*.
2. **List** Name four different reasons why teens become friends.
3. **Identify** What are four personal qualities good friends share?

Thinking Critically

4. **Apply** Describe how a friend might respond if people are laughing behind his or her friend's back.

5. **Distinguish** How does positive peer pressure differ from negative peer pressure?
6. **Explain** Why do refusal skills help you resist negative peer pressure?

Applying Health Skills

7. **Analyzing Influences** Write a paragraph in which you describe a friendship you had as a child. Name the ways, if any, that friendship has changed you as you have grown.

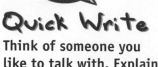

Quick Write

Think of someone you like to talk with. Explain why you like to talk to that person.

LEARN ABOUT...

- how people communicate.
- the best way to communicate your thoughts and feelings.
- how you can be a better speaker and listener.

VOCABULARY

- communication
- gesture
- body language

Communication: More Than Words

How Do We Communicate?

You get on the school bus and sit next to your friend, who tells you about something funny that happened in the hallway. You respond by sharing your friend's good feelings and maybe telling a story of your own. In short, you and your friend are communicating.

The sharing of thoughts and feelings between two or more people is **communication**. As **Figure 3.5** shows, communication requires a message, a sender, and a receiver. It is a two-way process that involves both sending and receiving messages.

FIGURE 3.5

THE COMMUNICATION PROCESS

When someone sends a message and another person receives it, communication occurs.

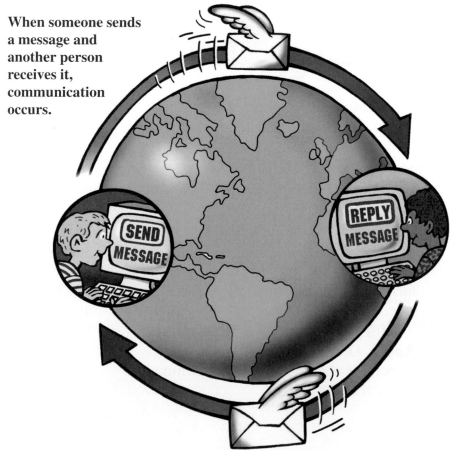

Types of Communication

People communicate by speaking and listening to one another. However, people often say more about their feelings with their faces or the way they move their bodies. Messages can involve all of the following:

- **Words.** The words you use help you communicate. How you say the words gives others clues about your feelings.
- **Facial Expressions.** The look on your face says a lot about how you feel. A smile suggests a person is happy. A raised eyebrow can mean someone is doubtful or suspicious.
- **Gestures.** People often use gestures, or *movements of the hands, arms, and legs,* when they communicate. A clenched fist suggests that a person is angry. People sometimes tap their fingers or feet when they are nervous.
- **Posture.** The way people hold their bodies can also communicate feelings. Standing or sitting straight with the head held high suggests that a person feels good. People who are sad might slouch or walk with their heads down.

Sometimes people send mixed messages—their words don't match their expression, gesture, posture, or tone of voice. For example, a friend might say, "I'm fine," but sound like she really wants to cry. Mixed messages are confusing for listeners.

Good Communication

Being a good communicator will help you build healthy relationships. The following skills will help you as a speaker:

1. **Use "I" messages.** Express your concerns in terms of yourself. You'll be less likely to make others angry or feel defensive.
2. **Make clear, simple statements.** Be specific and accurate. Stick to the subject. Give the other person a chance to do the same, too.
3. **Be honest with thoughts and feelings.** Say what you really think and feel but be polite. Respect the feelings of your listener.
4. **Use appropriate body language.** The term body language refers to *facial expressions, gestures, and posture.* Make eye contact. Show that you are involved as a speaker.

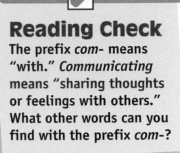

Reading Check

The prefix *com-* means "with." *Communicating* means "sharing thoughts or feelings with others." What other words can you find with the prefix *com-*?

The following skills will help you as a listener:

1. **Use appropriate body language.** Even if you disagree, listen to what the other person has to say. Make eye contact and don't turn away.
2. **Use conversation encouragers.** Say things like "No kidding!" or "Really?" to show you are paying attention.
3. **Mirror thoughts and feelings.** Pay attention to what is being said. Repeat what someone says to show that you hear them.
4. **Ask questions.** Show that you are listening by asking the speaker questions.

Hands-On Health

READING BODY LANGUAGE

As the photograph below shows, body language can tell you a lot about how a person feels. This activity will help you practice reading body language.

WHAT YOU WILL NEED
- newspapers, magazines
- scissors, tape, tacks
- paper, pen, sketch pad

WHAT YOU WILL DO
1. Find pictures or cartoons from newspapers and magazines that demonstrate various forms of body language.
2. Write a caption for each picture describing the body language you observe and what it is communicating. Attach your caption to the back of the picture.
3. Make a sketch or select a picture showing an effective example of body language that you have used or observed others using in the past week. Write a descriptive caption on the back of the sketch.

4. Share your pictures and sketches with your classmates. Ask them what caption they would choose for each picture. Compare their choices to yours.

IN CONCLUSION
1. How often did your interpretation of body language in a picture agree with your classmates' views?
2. How does understanding body language improve your communication with others?

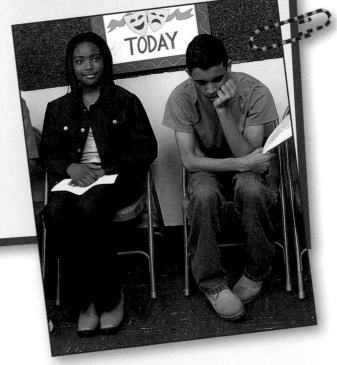

Developing Good Communication Skills

Whether you are sending or receiving messages, your speech and body language represent who you are to others. Like everyone else, you want others to see you in your best light. Improving your communication skills will help you reach that goal. It will also help you meet your need for healthy relationships.

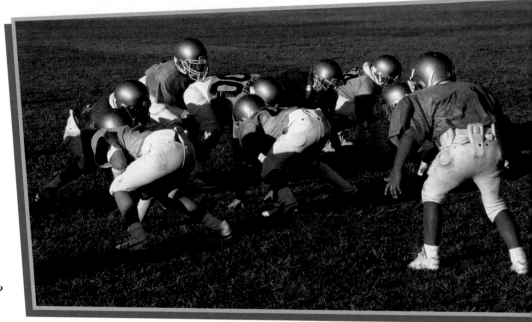

You use your communication skills in all kinds of situations. *What special methods do you use to communicate plays or strategies in a team sport?*

Lesson 3 Review

Using complete sentences, answer the following questions on a sheet of paper.

Reviewing Terms and Facts

1. **Vocabulary** Define the term *communication*. Use it in an original sentence.
2. **Recall** Name three ways in which people communicate with one another.
3. **Identify** List four speaking skills a good communicator uses.

Thinking Critically

4. **Apply** Write a paragraph describing a situation in which you or someone you know expressed his or her feelings in a healthy, thoughtful way.

5. **Predict** How might developing good communication skills help you in the future?

Applying Health Skills

6. **Communication Skills** Write a short story about a teen with a communication problem. Explain how he or she could solve the problem. Share your story with a classmate.

Resolving Conflicts

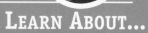

LEARN ABOUT...

- why conflicts occur.
- what to do if you are not getting along with someone.
- how you can protect yourself from violence.

VOCABULARY

- conflict
- tolerance
- compromise
- peer mediation
- violence

Why Does Conflict Occur?

Have you ever argued with a friend or family member? If you're like most people, you have done so many times. An argument is an example of **conflict**, or *a problem in a relationship.* Conflict is a normal part of life. However, when people do not resolve, or deal with, their conflicts, they might end up shouting at or not speaking to each other. An argument can even lead to pushing and shoving contests. **Figure 3.6** shows how some conflicts occur.

FIGURE 3.6

HOW CONFLICTS DEVELOP

Different situations can lead to conflict. *What situations in your life have led to conflict?*

A Differing Expectations
Mark and his sister can't agree on when each of them should get to use the home computer.

B Differing Values
Sita wants to be paid for babysitting her sister. Her mom thinks this is Sita's responsibility as a family member.

C Hurt Feelings
Jake never invites Manuel over to his house after school.

D Changing Roles
Now that Rachel's sister Gina is away at college, Rachel has to do more chores.

E Jealousy
Beth did not make the pep squad, but her friend Shira did.

F Possessions
Sam's friend Don borrowed his book two weeks ago and still hasn't returned it.

G Struggle for Power
Colleen's group of friends has always seen her as their leader. Now Keiko, a new girl, is challenging that role.

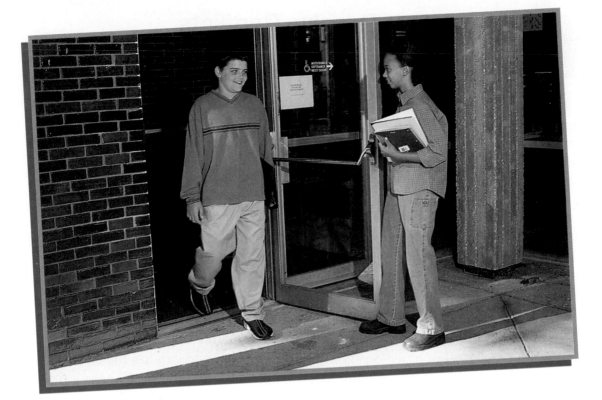

Some conflicts can be avoided by showing common courtesy. *What are other ways you can avoid conflict?*

How to Prevent Conflict

How do you handle conflict? One way is to prevent it from happening in the first place. There are a number of approaches you can take.

Practicing tolerance can prevent many conflicts. **Tolerance** (TAHL·er·ence) is *the ability to accept other people as they are.* People may not always behave the way you like. Use your communication skills. They can clear up a misunderstanding before it builds up and causes further trouble.

If you sense a conflict in the making, try to make the situation less tense. Put it in perspective. Tell a joke or change the subject. You might suggest a quick change of activity.

When a conflict gets out of hand, walk away and cool off. Angry words and insults will only make matters worse. You might say something in the heat of the moment that you will regret later. Also, ask yourself if the issue is worth the conflict. You may not want to waste your energy on something that's not so important to you.

How to Resolve Conflicts

What can you do if you are involved in a dispute? Almost every solution requires each side to give a little. **Compromise** means that *each person gives up something in order to reach a solution that satisfies everyone.*

Resolving Conflict Through Communication

Good communication can help resolve conflict as well as prevent it. Use your speaking skills to present your side of the argument. Use your listening skills when the other person explains his or her side. The T.A.L.K. strategy can also help you resolve conflicts.

- **Take a time-out.** Wait at least 30 minutes before you talk over the situation. This will give both of you a chance to calm down.
- **Allow each person to tell his or her side uninterrupted.** Each person should have the chance to explain his or her feelings without the other person breaking in. Choose a time and place to talk where you won't be interrupted.
- **Let each person ask questions.** Both people should have the chance to question each other. Stay calm and respectful. Also, stick to the issue. Don't bring up other problems at this time.
- **Keep brainstorming.** Try to see the situation from the other person's point of view. It will help you find a solution that will satisfy you both.

HEALTH SKILLS ACTIVITY

COMMUNICATION SKILLS

"You" and "I"

When resolving conflicts, choose your words wisely. Be careful how you use the little words "you" and "I." Sentences centered on "you" tend to place blame on the other person. Sentences stressing "I" show a willingness to work things out.

- **"YOU" MESSAGE:** "Why do you always get to pick where we'll hang out? Some of us deserve a chance to pick, too."

- **"I" MESSAGE:** "I feel frustrated that I never get to choose where we hang out."

WITH A GROUP

Write three sentences that use "you" messages to express anger or frustration. Then exchange lists with another student. Rewrite your partner's "you" messages as "I" messages. Compare your messages with your partner's.

Resolving Conflict Through Peer Mediation

A mediator can help resolve conflicts. Mediators are people who are not involved in the dispute. Counselors, parents, or other adults can be mediators. Many schools have peer mediation programs. **Peer mediation** (mee·dee·AY·shuhn) is *a process in which a specially trained student listens to both sides of an argument and then helps the opposing sides reach a solution.* **Figure 3.7** shows the steps a peer mediator might follow to help settle a conflict.

FIGURE 3.7

THE MEDIATION PROCESS

To help students resolve conflicts, peer mediators go through hours of training. If you are a mediator, here are the basic steps you take in any mediation situation:

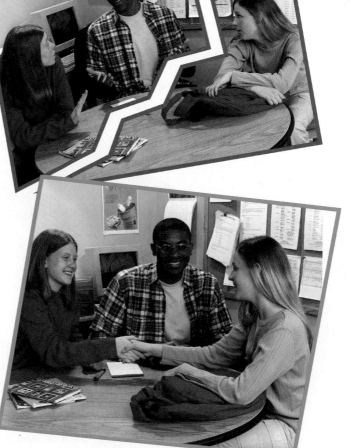

Step 1 **Establish neutrality.** Tell the opposing sides you will remain neutral. You will not take sides or decide who is right or wrong.

Step 2 **Set the ground rules.** Get the opposite sides to agree on rules for keeping the discussion fair and orderly. For example, you would want to prohibit name-calling and interrupting.

Step 3 **Listen to each side.** Allow each person to tell his or her view of the situation without interruption. Then allow each person to ask questions.

Step 4 **Search for possible solutions.** Brainstorm solutions together or ask each person to suggest a solution. Think of as many solutions as possible. Continue until you reach a solution that satisfies both sides.

Step 5 **Don't give up.** If the opposing sides can't reach an agreeable solution, ask for help from an adult trusted by both sides.

When Conflicts Get Out of Hand

Conflicts that get out of hand can lead to violence. **Violence**, or *the use of physical force to harm someone or something,* is a serious problem in the United States. Music lyrics, movies, television shows, and video games often show or suggest violent behavior. When people think that violence is an acceptable way to deal with conflict, they may attack or even kill other people. **Figure 3.8** shows some causes of violence.

Violent crime affects everyone. Victims of crime and their families are the first to suffer. People who witness crimes are often affected. Medical expenses, trials, and prisons make violent crimes costly for everyone.

FIGURE 3.8

WHY VIOLENCE ERUPTS

There are some common factors that contribute to violent acts.

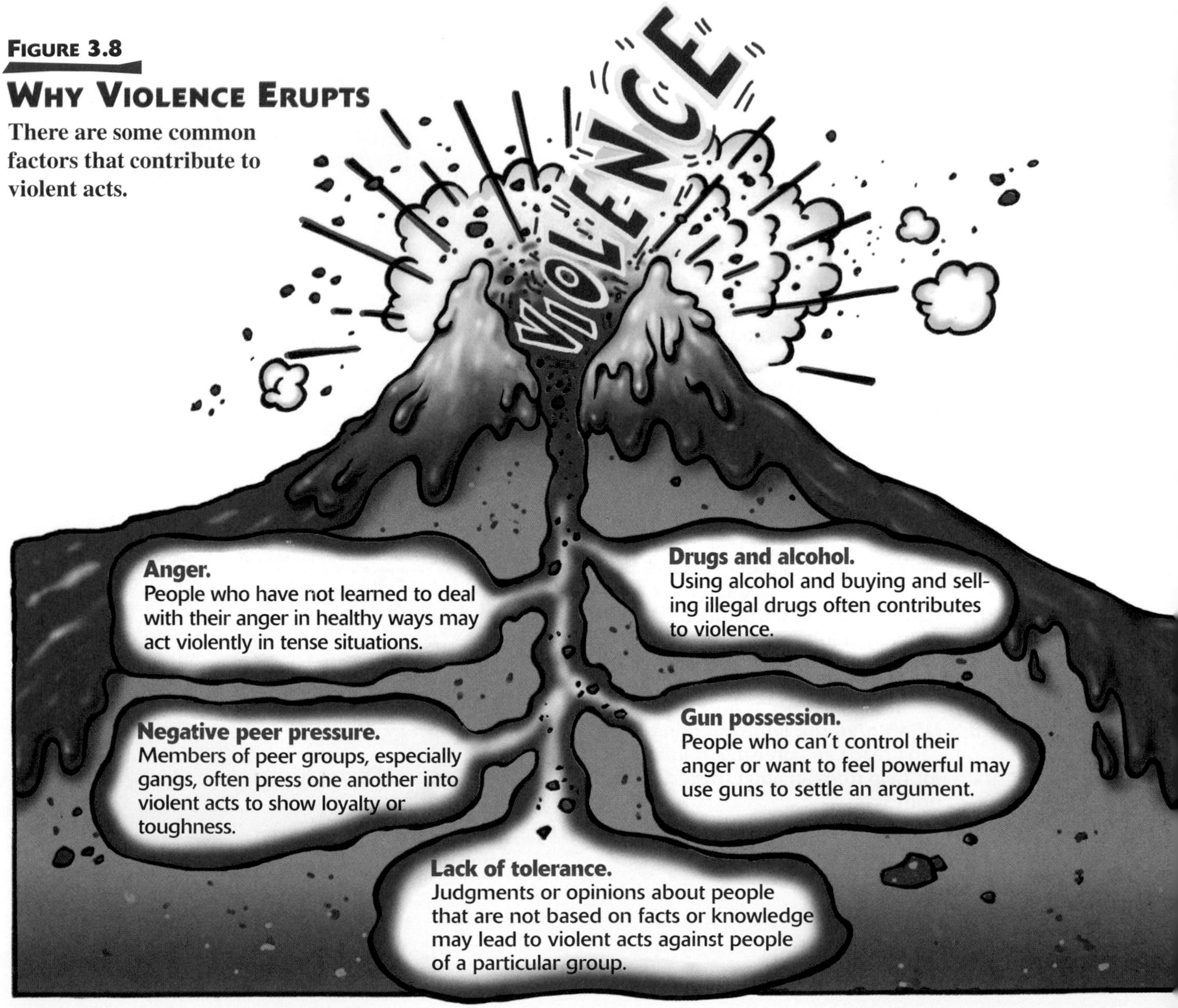

Anger.
People who have not learned to deal with their anger in healthy ways may act violently in tense situations.

Drugs and alcohol.
Using alcohol and buying and selling illegal drugs often contributes to violence.

Negative peer pressure.
Members of peer groups, especially gangs, often press one another into violent acts to show loyalty or toughness.

Gun possession.
People who can't control their anger or want to feel powerful may use guns to settle an argument.

Lack of tolerance.
Judgments or opinions about people that are not based on facts or knowledge may lead to violent acts against people of a particular group.

What You Can Do

You might ask, "What can one person do to stop violence?" You can start by believing in yourself and knowing that you deserve respect. Then, follow these steps to protect yourself.

- **Commit to nonviolence.** Do not fight or threaten others. Don't watch fights or encourage others to fight.
- **Dress for safety.** Do not wear T-shirts with offensive messages. Avoid wearing anything that could be mistaken for gang clothing. Avoid wearing expensive items like gold jewelry or leather jackets, which may put you in danger. If you use a purse, carry it with the strap across your chest.
- **Avoid weapons, gangs, and drugs.** Any contact with weapons, gangs, or drugs is likely to lead to trouble.
- **Use conflict resolution.** Recall the skills you've learned for settling disputes and practice them whenever possible.
- **Use good manners.** Being polite can help ease tensions that can lead to violence.
- **Accept differences.** Recognize that individuals and groups are entitled to have different ideas, beliefs, and values.
- **Advocate for peace.** Serve as a positive example. Become a peer mediator or volunteer with an anticrime group.

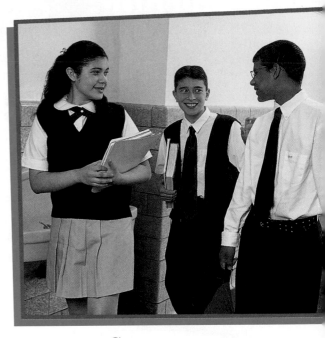

Some schools require students to wear uniforms. This eliminates gang colors and clothes. *Do you think school uniforms are a good idea?*

Lesson 4 Review

Using complete sentences, answer the following questions on a sheet of paper.

Reviewing Terms and Facts

1. **Vocabulary** Use *conflict* and *compromise* in two original sentences that show the meanings of the terms.
2. **Identify** Name two ways you can help prevent conflict from occurring.
3. **Recall** List the communication skills that help resolve conflict.

Thinking Critically

4. **Restate** In your own words, state the steps in the mediation process.

5. **Analyze** Name two factors that can lead to violence. Suggest ways to eliminate these factors or lessen their effects.

Applying Health Skills

6. **Analyzing Influences** Prepare a booklet in which you describe or place advertisements for movies or television programs that depict violence. Explain how you think these advertisements affect viewers.

LET'S TALK

Model

Communication is a skill. The more you practice it, the better you will become at it. Good communication will help you build healthy relationships with friends and family members. Read the following dialogue between Malik and Carly, two good friends who communicate well together.

"Is something wrong, Malik? You look upset."
CONVERSATION ENCOURAGER; BODY LANGUAGE

"Yeah, I'm really worried. My dog, Buster, got sick this weekend and we had to take him to the vet."
"I" MESSAGE; HONEST THOUGHTS AND FEELINGS

"Oh, I'm sorry. You must be really nervous about him. Does the vet know what's wrong?"
MIRROR THOUGHTS AND FEELINGS; ASK QUESTIONS

"Not yet. I hope my mom will know something when I get home from school today."
HONEST THOUGHTS AND FEELINGS

"I hope so, too. Let me know how it goes."
CLEAR, SIMPLE MESSAGE

Practice

Practice your conversation skills with a simple game. Form groups of three. One of you will be the speaker, one will be the listener, and one will keep score. The scorekeeper will write down the speaking and listening skills shown in the Coach's Box. Then the speaker will choose a topic to discuss with the listener. The scorekeeper will give the speaker a point each time he or she uses good speaking skills. The listener will get points for using good listening skills. When you are finished, trade roles: make the speaker the new listener and the listener the new scorekeeper. Play the game once more then rotate the roles again and play a third time.

Apply/Assess

Now try writing your own conversation. Choose one situation shown here or make up your own. Write a conversation using the speaking and listening skills you learned. Role-play your conversation with a partner. Have your classmates identify the speaking and listening skills you use as you role-play your conversation.

You and a friend are talking about plans for the weekend.

You are discussing a problem with your parent.

You are talking to a brother or sister about a family vacation.

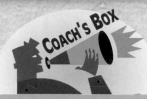

Communication Skills

Speaking skills
- "I" messages
- Clear, simple statements
- Honest thoughts and feelings
- Body language

Listening skills
- Body language
- Conversation encouragers
- Mirror thoughts and feelings
- Ask questions

Self-√ Check
- Did our conversation show good speaking skills?
- Did our conversation show good listening skills?

WORKING THINGS OUT

Model

Conflicts are common in relationships. A healthy way to resolve these conflicts is to communicate about the problem. Read about how two sisters, Kari and Samantha, resolved a conflict.

> "Samantha, I noticed something a while ago, and I'd like to talk about it."
>
> **T—TAKE A TIME-OUT.**

> "Sure, what's going on?"
>
> **L—LET EACH PERSON ASK QUESTIONS.**

> "I feel upset when you borrow my clothes without asking. I haven't even gotten to wear that sweater yet. Why did you borrow it?"
>
> **A—ALLOW EACH PERSON TO TELL HIS OR HER SIDE UNINTERRUPTED; L—LET EACH PERSON ASK QUESTIONS.**

> "I guess I wasn't thinking. I just opened your drawer and saw this great sweater. Do you want it back right now?"
>
> **A—ALLOW EACH PERSON TO TELL HIS OR HER SIDE UNINTERRUPTED.**

> "No, but I would like to have an agreement about this. What if we always ask before we borrow each other's stuff?"
>
> **K—KEEP BRAINSTORMING TO FIND A GOOD SOLUTION.**

> "Sure, I will if you will."

Practice

See what you have learned about resolving conflict. Read the following conversation between Carlos and Lee. This afternoon Lee found a CD that Carlos had lost. When Carlos asked for it back, Lee said, "Finders keepers." Can you identify the steps that the boys take to resolve their conflict? Write the conversation on your own paper and label the steps, T.A.L.K. Complete the conversation by writing an ending in which Carlos and Lee agree on a solution.

CARLOS: Lee, I'd like to talk about what happened this afternoon.

LEE: I'll listen, but I did find the CD. If I hadn't found it, someone else would have picked it up and taken it.

CARLOS: I know, and I'm glad you found it. But it's my favorite CD, and I would like to have it back.

LEE: So what should we do?

Apply/Assess

Adolescence is a good time to learn how to resolve conflicts. This ability helps keep relationships healthy. On your own paper, list several situations that lead to conflict for teens. Choose one of these situations and write a script showing how the conflict can be resolved. Remember to use the T.A.L.K. steps for conflict resolution and show a respectful tone.

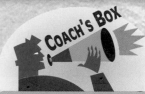

Conflict Resolution

T Take a time-out, at least 30 minutes.
A Allow each person to tell his or her side uninterrupted.
L Let each person ask questions.
K Keep brainstorming to find a good solution.

Self-√Check

- Did my script show how to use the T.A.L.K. steps for conflict resolution?
- Did my script show both sides and use a respectful tone?

SUMMARY

LESSON·1 Many types of family structures exist in the United States today. All types of families can be both happy and healthy.

LESSON·2 Friendships become increasingly important in the early teen years. Friends help meet many social and emotional needs.

LESSON·3 Effective communication skills help people express thoughts and feelings in healthy ways.

LESSON·4 Communication, compromise, and peer mediation are three ways to resolve conflicts peacefully.

Reviewing Vocabulary and Concepts

On a sheet of paper, write the numbers 1–10. After each number, write the term from the list that best completes each sentence.

- emotional
- empathy
- family
- nuclear
- nurture
- peer pressure
- peers
- refusal skills
- reliable
- sexual

Lesson 1

1. The _____ is the basic unit of society.
2. A(n) _____ family is made up of two parents and one or more children.
3. Healthy families _____ their members, or provide for their physical, mental/emotional, and social needs.
4. Yelling at and putting down a family member is an example of _____ abuse.
5. _____ abuse occurs when an adult engages in sexual activity with a child or teen.

Lesson 2

6. A(n) _____ person is dependable.
7. The ability to identify and share people's feelings is called _____ .
8. Your _____ are your friends and other people in your age group.
9. You experience negative _____ when your friends urge you to do something dangerous or unsafe.
10. Methods for saying no are called _____.

Lesson 3

On a sheet of paper, write the numbers 11–13. After each number, write the letter of the answer that best completes each statement.

11. The sharing of thoughts and feelings between two or more people is
    a. empathy.
    b. body language.
    c. mediation.
    d. communication.

12. Movements of the hands, arms, and legs, often used in communication, are called
a. speaking skills.
b. mixed messages.
c. gestures.
d. posture.

13. Body language involves
a. facial expressions.
b. gestures.
c. postures.
d. all of the above.

Lesson 4

On a sheet of paper, write the numbers 14–18. Write *True* or *False* for each statement below. If the statement is false, change the underlined word or phrase to make it true.

14. Conflict is a problem in a relationship.

15. Exercising tolerance, the ability to accept other people as they are, is a good way to prevent conflict.

16. Mediation occurs when each person in a conflict gives up something in order to reach a solution that satisfies everyone.

17. Peer pressure is a process in which a specially trained student listens to both sides of an argument and then helps the opposing sides reach a solution.

18. The use of physical force to harm someone is known as violence.

Thinking Critically

Using complete sentences, answer the following questions on a sheet of paper.

19. Describe What are three ways of refusing when you are experiencing negative peer pressure?

20. Interpret Why do you think it can be difficult for teens to resist negative peer pressure?

21. Suggest What are some ways to open lines of communication with someone who is reluctant to talk?

22. Analyze Describe some ways of resolving or preventing conflict that you have found to be effective.

Career Corner

Family Counselor

A family that is having problems can find help from a family counselor. These professionals teach family members how to listen to one another. They help families work together to find solutions. Family counselors need a four-year college degree plus two years of graduate work in counseling. To learn more, click on Career Corner at health.glencoe.com.

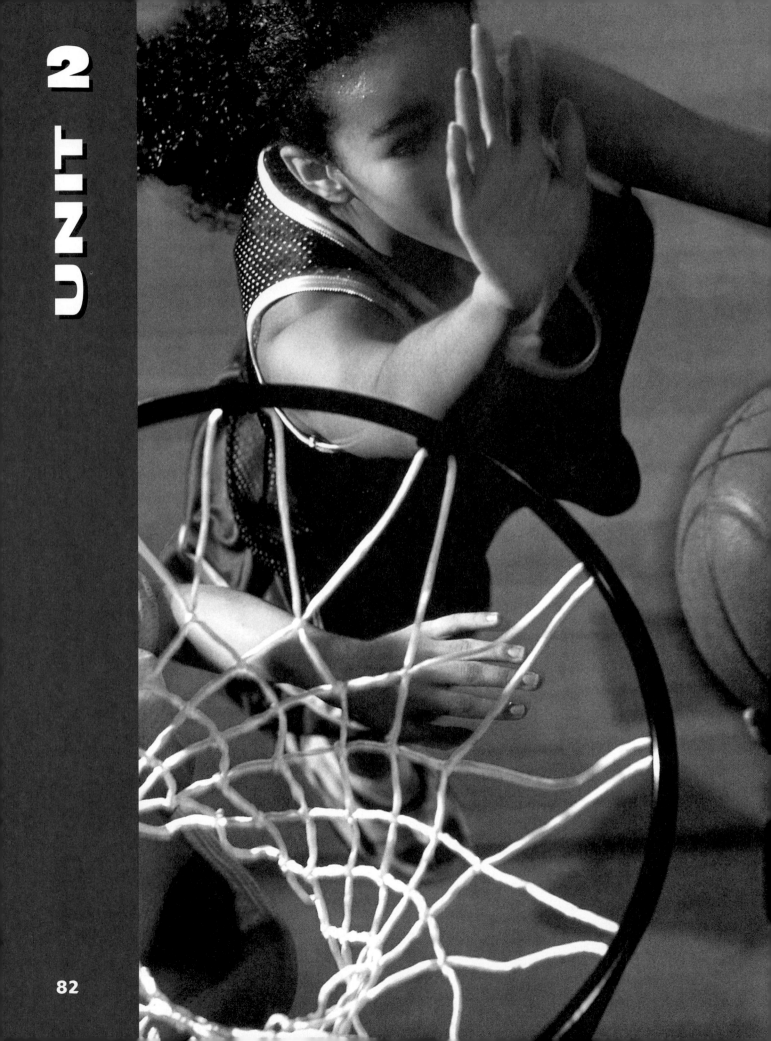

UNIT 2

Promoting Physical Health

Technology Project

Safe Internet Searches

Learn how to access accurate, reliable health information on the Internet.

- Log on to health.glencoe.com.
- Click on Technology Projects and find the "Safe Internet Searches" activity.
- Identify topics for your search and follow the guidelines to evaluate the sites you find.

In Your Home and Community

Communication Skills

During adolescence, your relationship with your parents may change. Write a letter to your parents that explains how you are changing as you go through adolescence. Describe the ways in which you see them differently. Express your feelings about how you would like your parents to treat you now that you are older and more mature.

Personal Health

Quick Write

Write down your responses to the following questions. How well do you take care of your personal health and appearance? Who or what influences you to practice these healthful behaviors?

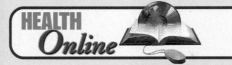

Go to health.glencoe.com and take the Health Inventory for Chapter 4 to rate how well you take care of your teeth, skin, eyes, and ears.

✔ Reading Check

Using each lesson title as a column heading, put the following words under the title where it best fits: *clinics, contact lenses, noise level, dandruff, comparison shopping, eyestrain, advertisements, orthodontists, health insurance, sunblock, plaque.*

Your Teeth, Skin, and Hair

Quick Write

List the things you do to take care of your teeth, skin, and hair.

LEARN ABOUT...

- how you can keep your teeth healthy.
- ways to take care of your skin.
- how you should care for your hair and nails.

VOCABULARY

- plaque
- tartar
- fluoride
- orthodontist
- epidermis
- dermis
- acne
- dermatologist
- cuticle
- dandruff

Healthy Teeth and Gums

Your teeth and gums help you eat, smile, and even talk. For these reasons and more, it is important to take care of your teeth and gums. Developing healthy dental habits now will help prevent tooth decay and loss throughout your life.

Tooth and gum problems start when plaque stays on the teeth too long. **Plaque** (PLAK) is a *soft, colorless, sticky film containing bacteria that grows on your teeth.* It is the main cause of both tooth decay and gum disease. It can also make your breath smell bad. **Figure 4.1** shows you how plaque causes tooth decay.

FIGURE 4.1

TOOTH DECAY

Tooth decay and gum disease usually result from poor dental care. *Do you know the correct way to brush your teeth?*

Stage 1
The bacteria in plaque combine with sugars to form a harmful acid. This acid eats into the enamel, the hard outer surface of the tooth.

Stage 2
Repeated acid attacks on the enamel cause a cavity, or hole, to form.

Stage 3
If the cavity grows and reaches the sensitive inner parts of the tooth, it can cause a toothache.

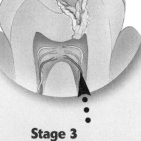

Preventing Tooth and Gum Problems

The best way to avoid tooth and gum problems is to clean your teeth correctly, as shown in **Figure 4.2**. If plaque is not removed by brushing, it can turn into a *hard material* called tartar (TAR·ter). Tartar threatens the health of your teeth and gums. Brushing cannot remove tartar. Only a dentist or dental hygienist can remove it with special instruments.

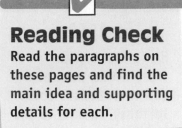

Reading Check
Read the paragraphs on these pages and find the main idea and supporting details for each.

FIGURE 4.2

BRUSHING AND FLOSSING

To reduce plaque, you should brush after eating whenever possible and floss at least once a day.

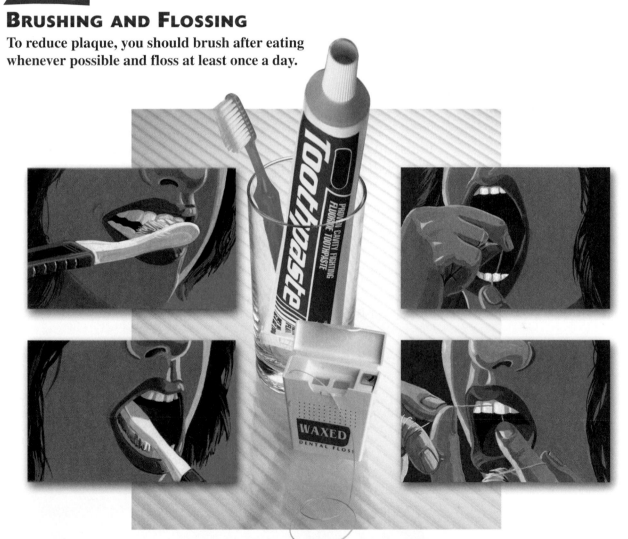

Brushing
Use a soft-bristled brush and toothpaste that contains **fluoride** (FLAWR·eyed), *a substance that fights tooth decay.* Brush the outer tooth surfaces first. Tilt the top of your toothbrush where your teeth and gum meet. Move your brush back and forth gently, using short strokes across your teeth. Then brush the inner tooth surfaces, your chewing surfaces, and your tongue.

Flossing
Take about 18 inches of dental floss and wrap the ends around the middle finger of each hand. Hold the floss tightly between your thumbs and forefingers and slide it gently between your teeth. Move it up or down to the gum line with a gentle sawing motion. Rub the side of the tooth and bring the floss back out gently. Repeat the process between all of your teeth.

More teens than ever can wear braces comfortably, thanks to the National Aeronautics and Space Administration (NASA). NASA was the first to develop tooth-moving wires. When activated by body heat, the wires become stronger and more flexible. This makes the braces more comfortable.

Keep your teeth strong and healthy by eating right. Fresh fruits and vegetables are especially good for your teeth. So are foods high in calcium, such as milk, cheese, and yogurt. If you eat sugary or starchy foods, it is best to eat them with a meal. Otherwise, brush your teeth right away.

Visiting the Dentist

To keep your teeth and gums healthy, see your dentist twice a year. The dentist or dental hygienist will clean your teeth thoroughly to prevent decay and disease. Then the dentist will look for signs of tooth decay and gum disease and provide treatment before problems occur.

In addition to your regular dentist, you may need to visit an orthodontist. An **orthodontist** is *a dentist who specializes in dealing with irregularities of the teeth and jaw.* Straightening teeth that are crooked does more than make them look better. It also makes them easier to clean. This reduces the chance that tooth decay or gum disease will develop.

To straighten teeth, an orthodontist will apply braces. This involves attaching a small bracket to each tooth and connecting the brackets with wires. Braces can be made of metal, ceramic, or plastic. Patients can also choose from a variety of colors.

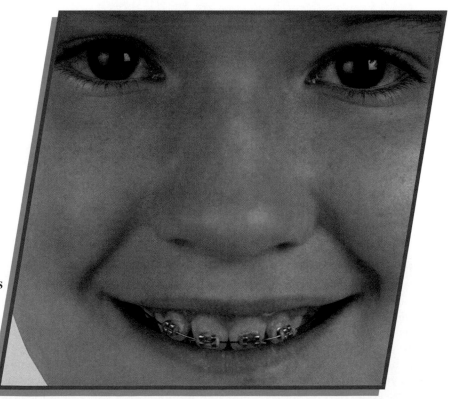

Choosing different colors makes wearing braces more fun. *Why do you think patients would choose colored braces?*

Healthy Skin

Your skin is your body's largest organ. Like your other body organs, your skin performs many important functions. It protects you from germs and helps control your body temperature. The nerve endings in your skin allow you to feel textures, temperatures, pressures, and pain.

Parts of the Skin

Your skin is a complex organ. It is made up of various tissues that work together to perform many functions. Your skin consists of two main layers. The *thinner outer layer of the skin* is called the **epidermis**. The *thicker inner layer of the skin* is known as the **dermis**. See **Figure 4.3**.

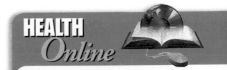
FIGURE 4.3

THE SKIN

Your skin has many more parts than just the outside surface.

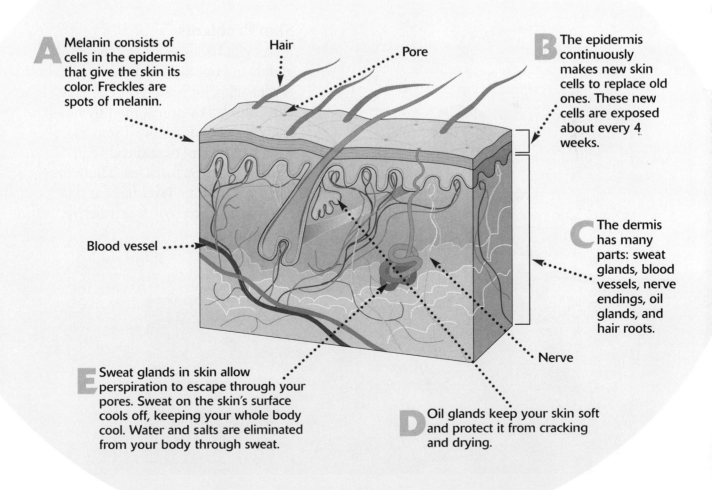

A Melanin consists of cells in the epidermis that give the skin its color. Freckles are spots of melanin.

Hair

Pore

B The epidermis continuously makes new skin cells to replace old ones. These new cells are exposed about every 4 weeks.

Blood vessel

C The dermis has many parts: sweat glands, blood vessels, nerve endings, oil glands, and hair roots.

Nerve

E Sweat glands in skin allow perspiration to escape through your pores. Sweat on the skin's surface cools off, keeping your whole body cool. Water and salts are eliminated from your body through sweat.

D Oil glands keep your skin soft and protect it from cracking and drying.

Caring for Your Skin

The best way to care for your skin is to keep it clean and protect it from the sun.

- **Keep your skin clean.** As your body develops, sweat glands increase their activity. When sweat mixes with bacteria that live on your body, it starts to smell. Washing sweat away keeps your skin clean and smelling fresh. To control odor, use a deodorant. This product slows the growth of bacteria.

- **Protect your skin from the sun.** Ultraviolet (UV) rays from the sun damage your skin. Over time, they can cause wrinkles or contribute to skin cancer. The lighter your skin is, the more easily these rays can harm you. UV rays are strongest between 10:00 a.m. and 4:00 p.m. in the summertime, or 9:00 a.m. and 3:00 p.m. in the wintertime. Try to stay out of direct sunlight during these hours. When you are in the sun, wear protective clothing, such as long-sleeved shirts and wide-brimmed hats. Cover exposed skin with sun-blocking agents or sunscreens with a sun protection factor (SPF) of 15 or higher. An SPF of 15 gives your skin 15 times its natural protection from sunburn. Read the label on the bottle to find out how often to apply sunscreen.

Skin Problems

As you become a teen, the oil glands in your skin start to work harder. This increased oil can clog hair follicles or pores, the tiny holes from which hairs grow. Pimples, whiteheads, and blackheads can form in blocked follicles. These are all forms of **acne** (AK·nee), a *skin condition caused by overly active oil glands.*

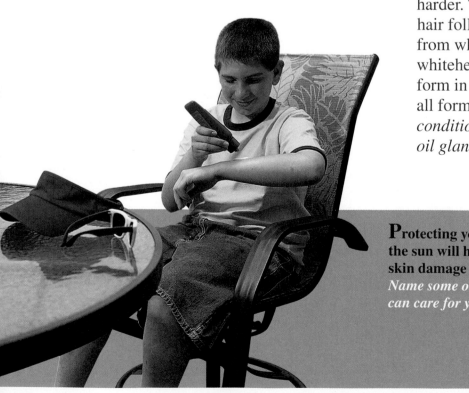

Protecting your skin from the sun will help you avoid skin damage in later life. *Name some other ways you can care for your skin.*

PRACTICING HEALTHFUL BEHAVIORS

Skin Care Strategies

To prevent acne, wash your skin twice a day with a mild soap or cleanser. Rinse with warm water and blot it dry gently with a clean towel. You can also help keep your skin healthy by following these tips:

- Eat sensibly.
- Drink plenty of water.
- Exercise regularly.
- Manage stress.
- Avoid greasy, oil-based makeup or creams.
- Get enough sleep.
- Wash bed linens and towels regularly.
- Keep your hair clean to prevent oil from spreading to your face.

- Keep your hands away from your face. Your fingers can spread bacteria.
- Resist the urge to pop, pick, or squeeze pimples. You could cause more skin irritation, leaving tiny pits and scars.

ON YOUR OWN

Create a personal routine for skin and face care. Follow your routine for a week. Do you notice any change in the appearance of your skin?

Most teens—about 90 percent—have some form of acne. Stress can make acne worse. Mild acne can usually be treated at home. For serious acne, see your regular doctor or a **dermatologist** (DER·muh·TAH·luh·jist), *a doctor who treats skin disorders.*

Skin decorations, such as tattoos and piercings, can also cause skin problems. If needles and other equipment are not perfectly clean and disinfected, they can spread serious infections. These include HIV (the virus that causes AIDS) and hepatitis, a dangerous inflammation of the liver.

The earlobe is the only body part generally considered safe for piercing. *Why might ear piercing be safer than other kinds of body piercing?*

Healthy Nails

Fingernails and toenails are dead cells that grow out of living tissue located in the dermis. A *nonliving band of epidermis* called the **cuticle** (KYOO·ti·kuhl) surrounds the nails. Well-kept nails make your hands look attractive and healthy. Follow these steps to care for your nails.

- Soften your hands with warm water and use a cuticle stick to push back the cuticle.
- Use a nail clipper or small scissors to trim your nails. Round the ends of your fingernails slightly. Cut your toenails straight across, with the nail at or slightly beyond skin level.
- Use an emery board or nail file to round out the ends of your fingernails. An emery board also smoothes out rough edges.

Healthy Hair

No part of your body grows faster than your hair. Hair shafts, the part of the hair you can see, consist of dead protein cells that overlap each other, like shingles on a roof. The shape of these hair shafts determines the overall appearance of your hair: wavy, straight, or curly. Your hair color comes from melanin, the same substance that gives your skin its color.

What Causes Hair and Scalp Problems?

If the scalp produces too much oil, hair may become flat, stringy, and greasy. If it produces too little oil, hair may be coarse and brittle. That's why you should always use the right shampoo for your hair type—dry, oily, or normal.

Sun exposure or excessive heat from hair dryers can make hair dry, brittle, and faded. Curling irons also can overdry hair and increase breakage. Dyeing or bleaching hair at home can cause disastrous results. Chlorine in pool water can damage and dry your hair shafts. Special shampoos can remove chlorine from your hair to prevent damage.

A common scalp problem is **dandruff**, *flaking of the outer layer of dead skin cells*. A dry scalp usually causes dandruff. Washing your hair regularly controls dandruff. If this does not work, use a dandruff shampoo. Sometimes head lice cause an itchy scalp. These tiny, wingless insects that live in the hair are very common and easy to catch from someone else. To

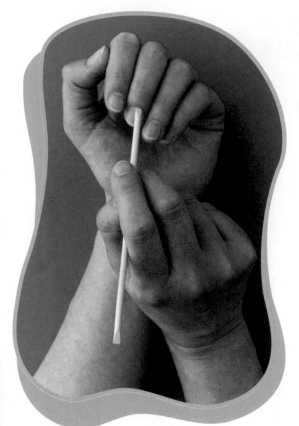

You can keep your cuticles looking neat by pushing them back with a cuticle stick. *What else can you do to improve the appearance of your nails?*

prevent lice from spreading, avoid sharing hats, combs, or brushes with other people. If you get lice, you can kill them with a medicated shampoo. You will also need to wash all your bedding, towels, combs, brushes, and clothing. Everyone else in your house will need to take these steps, too.

Caring for Your Hair

To keep your hair healthy and looking good, wash it regularly and comb or brush it carefully.

- **Washing.** Use a gentle shampoo and rinse completely with warm water to remove excess shampoo or conditioner. Oily hair may require a deep cleaning shampoo. If possible, let your hair dry by itself. If you use a blow dryer, use low heat. Avoid washing your hair too often, which can dry it out.

- **Brushing and combing.** Brushing or combing once a day helps spread natural scalp oils down the hair shaft. Too much brushing, though, can break the hair shaft or pull hair out. If you use a brush, choose one with rounded or balled tips so you do not scratch your scalp.

No matter what type of hair you have, taking good care of it is a healthful habit. *List three things you can do to take care of your hair.*

Oval shaft, wavy hair

Round shaft, straight hair

Flat shaft, curly hair

Lesson 1 Review

Using complete sentences, answer the following questions on a sheet of paper.

Reviewing Terms and Facts

1. **Vocabulary** Define *plaque* and *tartar*. How are the terms related?
2. **Vocabulary** Define the words *epidermis* and *dermis*.
3. **Recall** What is dandruff and how can you get rid of it?

Thinking Critically

4. **Explain** What can you do to keep the sun from damaging your skin?
5. **Apply** What can teens do to prevent acne?

Applying Health Skills

6. **Advocacy** Write and illustrate a persuasive pamphlet that explains how to brush or floss teeth. Be sure to convince the reader that brushing and flossing are important. Distribute the pamphlet to a younger class.

Protecting Your Eyes and Ears

Quick Write

Do you like studying with music on? Do you prefer quiet when you read or talk with friends? Write a paragraph about what level of sound feels most comfortable for you.

LEARN ABOUT...

- how to care for your eyes and vision.
- how to protect your ears and hearing.

VOCABULARY

- farsightedness
- nearsightedness
- astigmatism
- decibels
- sound waves

Healthy Eyes

Your eyes allow you to see your friends, read your favorite books, and do much more. Taking care of your eyes will help you look and feel good throughout your life. First, find out how the eye works by looking at **Figure 4.4**.

Caring for Your Eyes

The following tips will keep your eyes healthy.

- **Protect your eyes from eyestrain.** Reading, watching television, or using a computer for too long can strain your eyes. To avoid this, read and watch television in a well-lighted room. Place your reading lamp so it shines on your reading material. When you use a computer, keep the screen about two feet from your face and tilted slightly away from you. Take breaks whenever you watch TV, work on the computer, or do other close-up work.

Protecting your eyes is a good health habit that will help you maintain good vision throughout your life. *List some of the ways you can keep your eyes healthy.*

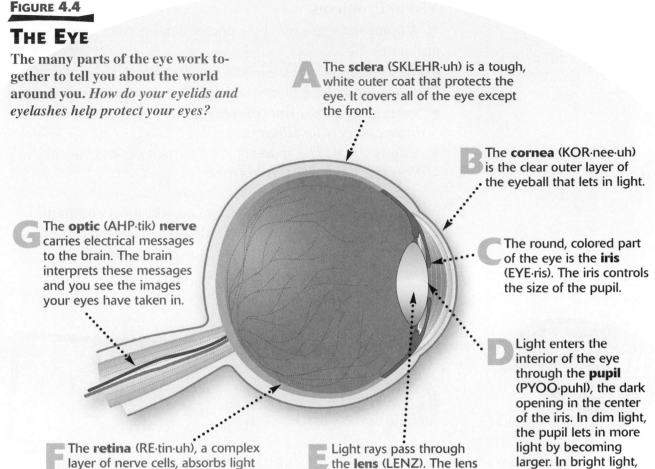

FIGURE 4.4

THE EYE

The many parts of the eye work together to tell you about the world around you. *How do your eyelids and eyelashes help protect your eyes?*

A The **sclera** (SKLEHR·uh) is a tough, white outer coat that protects the eye. It covers all of the eye except the front.

B The **cornea** (KOR·nee·uh) is the clear outer layer of the eyeball that lets in light.

G The **optic** (AHP·tik) **nerve** carries electrical messages to the brain. The brain interprets these messages and you see the images your eyes have taken in.

C The round, colored part of the eye is the **iris** (EYE·ris). The iris controls the size of the pupil.

D Light enters the interior of the eye through the **pupil** (PYOO·puhl), the dark opening in the center of the iris. In dim light, the pupil lets in more light by becoming larger. In bright light, the pupils keep out some light by becoming smaller.

F The **retina** (RE·tin·uh), a complex layer of nerve cells, absorbs light rays from the lens. It changes light rays into electrical images and sends them to the optic nerve.

E Light rays pass through the **lens** (LENZ). The lens adjusts to focus the light on the retina, like the lens of a camera.

- **Protect your eyes from injury.** Use safety eyewear when using power tools or playing certain sports. If you get something in your eye, do not rub it. Try to blink and let tears wash the object out. If this does not work, rinse the eye with water or an eye wash.
- **Protect your eyes from infection.** If your eyes hurt or itch, do not rub them. The discomfort could be caused by an infection. See your doctor for treatment. To avoid spreading infections, don't share eye makeup or eye care products.
- **Protect your eyes from the sun.** When in strong sunlight, wear a hat or visor and sunglasses. Make sure that your sunglasses protect your eyes from both kinds of ultraviolet light: UVA rays and UVB rays.
- **Get regular checkups.** If you wear glasses or contacts, get your vision checked every year. Otherwise, get a checkup every two years.

Vision Problems

A complete eye exam by a doctor can uncover these problems:

- **Farsightedness.** *You can see objects at a distance, but close objects look blurry.*
- **Nearsightedness.** *You can see objects close to you, but distant objects look blurry.*
- **Astigmatism.** *The shape of your cornea or lens causes objects to look wavy or blurred.*

Eyeglasses or contact lenses can correct most common vision problems. These devices help the lens of the eye focus light on the retina. Your doctor will suggest a type of lens depending on your vision problem.

Hands-On Health

OBSERVING THE EYE

Your eyes can adjust very quickly to different light levels. The muscles in the iris change so that the pupils let in more or less light. The eyes of most people can also distinguish the colors of different objects. However, about 1 in 12 men and 1 in 250 women have some problems with color vision. Try this activity to observe your eyes' reactions to light and color.

WHAT YOU WILL NEED
- a mirror

WHAT YOU WILL DO
1. Turn off the lights and sit in the dark for two to three minutes.
2. Turn the lights back on and quickly look in the mirror. Watch what your pupils do. You should be able to see them shrinking to block out some of the light.
3. After your eyes have adjusted to the light, do the color vision test. Look at the circle shown here. Can you see a number in the circle? If not, you may have trouble

distinguishing the colors red and green. This condition is not dangerous, but you should let an adult know about it.

IN CONCLUSION
As a class, make a chart or graph that compares the results for all students. What do your findings show?

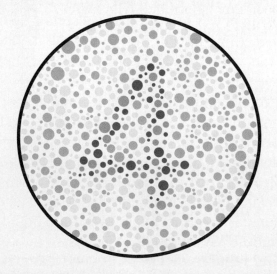

Most people find glasses easy to wear. They come in many attractive styles and colors. By law, prescription glasses must resist impact, but they are not shatterproof.

Some people prefer to wear contact lenses. These tiny lenses cling to the cornea, are nearly invisible, and often offer better sight than glasses. Compared to glasses, they take more time to properly clean and store. Also, users must follow wearing schedules and have more follow-up visits to maintain eye health.

✔
Reading Check
Create a Venn diagram. Use information from these pages and facts you already know to describe both eyeglasses and contact lenses. Write each fact in the diagram.

Healthy Ears

Your ears do not just enable you to hear. They also help keep your balance so you can stand upright or walk. Protecting your ears will help you hear better throughout your life. **Figure 4.5** shows the parts of the ear.

FIGURE 4.5

THE EAR

Your ears transmit sound to your brain and help you keep your balance. *Why is it important to protect your ears?*

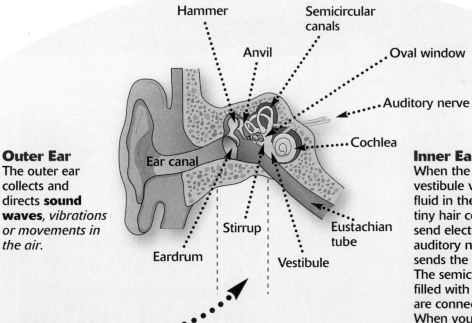

Hammer — Semicircular canals — Anvil — Oval window — Auditory nerve — Cochlea — Ear canal — Stirrup — Eustachian tube — Eardrum — Vestibule

Outer Ear
The outer ear collects and directs **sound waves**, *vibrations or movements in the air*.

Inner Ear
When the oval window in the vestibule vibrates, it moves the fluid in the cochlea. Thousands of tiny hair cells inside the cochlea send electrical messages to the auditory nerve. This nerve then sends the messages to the brain. The semicircular canals are also filled with fluid and hair cells that are connected to nerve endings. When you move, these hair cells tell your brain, helping you keep balanced.

Middle Ear • • • • • • •
Sound waves strike the eardrum, causing it to vibrate. As it vibrates, the eardrum moves three tiny bones called the hammer, anvil, and stirrup. Sound vibrations are carried to the oval window, which leads to the inner ear. The eustachian tube goes from behind the eardrum to the throat. This tube helps keep air pressure on either side of the eardrum equal. Without it, the eardrum would tear with sudden pressure changes.

Caring for Your Ears

What's the best way to care for your ears? Protect them from loud sounds. *Loudness of sound* is measured in **decibels**. Normal conversation measures about 60 decibels. **Figure 4.6** shows how louder noises can affect your hearing.

Sudden loud noises can injure the tiny hair cells in your inner ear. So can repeated exposure to sounds higher than 85 decibels. This can cause temporary or even permanent hearing loss. It can also cause a ringing in the ears called tinnitus (TI·nuh·tuhs). Many people hurt their ears by wearing earphones with the volume turned up too high.

Cold weather can also harm your ears. When cold air enters your ear canal, it can irritate your middle ear, causing pain. In the cold weather, wear earmuffs or a hat that covers your ears.

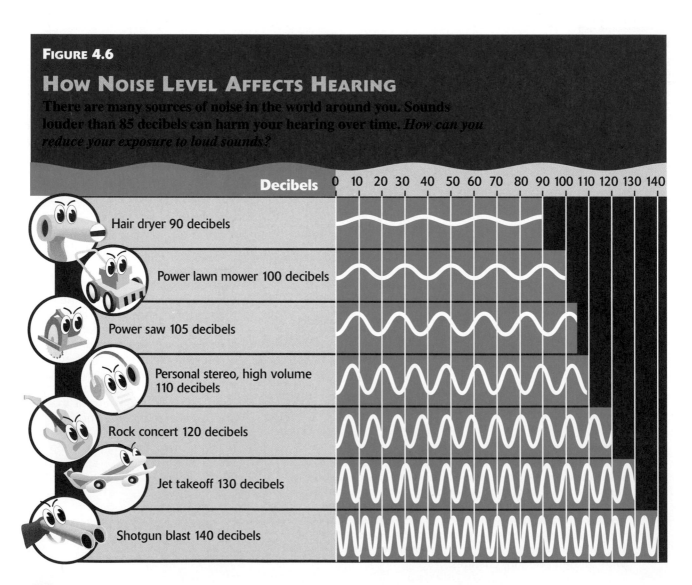

FIGURE 4.6

HOW NOISE LEVEL AFFECTS HEARING

There are many sources of noise in the world around you. Sounds louder than 85 decibels can harm your hearing over time. *How can you reduce your exposure to loud sounds?*

Decibels 0 10 20 30 40 50 60 70 80 90 100 110 120 130 140

Hair dryer 90 decibels

Power lawn mower 100 decibels

Power saw 105 decibels

Personal stereo, high volume 110 decibels

Rock concert 120 decibels

Jet takeoff 130 decibels

Shotgun blast 140 decibels

Ear Problems

Infections of the middle ear are the most common ear problems. A nose or throat infection can also lead to pain in the ear. Sometimes infections move from the throat up the eustachian tube to the ear. A doctor can treat these infections.

Hearing loss and deafness are the most serious ear problems. Too much wax in the ear canal, an ear infection, or nerve damage can cause partial hearing loss or ringing in the ears. A total hearing loss can result from ear injury, disease, or birth defects.

People with hearing problems often communicate using lipreading and sign language. Some may wear hearing aids that increase the loudness of sound waves. *What other ways can people communicate?*

Lesson 2 Review

Using complete sentences, answer the following questions on a sheet of paper.

Reviewing Terms and Facts

1. **Vocabulary** Define the words *farsightedness* and *nearsightedness*.
2. **Explain** What do glasses and contact lenses do?
3. **Recall** What part of the ear helps you maintain your balance?

Thinking Critically

4. **Analyze** How do loud noises harm hearing?

5. **Summarize** What changes could you make in your life that would give greater protection to your eyes and your ears?

Applying Health Skills

6. **Accessing Information** Survey at least six people who wear glasses or contact lenses. First find out why they need the glasses or lenses. Then find out how long they have worn them and what they think the advantages and disadvantages of each are. Prepare a chart of your findings.

Choosing Health Products

Quick Write

Think about the health products you used last week for your hair, skin, nails, eyes, and ears. Make a list of all of these products. How did you decide which products to use?

LEARN ABOUT...

- what influences your decisions about health products.
- how to decide which health products are best for you.
- how to choose health products wisely.

VOCABULARY

- consumer
- advertisement
- warranty
- discount store
- coupon
- generic
- fraud

Recognizing Influences

You are a **consumer**, *someone who buys products or services.* For example, you use health products such as toothpaste, sunscreen, and deodorant. You also use health services—the work of doctors, dentists, and other health professionals.

Sometimes choosing health products and services can be confusing. **Figure 4.7** shows the many thoughts a person might have before deciding to buy a product. Building consumer skills will help you choose wisely and be aware of what influences your choices.

FIGURE 4.7

MAKING AN INFORMED CHOICE

Many factors affect your buying decisions. *List the factors that this teen is considering.*

EXTERNAL INFLUENCES

INTERNAL INFLUENCES

I just saw a TV commercial about this shampoo. The girl who used it got a lot of compliments.

Maybe I should choose this brand to save money.

My friend Tanya really likes this shampoo.

I want a shampoo with natural ingredients that doesn't hurt the environment.

This shampoo comes in coconut fragrance—my favorite!

This ad says the shampoo has special secret ingredients. I wonder what that means?

Making Good Consumer Choices

A major influence on your consumer choices is advertising. **Advertisements** are *messages used to persuade consumers to buy goods or services.* Ads may claim that products will make you happier, healthier, more attractive, or more popular.

If an advertising claim sounds too good to be true, it probably is not true. Advertisements are meant to sell products, not to give you useful information. Seek advice from your parents or other knowledgeable adults.

Be cautious about buying products from an unfamiliar source. You may not be able to get your money back if the product does not work. This is especially important when you send away for products or buy from door-to-door salespeople.

Smart Shopping

Smart shopping can help you save money. One way to be a smart shopper is to compare products and prices before buying. You can also read and understand product labels, like the one shown in **Figure 4.8**.

FIGURE 4.8

WHAT LABELS CAN TELL YOU

Product labels give you important information. *How does the information on a product label help you make a wise choice?*

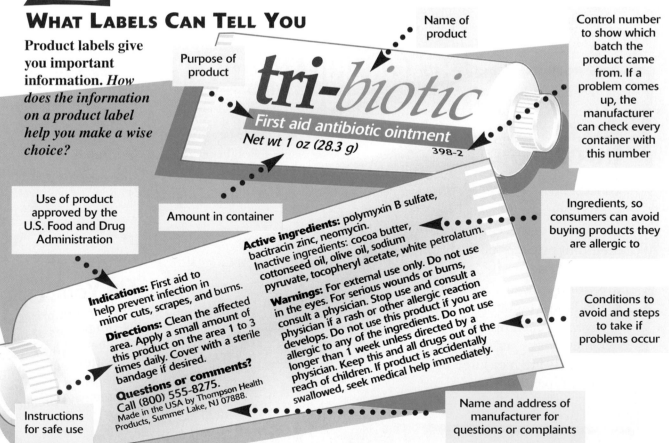

Purpose of product

Name of product

Control number to show which batch the product came from. If a problem comes up, the manufacturer can check every container with this number

Use of product approved by the U.S. Food and Drug Administration

Amount in container

Ingredients, so consumers can avoid buying products they are allergic to

Conditions to avoid and steps to take if problems occur

Instructions for safe use

Name and address of manufacturer for questions or complaints

tri-biotic
First aid antibiotic ointment
Net wt 1 oz (28.3 g)   398-2

Active ingredients: polymyxin B sulfate, bacitracin zinc, neomycin. **Inactive ingredients:** cocoa butter, cottonseed oil, olive oil, sodium pyruvate, tocopheryl acetate, white petrolatum.
Warnings: For external use only. Do not use in the eyes. For serious wounds or burns, consult a physician. Stop use and consult a physician if a rash or other allergic reaction develops. Do not use this product if you are allergic to any of the ingredients. Do not use longer than 1 week unless directed by a physician. Keep this and all drugs out of the reach of children. If product is accidentally swallowed, seek medical help immediately.

Indications: First aid to help prevent infection in minor cuts, scrapes, and burns.
Directions: Clean the affected area. Apply a small amount of this product on the area 1 to 3 times daily. Cover with a sterile bandage if desired.
Questions or comments? Call (800) 555-8275.
Made in the USA by Thompson Health Products, Summer Lake, NJ 07888.

Reading Check
Investigate word origin. Determine what the following words have in common: *warranty, cover, garage, guarantee.*

Comparison Shopping

When you compare brands, consider these factors:

- **Price.** How much can you afford to spend on this product?
- **Unit Price.** How much does the product cost per ounce or per gram? (See the Health Skills Activity for details.)
- **Benefits.** Does one brand offer more features than another?
- **Reputation.** Do people you know use and like this brand?
- **Warranty.** Does this brand come with a warranty? A **warranty** is *a promise to make repairs or refund money if the product does not work as claimed.*

Saving Money

Smart shoppers know how to save money. For example, they may buy personal products at **discount stores**. These are *stores that offer lower prices, but have fewer salespeople and services.* They may also clip and use **coupons**, *slips of paper that save you money on certain brands.* You can often save money by buying store brands or **generic** (juh·NEHR·ik) products, which are *products sold in plain packages.* These cost less because the packaging is cheaper and little money is spent on advertising. However, some generic drugs may not contain all of the same ingredients as name brands, so check with your pharmacist before using them.

HEALTH SKILLS ACTIVITY

ACCESSING INFORMATION

Understand Unit Pricing

To compare the value of two products, you need to compare their unit price, or cost per unit of weight or volume. To do this, follow these steps.

- Find the weight or volume given on each product container. Make sure that both products are measured in the same type of units.
- Divide the price of the product by its weight or volume. The result is the unit price.
- Compare the unit prices.

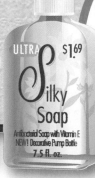

Silky Soap
Antibacterial Soap
$2.89
15 fl.oz

ULTRA $1.69
Silky Soap
Antibacterial Soap with Vitamin E
NEW! Decorative Pump Bottle
7.5 fl. oz.

ON YOUR OWN
Find the unit prices of the two bottles of soap shown here. Which costs less per fluid ounce? Why might a person buy the more expensive product?

FIGURE 4.9

False or Misleading Claims

These product labels make false or misleading claims. *What are other false claims you have read or heard in ads?*

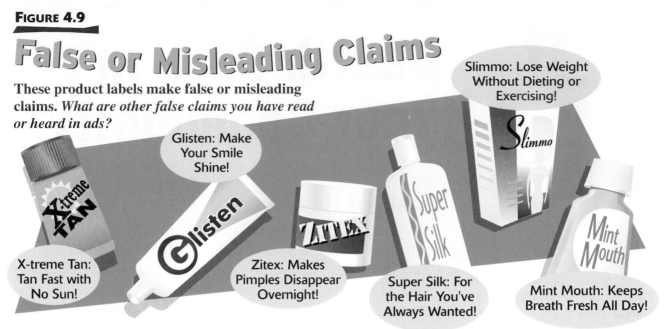

X-treme Tan: Tan Fast with No Sun!

Glisten: Make Your Smile Shine!

Zitex: Makes Pimples Disappear Overnight!

Super Silk: For the Hair You've Always Wanted!

Slimmo: Lose Weight Without Dieting or Exercising!

Mint Mouth: Keeps Breath Fresh All Day!

Spotting False Claims

All consumers need to beware of **fraud**, *deliberate deceit or trickery*. People who practice fraud make false claims about a product or service. **Figure 4.9** shows some examples of false and misleading claims.

Health fraud can be particularly dangerous. Some products falsely claim to cure dangerous diseases or cause rapid weight loss. It is unsafe to use any treatment that has not been approved by the U.S. Food and Drug Administration (FDA).

Lesson 3 Review

Using complete sentences, answer the following questions on a sheet of paper.

Reviewing Terms and Facts

1. **Vocabulary** Define the word *consumer.* Use it in an original sentence.
2. **Recall** Why is it a good idea to buy products that come with a warranty?
3. **List** Give three examples of ways to save money when shopping.

Thinking Critically

4. **Apply** Give two examples of how you could use the shopping tips in this lesson when purchasing a service, such as a haircut.
5. **Synthesize** List two reasons you might choose a more expensive product over a product with a lower unit price.

Applying Health Skills

6. **Analyzing Influences** Select a personal product that you use and would recommend to others. Prepare a presentation in which you explain to the class why you like it, where you bought it, and why it is worth its cost.

Health Care in Your Community

Quick Write

Think about the last time you went to see a health care professional. Write a paragraph about your experience there.

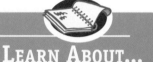

LEARN ABOUT...

- which health care professionals to see when you are sick.
- the importance of regular checkups for your health.
- groups that provide health care.

VOCABULARY

- specialist
- voluntary health group
- health insurance
- managed care

Goals of Health Care

Health care focuses on two areas: preventing health problems and treating problems when they arise. Many health professionals are involved in preventing problems. They include dietitians, dental hygienists, health teachers, nurses, and counselors. An important part of their job is to help you develop healthy habits. Practicing good health habits is easier and less costly than treating problems. When problems do arise, various health professionals identify and treat them. These people include doctors, dentists, nurses, pharmacists, and others.

When you feel ill, you probably go to see your family doctor. Sometimes your family doctor will send you to see a **specialist** (SPEH·shuh·list), *a doctor trained to handle particular health problems.* Some specialists treat specific types of people. For example, pediatricians treat children and teens. Other specialists treat specific conditions or body systems. **Figure 4.10** shows some of these specialists.

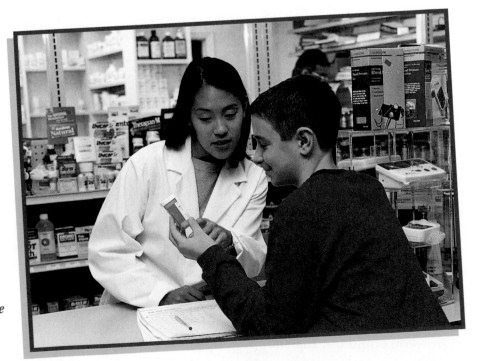

Your local pharmacist is a reliable source of information about health products. *What questions might this teen have for the pharmacist?*

Regular Checkups

Getting regular medical checkups is one way to avoid possible health problems. During a checkup, your doctor will measure your height and weight. He or she will check your heart and lungs. Your vision and hearing may also be tested. The doctor will give you whatever immunizations you need to help your body fight off diseases. You should see your doctor for a checkup about once a year. You might also have a checkup before you try any new sports or other physical activities. If you have a serious medical condition, you may need to visit the doctor more often.

FIGURE 4.10

THE SPECIALISTS

Each specialist treats a different type of person or condition. *Have you ever visited a specialist?*

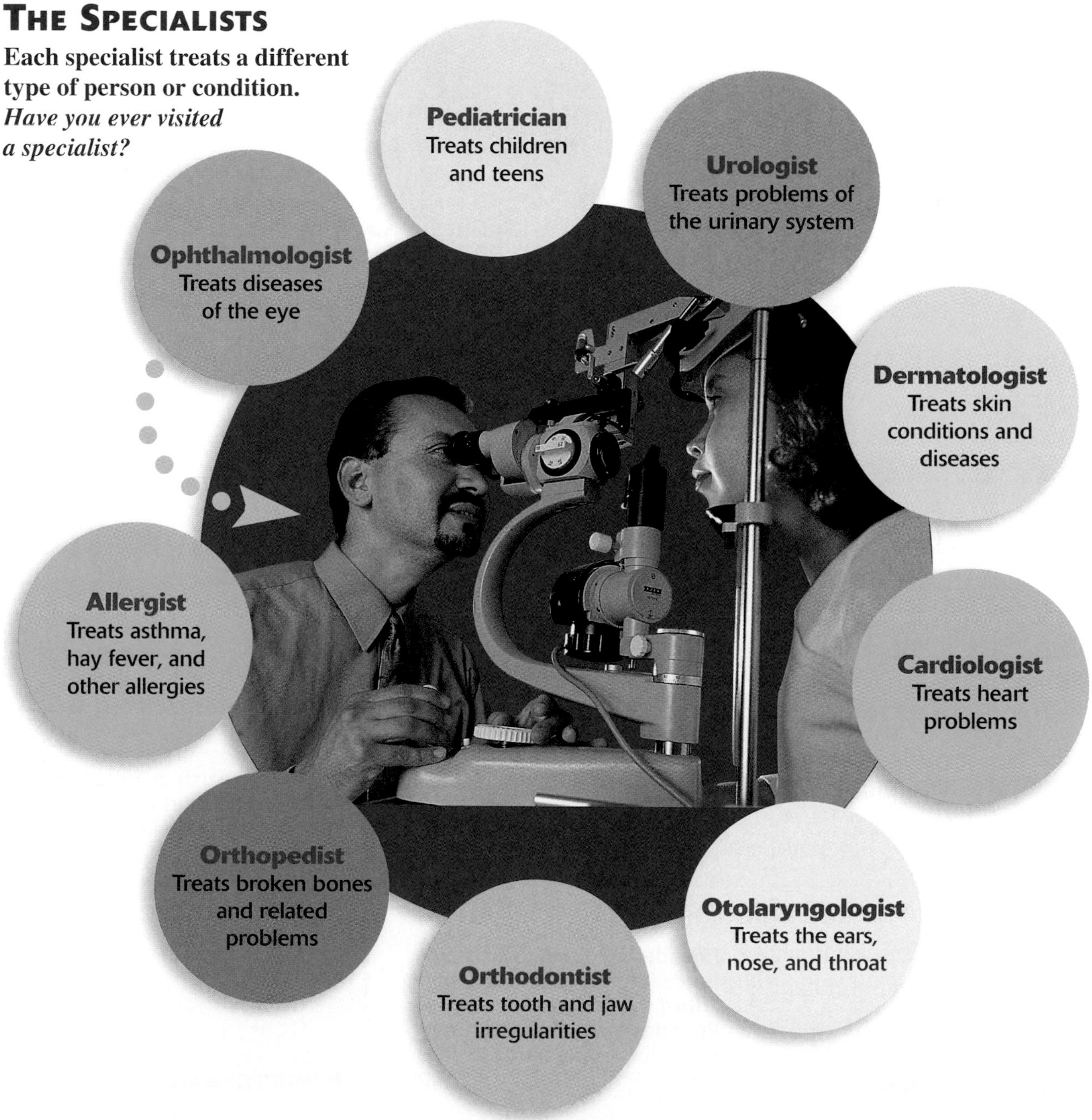

Pediatrician
Treats children and teens

Urologist
Treats problems of the urinary system

Ophthalmologist
Treats diseases of the eye

Dermatologist
Treats skin conditions and diseases

Allergist
Treats asthma, hay fever, and other allergies

Cardiologist
Treats heart problems

Orthopedist
Treats broken bones and related problems

Orthodontist
Treats tooth and jaw irregularities

Otolaryngologist
Treats the ears, nose, and throat

Sources of Health Care

You get health care from many sources, such as doctors' or dentists' offices, clinics, and hospitals. Your school nurse, if you have one, gives general advice and medical care. Other sources provide care for specific health problems. For example, counselors help people with mental and emotional problems.

The government also provides health care. **Figure 4.11** describes some of the health services performed by local, state, and federal governments.

Voluntary health groups are *organizations that work to treat and eliminate certain diseases.* Usually, these groups are run by volunteers. Instead of selling products, they ask people to donate money. Some of the money pays for research on disease. These groups also teach people how to prevent the disease and help those who have the disease.

Paying for Health Care

Many people use **health insurance** to help pay for health care. This means they pay *a monthly or yearly fee to an insurance company that agrees to pay for some or most costs of*

FIGURE 4.11

LOCAL, STATE, AND FEDERAL HEALTH SERVICES

Many government agencies work to protect the health of Americans. Look in the phone book to find out the location of your local health department.

	Preventing and Treating Disease	Information
Local and State Government	• Makes sure restaurant and hotel kitchens are clean • Collects and disposes of garbage • Makes sure water is safe to drink • Helps stop the spread of disease	• Teaches people how to care for their health • Keeps records of births, deaths, and diseases
Federal Government	• Helps support people who cannot work due to chronic illness or injury • Helps prevent and treat problems involving mental health, including alcohol and other drugs • Identifies and stops the spread of disease • Provides Medicaid (health care funds for people who cannot afford medical treatment) • Provides Medicare (health care funds for people over 65)	• Does research in areas such as cancer, heart disease, and the health of the elderly and children

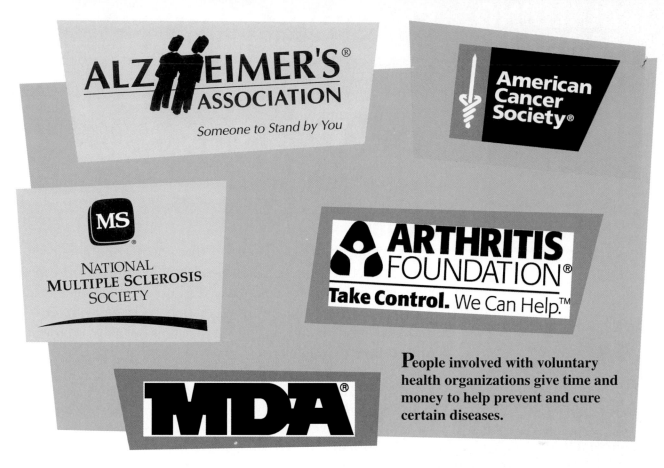

People involved with voluntary health organizations give time and money to help prevent and cure certain diseases.

medical care. One type of health insurance is **managed care**, *a health insurance plan that saves money by limiting people's choice of doctors.* It often costs less than traditional insurance plans. Many employers help pay for their employees' health insurance.

Lesson 4 Review

Using complete sentences, answer the following questions on a sheet of paper.

Reviewing Terms and Facts

1. **Vocabulary** Define the term *specialist* and give an example.
2. **List** Name four places that provide health care.
3. **Recall** How do managed care plans save money over other forms of health insurance?

Thinking Critically

4. **Speculate** Why do many health care providers emphasize disease prevention?
5. **Analyze** Why do you think the government takes responsibility for certain areas of health care?

Applying Health Skills

6. **Accessing Information** Contact a voluntary health group in your area to learn more about what it does. Find out whether it offers any volunteer opportunities for teens. Share your findings with the class.

ARE YOU SUN SMART?

Model

It's so much fun being outdoors that you may not think about protecting your skin and eyes from the sun. This is especially true on cloudy or cold days. It's important to plan ahead in order to protect yourself from UV rays every day you are outdoors. Read about Ken and list the steps he takes to protect himself from the sun's rays.

Ken's friends are going to the lake for the afternoon. Ken knows that too much sun can damage his skin. Before leaving his house, Ken applies a broad-spectrum sunscreen with an SPF of 30. When his friends arrive, Ken puts on his hat and sunglasses. At the lake, Ken spreads his towel out in the shade before he takes a swim. After swimming, he reapplies sunscreen and offers some to his friends. Around 4:00 p.m., Ken enjoys a game of volleyball and another swim. He has a great time and stays safe in the sun.

Practice

Increase your sun care basics by learning what other people know about UV protection. Interview three classmates. Ask them this question: "How do you protect yourself from the sun's damaging rays?" Record their answers on notebook paper.

1. How many different responses did you get to your question?
2. Which responses are good ways to protect the skin and eyes from UV rays?
3. Can you add to this list?

Apply/Assess

Here's your chance to spread the word about sun safety. Compose a poem or song about the importance of protecting skin and eyes from the sun. In your composition, name at least four ways people can protect themselves from UV rays. Focus on the importance of developing good sun safety habits early in life. Explain how the decisions you make now about sun protection affect your health throughout your life.

Practicing Healthful Behaviors

To protect yourself from the sun:
- stay out of direct sunlight between 10:00 a.m. and 4:00 p.m. in the summertime.
- use broad-spectrum sunscreens with an SPF of at least 15.
- wear protective clothing and a hat.
- wear sunglasses.

Self √ Check

- Did my poem or song focus on sun protection?
- Did it include at least four ways to protect skin and eyes?
- Did it explain the lifelong importance of good sun safety habits?

THINK BEFORE YOU BUY

Model

With so many health care products available, how do you choose the best one for you? You have many sources of information. The product label is a good place to start. It will tell you if a product's health claims have been reviewed by the Food and Drug Administration. A pharmacist can also answer your questions. Read about how Sandra decides which skin cleanser to buy.

Sandra is looking for a product that will clean and moisturize at the same time. She begins by reading the labels of several skin cleansers. She looks at the directions to see what the product is supposed to do and how to use it. She reads the list of ingredients in each product. If she isn't sure how the different ingredients work, she asks the pharmacist. Finally, she calculates the unit price. With all this information, she can make a confident choice.

Practice

You have learned how to find useful information about health products. You should also remember that advertisements are not good sources of information. They often exaggerate a product's effectiveness, promising "miracle" results in "no time at all." Compare the product claims below.

- *"Dynodent makes teeth whiter and brighter—instantly!"*
- *"Acnex cleanser is guaranteed to wash your pimples away."*
- *"Winter Cool mouthwash kills the germs that cause tooth decay."*
- *"Drink away 10 pounds in no time with Choco-Slim!"*
- *"So-Soft conditioner contains natural oils that add moisture to your hair."*

1. Which claims appear to be genuine?
2. Which ones may be inaccurate or misleading?
3. Where could you find more information to help you evaluate these product claims?

Apply/Assess

Look through teen magazines for advertisements that include product claims. Write them down on a sheet of paper. Which claims appear genuine? Which are inaccurate or misleading?

Write a statement identifying two sources where teens could find reliable information about health products. Explain why you would choose these resources.

COACH'S BOX

Accessing Information

Smart shopper tips:
- Read labels to learn what products contain, how they work, and how to use them.
- Be cautious about product claims made in advertisements.
- If you want more information about a product, talk to your parents, your family doctor, or your local pharmacist.

Self-√Check

- Did I identify health claims as genuine or misleading?
- Did I name two sources of reliable information about health products?
- Did I explain why these sources are reliable?

SUMMARY

LESSON·1 For healthy teeth, you should brush and floss correctly and see a dentist regularly. To keep skin healthy, wash it and protect it from the sun. Washing and brushing your hair will keep it healthy.

LESSON·2 For healthy eyes, protect them from strain, injury, and infection, and get regular eye checkups. To keep ears healthy, protect them from loud sounds and cold weather.

LESSON·3 Wise consumers compare brands, read product labels, and check unit pricing when they purchase health products. It is important to beware of false or misleading advertisements.

LESSON·4 Many people and places provide health care. To stay healthy, it is important to have regular checkups. Health insurance can help pay for medical care.

Reviewing Vocabulary and Concepts

On a sheet of paper, write the numbers 1–10. After each number, write the term from the list that best completes each statement.

- astigmatism
- cavity
- cuticle
- decibels
- dermatologist
- farsightedness
- melanin
- nearsightedness
- orthodontist
- sound waves

Lesson 1

1. A(n) _____ forms as a result of repeated acid attacks on the tooth enamel.
2. A nonliving band of epidermis that surrounds a fingernail is called the _____.
3. A(n) _____ is a doctor who treats skin disorders.
4. Freckles are spots of _____.
5. If you needed your teeth straightened, you would visit a(n) _____.

Lesson 2

6. If you have _____, close objects look blurry.

7. If you have _____, you have trouble seeing objects far away from you.
8. Vibrations or movements in the air are known as _____.
9. If you have _____, the shape of your cornea causes objects to look wavy or blurred.
10. Sound waves are measured in _____.

On a sheet of paper, write the numbers 11–20. Write *True* or *False* for each statement below. If the statement is false, change the underlined word or phrase to make it true.

Lesson 3

11. The goal of <u>advertisements</u> is to persuade you that one particular product is better than others.
12. Three ways to save money on health products are to use coupons, shop in discount stores, and buy <u>brand name</u> products.

13. A discount store has lower prices and <u>fewer</u> salespeople and services than other kinds of stores.
14. Generic products cost <u>more</u> than brand name products because of the difference in packaging costs.
15. People who practice <u>fraud</u> make false claims about a product or service.

Lesson 4

16. <u>Otolaryngologists</u> treat heart problems.
17. Teens need to have medical checkups every <u>two years</u>.
18. Voluntary health groups are usually run by <u>volunteers</u>.
19. <u>Health insurance</u> allows people to pay a monthly or yearly fee to an insurance company, which then pays part of their medical bills.
20. People in managed care plans usually pay <u>more</u> for their medical treatment than people with traditional insurance plans.

Thinking Critically

On a sheet of paper, write the numbers 21–25. Using complete sentences, answer the following questions.

21. **Explain** Give an example of a habit that will help you maintain the health of your teeth, skin, hair, eyes, or ears. Explain how developing this habit now will benefit your health throughout your life.
22. **Predict** How might allowing eye or ear problems to go untreated affect other areas of your health?
23. **Speculate** Why do you think many young people listen to loud music even though they know that it might damage their hearing?
24. **Interpret** Why should consumers evaluate claims made in advertisements before they buy health products?
25. **Hypothesize** Why do many people pay for health insurance?

Career Corner

Dental Hygienist

Would you like to help improve people's smiles? With just one to two years of training at a college or vocational/technical school, you could become a dental hygienist. These professionals assist dentists. They help clean teeth and gums, insert fillings, and take X-rays. Hygienists work with a variety of special tools. They also have lots of contact with people. Learn more about this and other health careers by clicking on Career Corner at health.glencoe.com.

Chapter 5

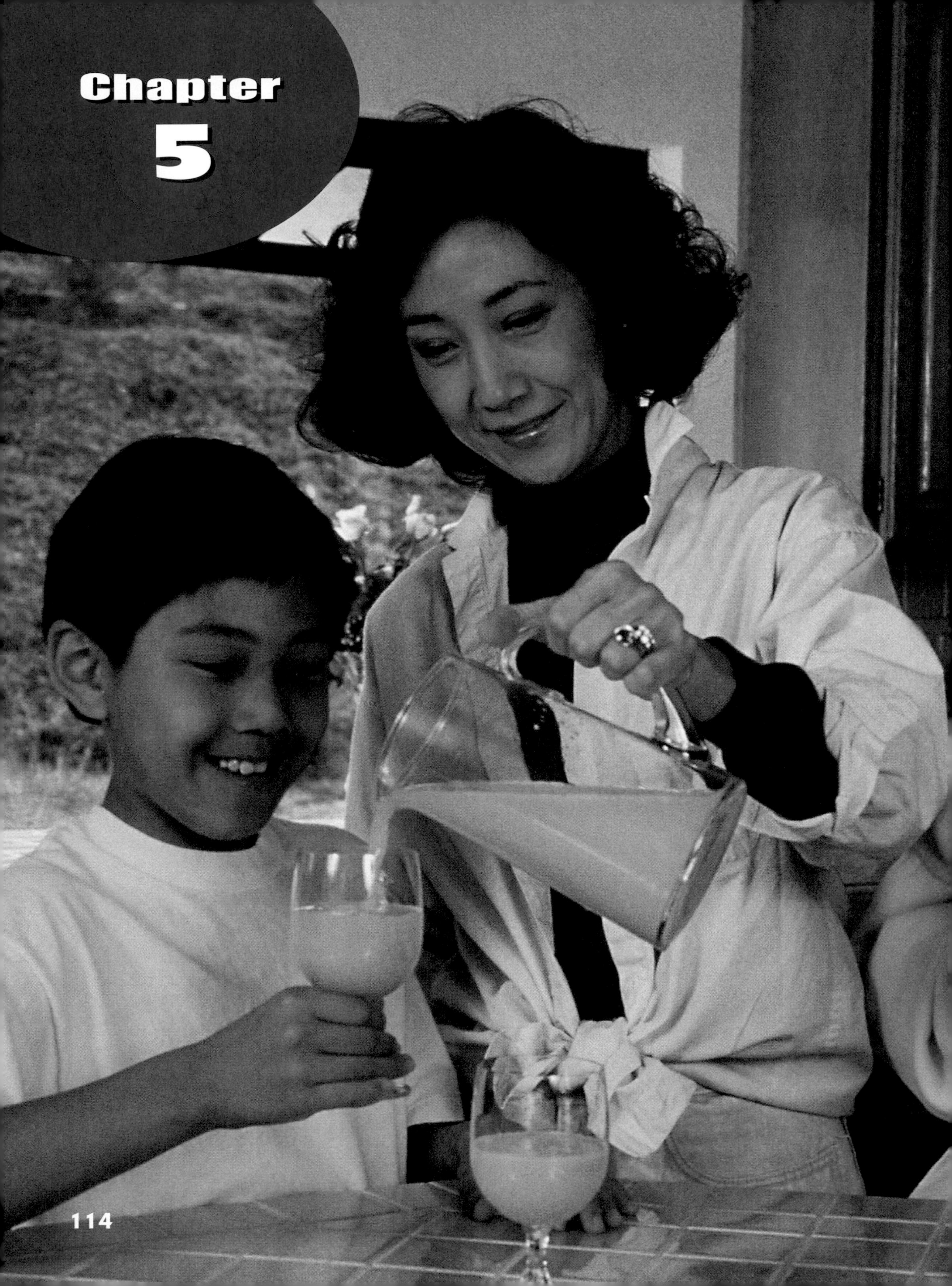

Nutrition and Physical Activity

Quick Write

Make a list of questions you have about teen nutrition and physical activity. When you have finished this chapter, see how many of your questions have been answered.

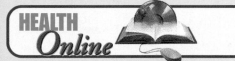

Do you practice healthy nutrition and fitness habits? Take the Health Inventory at health.glencoe.com to find out how your habits score.

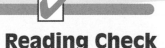

Reading Check

Make predictions. Complete these sentences in as many ways as you can.
If I eat nutritious food, then...
If I increase my physical activity, then...

Why Your Body Needs Nutrients

Quick Write

Write a menu of your favorite meal. Then explain why you think the foods belong in a healthful eating plan.

LEARN ABOUT...

- why your food choices are important.
- what kinds of food your body needs.
- how various kinds of foods affect your body.

VOCABULARY

- nutrition
- nutrient
- carbohydrate
- fiber
- protein
- fat
- vitamin
- mineral

Food Is Fuel

When you feel hungry, your body is sending you the message that you need more fuel. To your body, food is fuel because it gives your body the energy it needs to operate. It also provides the building blocks that allow your body to grow and to repair itself. **Figure 5.1** illustrates the steps in fueling and refueling your body.

During your teen years, your body grows more rapidly than it has since you were an infant. This means you need to provide your body with the kinds of foods it needs. Understanding nutrition will help you do this. **Nutrition** (noo·TRI·shun) is *the science that studies the substances in food and how the body uses them.*

FIGURE 5.1

Food: The Body's Fuel

Food gives your body the energy you need to move and do your daily activities. Nutritious foods help you grow, feel your best, and perform at your peak.

1 Morning is an important time to refuel.

2 An empty stomach tells your brain you need to eat. That signal is hunger.

The Nutrients in Foods

Nutrients (NOO·tree·ents) are *substances in food that your body needs.* You could think of nutrients as members of a team. Each one has a special job to do, and each one is important to the team. Together, nutrients keep you healthy, help you grow, and set the foundation for lifelong health and wellness.

Altogether there are more than 40 kinds of nutrients. They are grouped into the following six categories:

- Carbohydrates
- Proteins
- Fats
- Vitamins
- Minerals
- Water

Carbohydrates

Carbohydrates (kar·bo·HY·drayts) are *the main source of energy for your body.* Simple carbohydrates, or sugars, are found in fruits, milk, and table sugar. Starchy foods such as bread, rice, pasta, and potatoes contain complex carbohydrates. Your body breaks them down into simple sugars. Many starchy foods also contain fiber. **Fiber** is *the tough, stringy part of raw fruits, raw vegetables, whole wheat, and other grains, which you cannot digest.* Fiber helps carry wastes out of your body.

Reading Check

Learn more about the word *carbohydrate.* Use a dictionary to determine what the following words have in common: *carbohydrate, coal, water, fuel.*

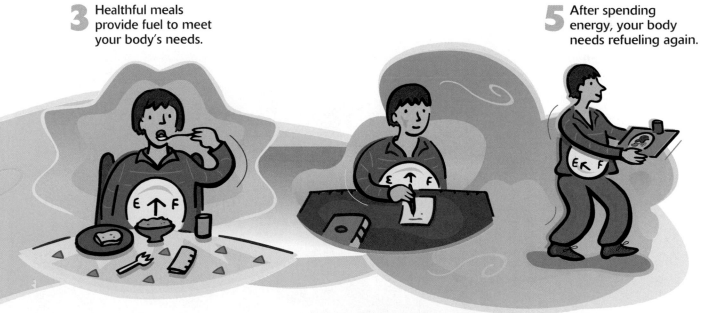

3 Healthful meals provide fuel to meet your body's needs.

4 Your body burns food energy to perform everyday activities, such as taking a test.

5 After spending energy, your body needs refueling again.

Proteins

Proteins (PRO·teens) are *essential for the growth and repair of all the cells in your body.* Meat and other animal products, such as eggs and dairy products, provide "complete" proteins. This means that they contain all the building blocks your body needs to build and maintain strong muscles. However, you can also get complete proteins by combining certain plant foods, such as rice and beans. You don't need to eat these foods at the same meal; any time during the day is fine.

Fats

Fats are *another source of energy.* Fats also carry certain vitamins in your bloodstream and help keep your skin healthy. However, eating too much fat can contribute to weight gain and other health problems, such as heart disease and cancer. These conditions usually appear later in life, but often result from poor health habits that began at an early age. Salad dressing and such popular fast foods as doughnuts and fries tend to be high in fat.

Vitamins

Vitamins (VI·tuh·mins) are *substances that help regulate body functions.* Vitamins help you in many ways. For example, they help your body use other nutrients and fight disease. Fruits, leafy green vegetables, whole-grain breads, and some meats are especially rich in vitamins.

Many delicious foods offer the nutrients your body needs. *Which of these foods provide complete proteins?*

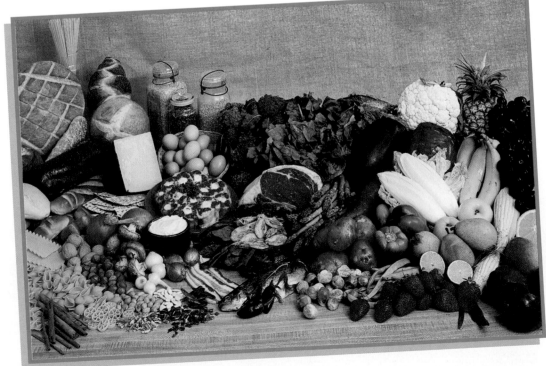

Some vitamins, such as vitamin C and the B-complex vitamins, dissolve in water. You must replace these water-soluble vitamins every day. Other vitamins, including vitamins A, D, E, and K, dissolve only in droplets of fat. Your body can store fat-soluble vitamins for longer periods. Because your body stores these vitamins instead of quickly releasing them, consuming very large amounts can be harmful.

HEALTH SKILLS ACTIVITY

ACCESSING INFORMATION

Reading a Food Label

Packaged foods have labels like the one shown here. Learning to read food labels can help you choose foods that will give you enough of different nutrients.

Nutrition Facts

Serving Size 1 cup (240 mL)
Servings Per Container About 2

Amount Per Serving	
Calories 130	Calories from Fat 30
	% Daily Value*
	5%
Total Fat 3g	5%
Saturated Fat 1g	2%
Cholesterol 5 mg	30%
Sodium 720 mg	7%
Total Carbohydrate 21g	12%
Dietary Fiber 3g	
Sugars 11g	
Protein 4g	

Vitamin A 40%	Vitamin C 2%
Calcium 6%	Iron 8%

*Percent Daily Values are based on a 2,000 calorie diet. Your daily values may be higher or lower depending on your calorie needs:

	Calories:	2,000	2,500
Total Fat	Less than	65g	80g
Sat Fat	Less than	20g	25g
Cholesterol	Less than	300mg	300mg
Sodium	Less than	2,400mg	2,400mg
Total Carbohydrate		300g	375g
Dietary Fiber		25g	30g

Calories per gram:
Fat 9 • Carbohydrate 4 • Protein 4

INGREDIENTS: TOMATO PUREE (WATER, TOMATO PASTE), CHICKEN STOCK, ZUCCHINI, CARROTS, DICED TOMATOES, CELERY, WATER, HIGH FRUCTOSE CORN SYRUP, ENRICHED MACARONI PRODUCT (WHEAT FLOUR, EGG WHITE SOLIDS, NIACIN, FERROUS SULFATE, THIAMINE MONONITRATE, RIBOFLAVIN).

- **SERVING SIZE** is the amount of food in one serving.
- **SERVINGS PER CONTAINER** is the number of servings the package contains.
- **CALORIES PER SERVING** is a measure of how much energy your body gets from one serving of the food.
- **DAILY VALUE** is the amount of a nutrient a typical person needs in one day. The label shows a percentage of the Daily Value for each nutrient in a serving of the food. This lets you compare nutrients in different products.
- **INGREDIENTS** in the food are listed in order. The first ingredient makes up the largest portion of the food. The last one listed makes up the smallest portion.

WITH A GROUP

With three or four classmates, compare food labels from different products. Analyze each one for nutritional value. Compare your findings with other groups of classmates.

Minerals

Minerals (MIN·uh·ruhls) are *elements in foods that help your body work properly.* For example, the minerals calcium and phosphorus aid many body functions. They strengthen growing bones, keep muscles healthy, and help your heart beat regularly. Several minerals allow the body to use the other types of nutrients. Most foods contain minerals, especially milk, meat, dried beans, vegetables, fruits, and whole-grain cereals. Different foods contain different minerals.

Some people take supplements, such as pills, to get extra vitamins and minerals. However, food sources are always better. Food has other nutrients that supplements don't have.

Water

Water carries nutrients around your body, and so is essential to life. It also helps with digestion, removes waste, and cools you off. You need six to eight cups of water every day (plus two to four more cups in hotter weather). Your body can also get water from juices, milk, and some fruits and vegetables.

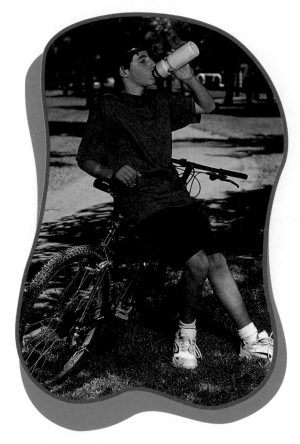

Your body needs six to eight cups of water each day to function properly. *Why do you think your body needs more water during exercise?*

Lesson 1 Review

Using complete sentences, answer the following questions on a sheet of paper.

Reviewing Terms and Facts

1. **Vocabulary** Define the term *nutrition.* Use it in an original sentence.
2. **Identify** List three things that food does for you.
3. **List** Name the six categories of nutrients.

Thinking Critically

4. **Predict** Describe how your knowledge of nutrients might affect your choice of snack foods in the future.

5. **Analyze** Record what you eat for one day. Then analyze the nutrients you have eaten. Remember to count the cups of water you drink. What improvements, if any, could you make?

Applying Health Skills

6. **Accessing Information** Analyze the ingredients in a recipe from a magazine or newspaper. Explain which of the six nutrient categories, if any, are missing. Suggest other foods that could be served at the same meal to provide a variety of nutrients.

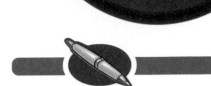
Following a Balanced Food Plan

The Food Guide Pyramid

Two government departments, the U.S. Department of Agriculture (USDA) and the Department of Health and Human Services, have provided a handy tool to help you plan nutritious meals. This tool is the **Food Guide Pyramid**, which provides *a daily guideline to help you choose what and how much to eat to get the nutrients you need.*

The Food Guide Pyramid divides foods into six groups. Five of these are basic food groups. Eating foods from all five basic groups each day gives you the nutrients and energy you need to grow and stay healthy. The sixth group contains fats, oils, and sweets, which you should only eat in small amounts.

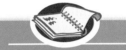

Quick Write

List two or three reasons you think people should try to avoid eating too many fats and sugary foods.

LEARN ABOUT...

- how to use the Food Guide Pyramid.
- the names of the five food groups.
- how much of the different kinds of food you should eat.

VOCABULARY

- Food Guide Pyramid

You can enjoy nutritious foods in many different settings. *What foods do you choose when you have a variety of options?*

You will find many of your favorite foods in **Figure 5.2**, which shows the Food Guide Pyramid. The size of each section in the Pyramid gives you a good idea of how much of each kind of food to eat every day. You should eat the most servings from the Bread, Cereal, Rice, and Pasta Group—the largest section of the Pyramid. Growing teens should get three full servings from the Milk, Yogurt, and Cheese Group. Notice that no number of servings from the smallest section—Fats, Oils, and Sweets—is recommended. Foods in this group provide energy but few nutrients.

FIGURE 5.2

THE FOOD GUIDE PYRAMID

Eating enough foods from the five basic food groups every day provides you with the nutrients you need to grow and stay healthy.

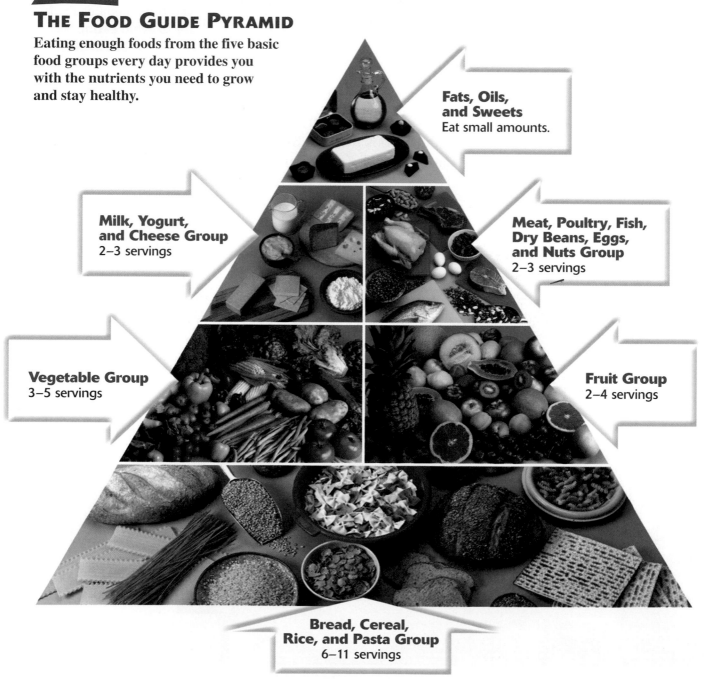

Fats, Oils, and Sweets
Eat small amounts.

Milk, Yogurt, and Cheese Group
2–3 servings

Meat, Poultry, Fish, Dry Beans, Eggs, and Nuts Group
2–3 servings

Vegetable Group
3–5 servings

Fruit Group
2–4 servings

Bread, Cereal, Rice, and Pasta Group
6–11 servings

The Food Groups

Which nutrients does each food group provide? Use **Figure 5.3** to find out. It shows the nutrients in each Pyramid section.

FIGURE 5.3

NUTRIENTS IN THE FOOD GROUPS

Bread, Cereal, Rice, and Pasta Group
6–11 servings

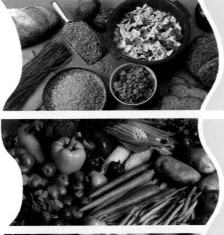

These foods are rich in complex carbohydrates, which provide energy. They supply certain vitamins and minerals. Combined with beans, or other foods such as peanut butter, they provide some protein. Whole-grain foods are also high in fiber.

Vegetable Group
3–5 servings

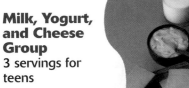

Most foods from these two groups are low in fat and high in carbohydrates. They provide many important vitamins, such as vitamins A and C, plus fiber and some minerals. Dark-green, leafy vegetables and dark-colored fruits are especially rich in nutrients. For good health, choose a variety of fruits and vegetables each day.

Fruit Group
2–4 servings

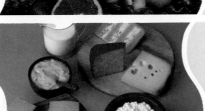

Milk, Yogurt, and Cheese Group
3 servings for teens

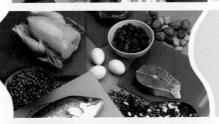

Foods in this group are a major source of calcium. They also offer protein, carbohydrates, and some vitamins. Some are high in fat. Choose mostly low-fat or fat-free milk, cheese, and yogurt.

Meat, Poultry, Fish, Dry Beans, Eggs, and Nuts Group
2–3 servings

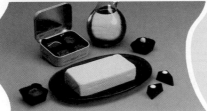

All foods in this group are high in protein. Most also contain B vitamins and minerals such as iron. However, they can also be high in fat. Eat mostly leaner meats, poultry, and fish. Cooked dry beans, combined with grain products, are another good choice.

Fats, Oils, and Sweets
Eat in small amounts.

This section contains foods that are high in fat or sugar and contain few other nutrients. Enjoy them in small amounts. They should not take the place of more nutritious foods in your meals and snacks.

Using the Food Guide Pyramid

The Food Guide Pyramid shows a range of daily servings for each food group. The number of servings recommended for you depends on your age, gender, body size, and activity level. But how much is a serving? Use **Figure 5.4** to find out. Keep in mind that many foods, such as pizza, contain servings from several different groups.

FIGURE 5.4

SERVING SIZES

These guidelines can help you eat enough of each type of food each day. List the foods you ate today. *How many servings did you eat from each food group?*

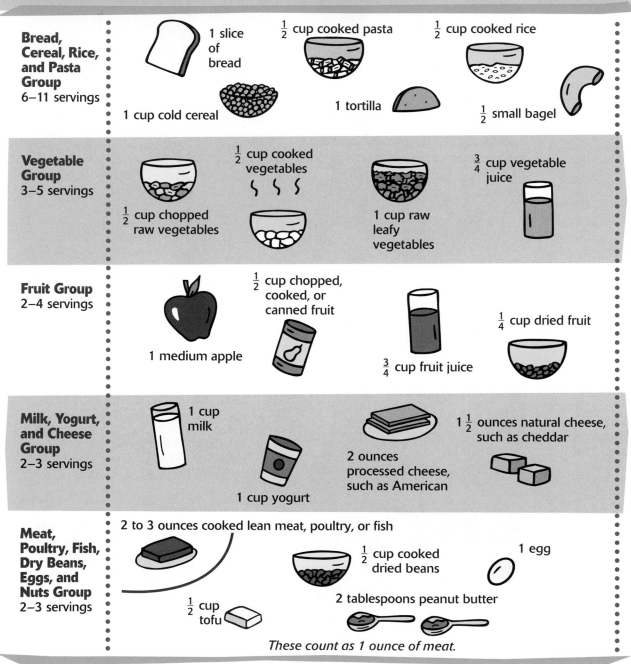

Bread, Cereal, Rice, and Pasta Group
6–11 servings

1 slice of bread
$\frac{1}{2}$ cup cooked pasta
$\frac{1}{2}$ cup cooked rice
1 cup cold cereal
1 tortilla
$\frac{1}{2}$ small bagel

Vegetable Group
3–5 servings

$\frac{1}{2}$ cup cooked vegetables
$\frac{3}{4}$ cup vegetable juice
$\frac{1}{2}$ cup chopped raw vegetables
1 cup raw leafy vegetables

Fruit Group
2–4 servings

$\frac{1}{2}$ cup chopped, cooked, or canned fruit
$\frac{1}{4}$ cup dried fruit
1 medium apple
$\frac{3}{4}$ cup fruit juice

Milk, Yogurt, and Cheese Group
2–3 servings

1 cup milk
$1\frac{1}{2}$ ounces natural cheese, such as cheddar
2 ounces processed cheese, such as American
1 cup yogurt

Meat, Poultry, Fish, Dry Beans, Eggs, and Nuts Group
2–3 servings

2 to 3 ounces cooked lean meat, poultry, or fish
$\frac{1}{2}$ cup cooked dried beans
1 egg
$\frac{1}{2}$ cup tofu
2 tablespoons peanut butter
These count as 1 ounce of meat.

ANALYZE YOUR FOOD CHOICES

Once you know how well your eating plan matches the Food Guide Pyramid, you will know what changes you need to make to eat more healthfully. This activity will help you make a detailed analysis of your food choices for the next two days.

WHAT YOU WILL NEED
- paper and pencil or pen
- ruler

WHAT YOU WILL DO
1. Mark off three vertical columns on your paper.
2. In the first column, list all the foods you eat in the next two days. Use a separate record for each day.
3. In the second column, write down the amount of each food you eat.

4. In the third column, list the number of servings from each food group that each food provided.
5. Add up the total number of servings you ate from each food group.

IN CONCLUSION
1. How well does your list for each day match the guidelines provided by the Food Guide Pyramid?
2. How could you improve your food choices?

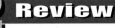

Lesson 2 Review

Using complete sentences, answer the following questions on a sheet of paper.

Reviewing Terms and Facts
1. **Vocabulary** What is the *Food Guide Pyramid*?
2. **Match** For each food group, list the number of daily servings recommended for a teen.
3. **Give Examples** Give an example of one serving from each of the five basic food groups.

Thinking Critically
4. **Recommend** Working in small groups, make a list of tasty and nutritious snack foods from each of the food groups.

Compare lists with other groups to get more ideas.
5. **Synthesize** Describe a low-fat meal that has one-third of the daily servings for all five food groups.

Applying Health Skills
6. **Analyzing Influences** Collect food ads from several teen magazines. Make a chart categorizing the ads into the five food groups plus fats, oils, and sweets. (Some ads will fit into several groups.) Decide which group is advertised most and explain how you think this affects the food choices of a typical teen.

Making Healthful Food Choices

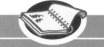
LEARN ABOUT...

- making responsible food choices.
- foods that are especially nutritious.
- what foods to limit or avoid in your eating plan.
- how to maintain a healthy weight.

VOCABULARY

- calcium
- saturated fat
- cholesterol
- sodium
- calorie
- anorexia nervosa
- bulimia nervosa

Influences on Your Food Choices

Why do you choose the foods you do? It may be simply because you enjoy eating a certain food, or perhaps because your friends eat it. Some foods may be family favorites or part of your cultural heritage. You may choose some foods because they are a good value or because they are convenient. You may choose other foods because they are in season or popular in your part of the country. Finally, advertisements can influence your food choices.

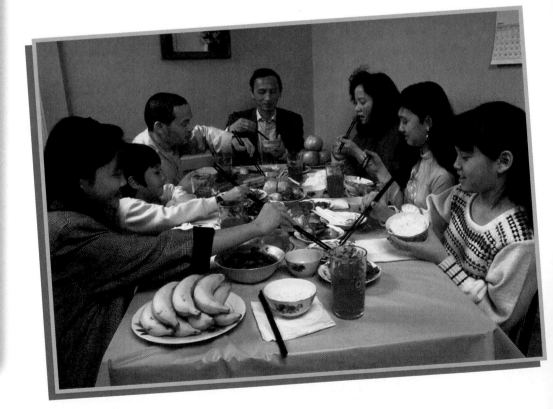

Food preferences in your family can influence your food choices all your life. *What are some of your family's favorites?*

Nutrition During the Teen Years

No matter what influences your choices, you want the foods you eat to help you stay healthy. During your teen years, your nutrient and energy needs are as high as they'll ever be. That's why you need to choose foods wisely. Eat plenty of foods high in complex carbohydrates. These starchy foods give you most of your food energy.

Another important nutrient for teens is calcium. **Calcium** is *a mineral that helps your body build healthy teeth and bones.* It is also important for muscle function. Dairy products are excellent sources of calcium. Canned fish with soft bones (such as salmon or sardines) and dark green leafy vegetables are other good sources. Calcium is also added to some breakfast cereals.

Planning for Good Nutrition

Maybe you're so busy that it seems hard to fit healthful eating into your schedule. Try tucking some healthy snacks into your school or lunch bag. Along with the usual selection of fruit, nuts, and raisins, you can also experiment with foods from around the world, such as pita bread and hummus. Make time for breakfast; ask someone to set aside a plate of food for you if you have to miss a family dinner. When you eat at a fast-food restaurant, try having a salad instead of something high in fat, and order juice or milk to drink.

It is best to get your food energy from foods high in carbohydrates and low in fat. *Name some high-carbohydrate foods that are good choices for teens.*

Developing Good Character

Citizenship

Many communities maintain free food banks to help people who cannot afford the food they need. Collecting food for food banks is a way to help your fellow citizens. It shows that you care about the health of others.

WORTH YOUR SALT
People today don't
think of salt as
important or precious.
The ancient Chinese,
however, used salt as
a basis of the tax sys-
tem. Roman soldiers
received their pay, or
salarium, in the form
of salt. This is the
source of the English
word *salary. Why
might salt have been
useful in ancient
times?*

Guidelines for Healthy Teens

Using the Food Guide Pyramid is just one way to choose healthy foods. There are several other steps you can take to get all the nutrients you need. The USDA has summarized these steps in the Dietary Guidelines for Americans.

Following the Dietary Guidelines is as easy as A-B-C. There are three basic points to follow:

- **A**im for Fitness
- **B**uild a Healthy Base
- **C**hoose Sensibly

Aim for Fitness

The first part of the Dietary Guidelines focuses on balancing the food you eat with physical activity. Being physically active every day, throughout your life, is one of the best things you can do for your body. You will be stronger and have more energy. It will also help you maintain a healthy weight.

Build a Healthy Base

The second part of the Dietary Guidelines advises you to build your eating plan on a healthy base. This means eating enough foods from the bottom three sections of the Food Guide Pyramid. Letting the Pyramid guide your food choices is the first step to building a healthy diet. Another important key to remember is variety. Choosing a variety of different foods will help you get all the nutrients you need. Lastly, keep the food you eat clean and safe. If you don't, your food may contain harmful substances that make you sick. To protect yourself, keep hot foods hot and cold foods cold. Always wash your hands before handling food.

Low-fat or nonfat milk is a healthy food choice. It is an important source of calcium during your teen years, when your bones are still growing.

Choose Sensibly

Finally, the Dietary Guidelines advise you to choose your foods sensibly. This means choosing the foods you know are healthful. It also means going easy on foods that can increase your risk of health problems. For example:

- **Moderate your intake of fats, especially saturated fats.** **Saturated** (SAT·chur·a·tuhd) **fats** are *fats found mostly in animal products such as butter, meat, milk, and egg yolks.* Eating too much saturated fat can increase your body's level of cholesterol. **Cholesterol** (kuh·LES·tuh·rawl) is *a waxlike substance our bodies produce and need in small amounts.* Eating less saturated fat helps you lower your risk of heart disease, cancer, and other serious diseases.

- **Watch for added sugar.** Foods with a lot of added sugar are often low in other nutrients. A little added sugar is fine, but sugary foods should not take the place of more nutritious ones, such as fruits or low-fat milk.

- **Watch your intake of salt.** Salt contains **sodium**, *a mineral that helps control the amount of fluid in your body.* Too much sodium can promote high blood pressure in some people. Read food labels to find foods with less sodium.

Smart snacking can help you meet the extra nutritional needs of your teen years. Time your snacks for two or three hours before mealtime so you won't feel like skipping a meal.

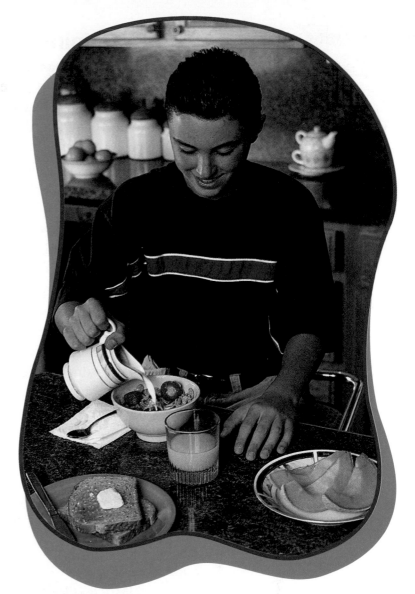

Toast, **English muffins, and hot cereal are popular breakfast foods. However, a bagel pizza or a bowl of leftover rice and beans will also get you off to a good start in the morning.** *What is your favorite breakfast food?*

Reading Check

Decide whether you agree or disagree with the following statements. *Everyone at the same height should weigh the same. Eating too many calories makes a person gain weight.*

Maintaining a Healthy Weight

Many growing teens fear that they weigh too much or too little. However, at your age, weight differences are normal. Trying to gain or lose a lot of weight can interfere with your normal growth and development. If you have serious weight concerns, however, ask your doctor for advice. He or she will assess your weight and, if necessary, suggest a plan that is just right for you.

The Role of Calories

The amount you weigh is related to how many calories you consume and how many you use. A **calorie** is *a unit of heat that measures the energy available in foods.* Your body uses this energy as you go about your daily activities. If you use up as many calories as you take in by eating, your weight will stay the same. If you consume more calories than your body uses, your body stores the extra calories as fat. About 3,500 extra calories per week add 1 pound to your weight. Similarly, if your body needs more calories than you are taking in, it will turn its stored fat into energy. As a result, you will lose weight.

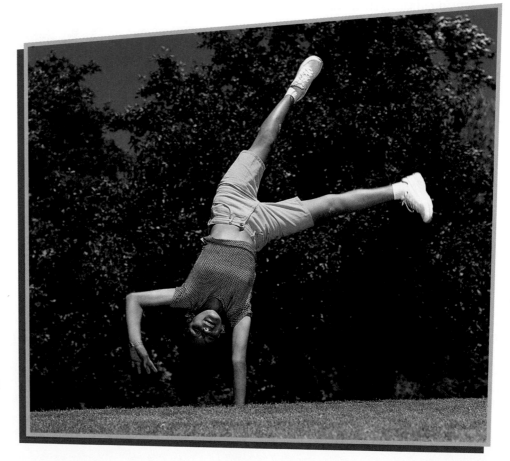

Feeling good about your body is much more important than the numbers on a scale. *Write down five things you like about your body.*

You can maintain a healthy weight by eating right and being physically active. Consume as many calories as your body needs for the activities you are doing. Don't worry too much about what the scale says. Instead, try to be comfortable with your body. Your growing years are not a good time to try to lose weight. A healthy body is a wonderful thing, no matter what size it is. Here are some more tips for maintaining a healthy weight.

- Choose your foods wisely. A slice of bread with peanut butter has about as many calories as a bag of potato chips, and it is more nutritious.
- Snack mostly on healthy foods.
- Eat enough to take away feelings of hunger. Eat slowly and take the time to enjoy your food. Stop when you feel full.
- Always eat breakfast.
- Try not to eat too many foods that are high in fat. These foods are usually high in calories and can also contribute to health problems.
- Drink plenty of water.
- Stay physically active.

Eating Disorders

Many people's self-images are closely tied to their body weight. Some people think they need to be thin to feel good about themselves. People who become overly concerned with their weight may develop eating disorders—extreme eating behaviors that can seriously damage the body. These are most common among teen girls and young women, but occur in males as well. There are three main types of eating disorders.

- **Anorexia nervosa** (an·uh·REK·see·uh ner·VOH·suh) is *an eating disorder in which a person has an intense fear of weight gain and starves himself or herself.* Victims with this disorder are obsessed with the idea of controlling their bodies. They eat far fewer calories than they need to stay healthy. They often exercise excessively and become dangerously thin, but still see themselves as overweight.

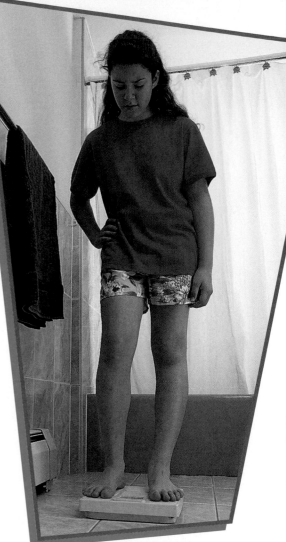

People with eating disorders may become obsessed with their weight. *Why might a person with a healthy weight believe that she or he is overweight?*

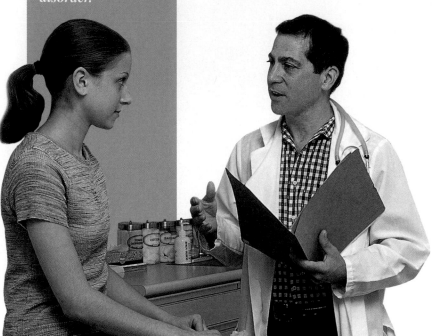

The first step in treating an eating disorder is to seek professional help. *Name some health professionals who could help a person with an eating disorder.*

- **Bulimia nervosa** (boo·LEE·mee·uh ner·VOH·suh) is *an eating disorder in which a person repeatedly eats large amounts of food and then purges by vomiting or using laxatives.* Victims also may exercise excessively, even though their weight is often normal.
- Binge eating is an eating disorder in which a person binges but does not purge or exercise excessively. Victims may be overweight. Often they "seesaw" from losing to gaining weight.

Eating disorders are a mental health problem. If you or anyone you know has symptoms of an eating disorder, talk to a trusted adult about getting professional help. The sooner a person receives treatment for an eating disorder, the likelier he or she is to recover from it.

Lesson 3 Review

Using complete sentences, answer the following questions on a sheet of paper.

Reviewing Terms and Facts

1. **List** Name five factors that influence your food choices.
2. **Vocabulary** Define the word *calcium* and name one food that contains calcium.
3. **Match** Which of the following items should you try to increase in your diet: saturated fat, fiber, cholesterol, calcium, sodium?
4. **Give Examples** Explain what an eating disorder is and name the three main types.

Thinking Critically

5. **Apply** Use the word *calorie* in a sentence about body weight.
6. **Analyze** How is physical activity important for maintaining a healthy body weight?

Applying Health Skills

7. **Goal Setting** Create an illustrated chart showing a plan for one week of healthy eating. You will want to refer to food labels and the information in this chapter. Make sure your choices result in a healthful diet.

The Benefits of Physical Activity

Physical Activity and Your Health

If you enjoy sports, you already know that exercising can make you feel good. Physical activity has many other benefits as well. **Physical activity** is *any kind of movement that causes your body to use energy.* Every kind of physical activity, vigorous or moderate, can help keep you healthy. **Figure 5.5** shows some of the health benefits of regular physical activity.

FIGURE 5.5

HOW PHYSICAL ACTIVITY BENEFITS YOUR HEALTH

Physical activity benefits your physical, mental/emotional, and social health. *What types of physical activity do you enjoy?*

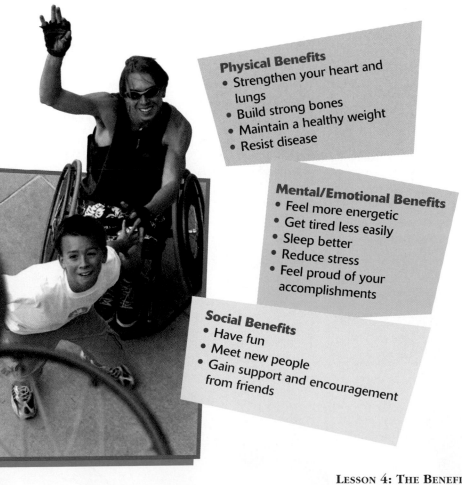

Physical Benefits
- Strengthen your heart and lungs
- Build strong bones
- Maintain a healthy weight
- Resist disease

Mental/Emotional Benefits
- Feel more energetic
- Get tired less easily
- Sleep better
- Reduce stress
- Feel proud of your accomplishments

Social Benefits
- Have fun
- Meet new people
- Gain support and encouragement from friends

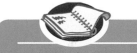

Quick Write

Describe your favorite physical activity and how you think it benefits your physical, mental/emotional, and social health.

LEARN ABOUT...

- the benefits of regular physical activity.
- the different ways physical activity can improve your health.
- the importance of aerobic exercise.

VOCABULARY

- physical activity
- strength
- endurance
- aerobic exercise
- anaerobic exercise
- flexibility
- physical fitness
- exercise

CONNECT TO Social Studies

STARTING THE DAY OFF RIGHT
People in many Japanese offices, factories, and schools start the day with group activity. Students in Japanese schools may learn traditional martial arts such as judo and karate. Share what you know about a physical activity or sport that is popular in a foreign country.

Strength, Endurance, and Flexibility

Different kinds of physical activity benefit your health in different ways. Some activities build **strength**, which is *the ability of your muscles to exert a force.* To build muscle strength, you need to push or pull against a force, such as gravity. Pull-ups, for instance, build muscle strength in your arms.

Activities that build strength may also increase your endurance. **Endurance** (en·DER·uhns) means *how long you can engage in physical activity without becoming overly tired.* There are two kinds of endurance. Muscular endurance is how well your muscles can perform a task without tiring. Heart and lung endurance is how well your heart and lungs can provide your body with oxygen. See **Figure 5.6**.

Aerobic exercise, *rhythmic, nonstop, moderate to vigorous activities that work the heart,* will build endurance. **Anaerobic exercise**, by contrast, is *intense physical activity that requires short bursts of energy.* Jogging 10 miles is aerobic exercise, while sprinting 50 meters at top speed is anaerobic exercise. It is a good idea to do both aerobic and anaerobic activities.

FIGURE 5.6

ACTIVITIES THAT BUILD ENDURANCE

This chart groups activities according to how well they build endurance. *Which of these exercises would you choose?*

Vigorous Activities
(Do at least 20 minutes three times a week.)
- Aerobic dancing
- Cycling
- Cross-country skiing
- Ice hockey
- In-line skating
- Running
- Skateboarding
- Swimming

Moderately Vigorous Activities
(Do at least 30 minutes three times a week.)
- Basketball
- Calisthenics
- Field hockey
- Handball
- Tennis
- Walking

Occasionally Vigorous Activities
(These activities will build muscle strength and flexibility.)
- Baseball
- Downhill skiing
- Football
- Snowboarding
- Softball
- Volleyball

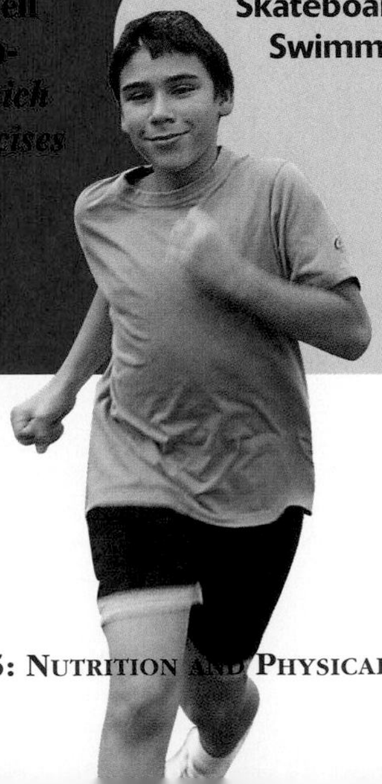

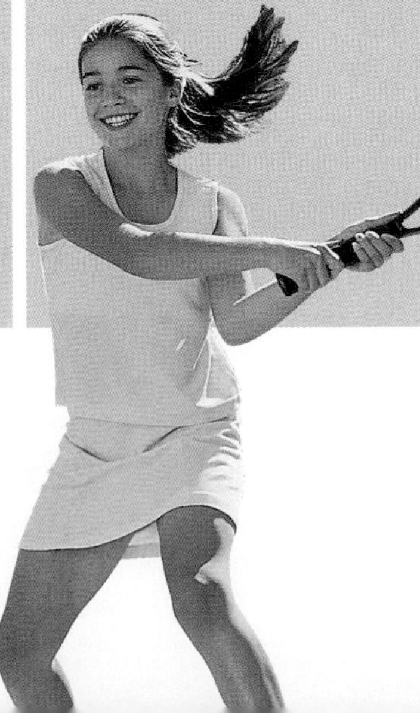

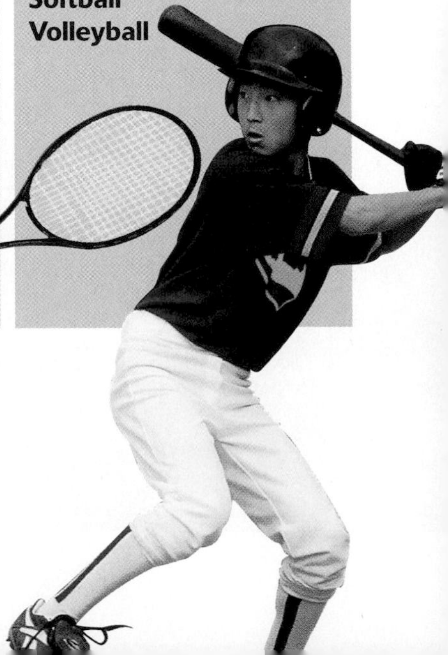

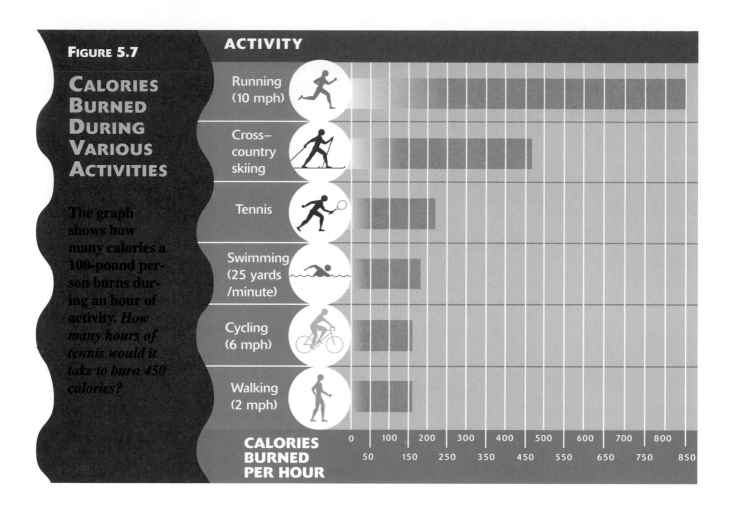

FIGURE 5.7

CALORIES BURNED DURING VARIOUS ACTIVITIES

The graph shows how many calories a 100-pound person burns during an hour of activity. *How many hours of tennis would it take to burn 450 calories?*

ACTIVITY

Running (10 mph)

Cross-country skiing

Tennis

Swimming (25 yards /minute)

Cycling (6 mph)

Walking (2 mph)

CALORIES BURNED PER HOUR

0   100   200   300   400   500   600   700   800
  50   150   250   350   450   550   650   750   850

Finally, physical activity can promote flexibility. **Flexibility** is *the ability to move body joints through a full range of motion.* It helps you with everything from dancing to playing football, and it may help prevent injuries. You can improve your flexibility by stretching your muscles and joints. Ballet, yoga, swimming, and volleyball are all good ways to build flexibility.

Other Benefits

Physical activity can loosen up your muscles and help you relax. During aerobic activities, your brain releases chemicals that calm you down. Vigorous activity can also release stress. You may even find that you sleep better after an active day.

During physical activity, your body burns calories. **Figure 5.7** shows the number of calories you use doing different types of activities. Regular activity can help you maintain a healthy weight. Physical activity can also help firm up your muscles. When you are active, you look better and feel better.

Reading Check
Sort the following words into three groups: *running, basketball, swimming, stair climbing, weightlifting, soccer, karate, softball, dancing.* Label each group.

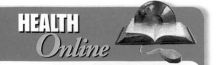
What Is Fitness?

Staying physically active keeps you physically fit. **Physical fitness** is *the ability to handle everyday physical work and play without becoming tired.* Physical fitness gives you enough energy to carry you through the day. It makes you more confident and helps you deal with stress. It also helps you maintain a healthy weight level. In short, it makes your life better!

You can improve or maintain your physical fitness by exercising. **Exercise** is *planned, structured, repetitive physical activity that improves or maintains physical fitness.* An ideal exercise plan includes a variety of different activities. Types of physical activity include:

- **Lifestyle activities.** Every day, try to keep your body moving as much as possible. There are lots of ways to do this. You can

---

HEALTH SKILLS ACTIVITY

STRESS MANAGEMENT

Tension Tamers

Physical activity is a good way to keep stress under control. If you feel stress building up, any kind of activity, even cleaning your room, will help. Here are several activities that can help relieve tension:

- **SHOULDER LIFT.** Hunch your shoulders up to your ears for a few seconds, then release. Repeat.
- **ELASTIC JAW.** Take a few deep relaxing breaths. Open your mouth and shift your jaw to the right as far as you can without discomfort. Hold for a count of three. Repeat on the left side. Do this exercise ten times.

- **SLEEPER.** Lie on your side, arms over your head. Stiffen your body, then relax, letting your body fall where it wants to. Repeat on the other side.
- **TENSE-RELAX.** Make a fist and tense the muscles in your hand and forearm, then release. Repeat with the other hand. You can do the same with your abdomen, thigh, buttocks, and toes.

ON YOUR OWN

Estimate your current level of body tension or stress on a scale of one to ten. Then perform one of the exercises listed here. Write down your estimated level of body tension afterward. Repeat for each of the other exercises. How did each exercise affect your tension level? Compare your results as a class.

walk or ride your bike to school, if it's not too far. You can take a walk for fun—with your dog, with a friend, or by yourself. Games such as tag or jump rope can also boost your activity level. Even cleaning your room is a way to get your body moving!

- **Aerobic activities.** Try to get some aerobic activity three to five times a week. Riding your bike, skateboarding, and in-line skating can give you exercise on the go. You can also try swimming, hiking, or running around the block. You will benefit most if you do these activities for at least 20 minutes at a time. You can get some of your aerobic activity from organized sports, such as soccer, basketball, or skiing.
- **Strength and flexibility activities.** Two to three times a week, work on your strength and flexibility. Such exercises as push-ups and pull-ups will help you develop strength. Dancing, rope climbing, or karate will help you build flexibility.

Try to cut down on the amount of time you spend sitting still. Obviously, you have to sit still some of the time—when you're in class, doing homework, or eating meals. However, you can reduce the amount of time you spend watching television or playing video games. Replace some of these idle hours with active games and sports, and you may find you're having more fun than ever.

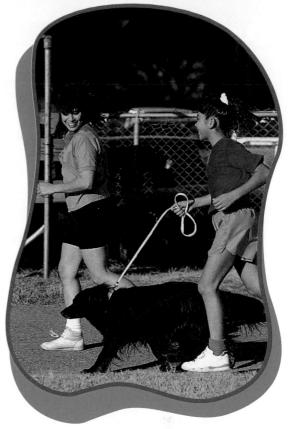

Going for a walk is an easy way to add some physical activity to your day. *What are some other ways you can be physically active every day?*

Lesson 4 Review

Using complete sentences, answer the following questions on a sheet of paper.

Reviewing Terms and Facts

1. **Vocabulary** Define the terms *strength, endurance,* and *flexibility.*
2. **Identify** What kind of exercise is best for building endurance?
3. **Describe** In an original sentence, explain what *physical fitness* means.

Thinking Critically

4. **Analyze** Which type of physical activity should you perform more often:

lifestyle activities such as household chores, or recreational activities such as soccer? Explain why.

5. **Apply** Describe your current level of physical activity. Based on this lesson, can you use more or less activity? Explain your response.

Applying Health Skills

6. **Advocacy** As a class, brainstorm ways teens can be physically active. Assign each idea to a team. The team should explain how the activity can become a daily habit for teens.

Setting Fitness Goals

Quick Write

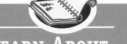

List all the ways you exercise regularly. Do you need to increase your level of activity? If so, what can you do?

LEARN ABOUT...

- how you can set goals to improve your fitness level.
- how to get the most out of exercise.
- how to avoid injuries during exercise.

VOCABULARY

- warm-up
- target pulse rate
- cool-down

Creating a Personal Fitness Plan

You can make sure that you get all the exercise and physical activity you need by creating a personal fitness plan. Before you make your plan, however, you need to decide the answers to these questions:

- **What do you hope to accomplish?** Are you looking for muscle tone or strength, greater endurance, or increased flexibility? Maybe you have several results in mind. Determine your goals and consider your abilities to achieve them.
- **Where should you begin?** Start small. If you have never run before, you're probably not ready to run a 5-kilometer race. Begin by running short distances—several hundred yards or one city block—every other day for a week. Increase your distance gradually. You can also start by walking instead of running, then gradually increase your speed.
- **What do you enjoy?** Choose activities that are fun for you. Doing something you like makes it easier for you to meet your fitness goals.

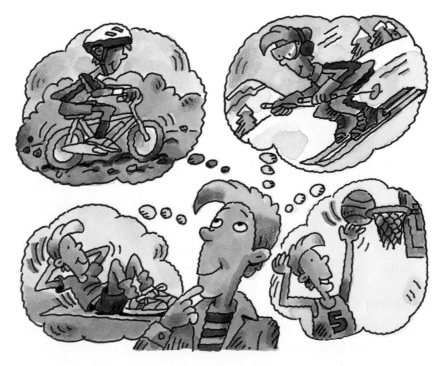

You can reach your fitness goals if you think carefully about your exercise program before you begin. *What fitness goals are you most eager to achieve?*

Choosing Activities

Now that you have a clear view of your goals, you're ready to create your fitness plan. As you form your plan, you will decide which exercises to include and when you will perform them. You will also consider ways to avoid injury.

Different types of exercise will help you to meet different fitness goals. The information in **Figure 5.8** can help you choose appropriate exercises. You should also consider

- whether you want to exercise alone or with others.
- what equipment you will need.
- how much money you or your parents are willing to spend.

FIGURE 5.8

Fitness Ratings for Different Activities

Different activities can promote muscular strength and endurance, heart-lung endurance, and flexibility. *Which exercises are good for achieving all three fitness goals?*

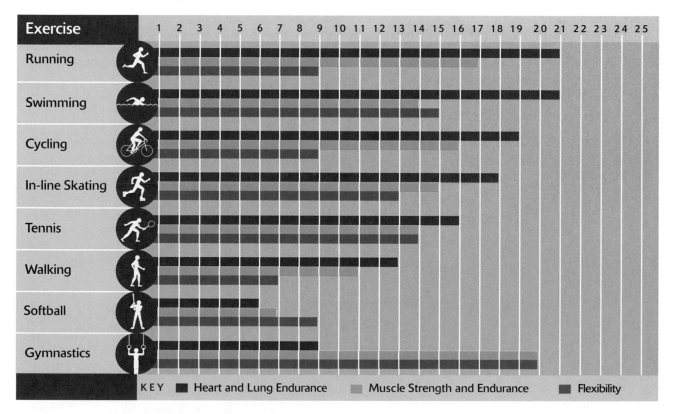

Exercise	1	2	3	4	5	6	7	8	9	10	11	12	13	14	15	16	17	18	19	20	21	22	23	24	25
Running																									
Swimming																									
Cycling																									
In-line Skating																									
Tennis																									
Walking																									
Softball																									
Gymnastics																									

KEY ■ Heart and Lung Endurance   ■ Muscle Strength and Endurance   ■ Flexibility

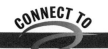
Making Time for Exercise

One way to make exercise a regular part of your life is to set aside a regular time for it. For example, if you do outdoor activities, you would choose a time during the daylight hours. One time you should not exercise is right after a meal. Exercise can interfere with your digestion.

Exercising Safely

When exercising, you need to take steps to avoid injuring yourself (see **Figure 5.9**). Start with a **warm-up**, *some gentle activity that prepares your body for exercise.* Next, stretch your muscles and joints to loosen them. Then work up to your **target pulse rate**, *the level at which your heart and lungs receive the most benefit from a workout.* It is 60 to 80 percent of the heart's maximum rate, which you can estimate by subtracting your age from 220. A 12-year-old's target pulse rate is 125 to 167 beats per minute.

HEALTH SKILLS ACTIVITY

GOAL SETTING

Increasing Your Activity Level

How can busy teens find the time to get active? Here are a few possibilities.
IF YOU ARE RARELY ACTIVE, increase your everyday activities by

- taking the stairs whenever possible.
- reducing your television time.
- walking whenever you can.

IF YOU ARE ACTIVE SOME OF THE TIME, work to become more consistent by

- choosing activities you enjoy.
- planning your daily activities.
- setting goals you can meet.

IF YOU ARE ALREADY ACTIVE AT LEAST FOUR DAYS EACH WEEK, keep your activity level up by

- changing your routine if you feel bored.
- exploring new activities.

Lifestyle activity	about 1 hour every day	
Aerobic activity	about 20 minutes per week	walk to school 2–3 times per week
Recreational activity	soccer practice twice a week	go skating with friends on weekend
Flexibility and strength exercise	none	do 10 push-ups and 10 sit-ups three days a week
Inactivity	about 15–20 hours a week	watch TV only 1 hour a day

ON YOUR OWN
Draw a 3-column table. In the first column, list the types of physical activity described in Lesson 4. In the second column, list the time you spend on each every week. If you fall short in any area, use the third column to list ways to improve.

Adjust for the weather. On hot, humid days, work out for a shorter time in the early morning or the evening. On cold days, wear layers of clothing to remove as you get warm. Always drink water as you exercise. Listen to your body's signals: if you feel pain, stop. End your workout with a **cool-down**—*some gentle activity to slow down after exercise*—and some more stretching.

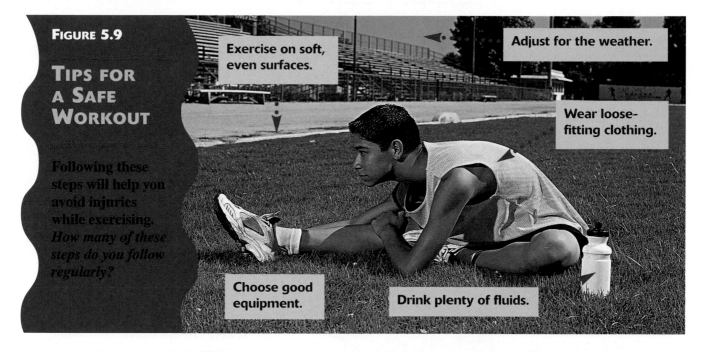

FIGURE 5.9

TIPS FOR A SAFE WORKOUT

Following these steps will help you avoid injuries while exercising. *How many of these steps do you follow regularly?*

Exercise on soft, even surfaces.

Adjust for the weather.

Wear loose-fitting clothing.

Choose good equipment.

Drink plenty of fluids.

Lesson 5 Review

Using complete sentences, answer the following questions on a sheet of paper.

Reviewing Terms and Facts

1. **Identify** Name two good activities for building heart and lung endurance, two for building muscle strength and endurance, and two for building flexibility.
2. **Recall** Why is it unwise to exercise right after eating a meal?
3. **Vocabulary** Use the terms *warming up, target pulse rate,* and *cooling down* in an original paragraph about planning a workout. Make sure you explain the meanings of these terms in your paragraph.

Thinking Critically

4. **Apply** Identify three questions you should ask yourself as you think about what exercises to include in your fitness program.
5. **Describe** How can you prepare for exercise on a warm, humid day? On a cold day?

Applying Health Skills

6. **Goal Setting** Select an activity that will help meet one of your fitness goals. Write a plan that shows when and where you will do this activity. Set goals for improving your performance in this activity over a four-week period. Keep a record of your progress.

FUELING YOUR BODY

Model

Every day, you make many food choices that affect your health. You may choose foods at home, in the school cafeteria, or when eating out. Read about Paola, who was at the mall with her friends one weekend around lunchtime. The food court offered a variety of fast-food meals. Paola used the six-step decision-making process to consider her options.

STEP 1. STATE THE SITUATION.
I want to eat something that tastes good and is good for me.

STEP 2. LIST THE OPTIONS.
I could get a couple of slices of cheese pizza, a burger and fries, or a bean burrito.

STEP 3. WEIGH THE POSSIBLE OUTCOMES.
The pizza has a lot of protein, but the cheese is high in fat. The burrito has the least fat, and the most fiber. The burger and fries are my friends' favorite, but they have a lot of calories and fat.

STEP 4. CONSIDER YOUR VALUES.
I am a vegetarian, so I don't want to eat meat.

STEP 5. MAKE A DECISION AND ACT.
I will get a bean burrito. It's something I like that is good for me and doesn't include meat.

STEP 6. EVALUATE THE DECISION.
I feel satisfied. The burrito tasted good and I gave my body the nutrients it needs without eating meat.

Practice

Antonio is late and has to eat on the run. In the kitchen he finds granola bars, peanut butter crackers, raisins, and string cheese. He wants something that is filling (contains protein) and provides energy (carbohydrates) but is low in fat. Look at the four food labels on this page. Each label provides information for one serving. Write out the decision-making steps on a sheet of paper to help Antonio choose a snack.

Apply/Assess

Imagine that you are hungry for an after-school snack. There are four snack foods that you like: granola bars, peanut butter crackers, raisins, and string cheese. Take another look at the nutrition labels on this page. This time, think about what you usually eat for breakfast and at school. How many servings from each food group have you already consumed? Which of these snacks come from the food group(s) that you still need? Write your decision-making steps on a sheet of paper. Be prepared to justify your choice.

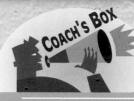

Nutrition Facts

Serving Size: 2 bars (42g)

Amount Per Serving:

Calories 180 Calories from Fat 60

	% Daily Value*
Total Fat 6g	**10%**
Saturated Fat 0.5g	**3%**
Cholesterol 0mg	**0%**
Sodium 160mg	**7%**
Total Carbohydrate 29g	**10%**
Dietary Fiber 2g	**9%**
Sugars 11g	
Protein 4g	

Vitamin A 40% • Vitamin C 0%
Calcium 0% • Iron 6%
*Percent Daily Values are based on a 2,000 calorie diet.

Granola bar

Raisins

Nutrition Facts

Serving Size: 1 box (42g)

Amount Per Serving:

Calories 130   Calories from Fat 0

	% Daily
	0%
Total Fat 0g	**0%**
Saturated Fat 0g	**0%**
Cholesterol 0mg	**7%**
Sodium 180mg	**10%**
Total Carbohydrate 31g	**9%**
Dietary Fiber 2g	
Sugars 29g	
Protein 1g	

Vitamin A 0% • Vitamin C 0% • Calcium 2% • Iron 6%
*Percent Daily Values are based on a 2,000 calorie diet.

Nutrition Facts

Serving Size: 1 package (39g)

Amount Per Serving:

Calories 200   Calories from Fat 100

	% Daily Value*
Total Fat 11g	**17%**
Saturated Fat 2g	**10%**
Cholesterol 0mg	**0%**
Sodium 290mg	**12%**
Total Carbohydrate 22g	**7%**
Dietary Fiber 1g	**4%**
Sugars 3g	
Protein 4g	

Vitamin A 0% • Vitamin C 0% • Calcium 0% • Iron 8%
*Percent Daily Values are based on a 2,000 calorie diet.

Peanut butter crackers

Nutrition Facts

Serving Size: 1 piece (24g)

Amount Per Serving:

Calories 70   Calories from Fat 45

Total Fat 5g	**7%**
Saturated Fat 3g	**15%**
Cholesterol 15mg	**5%**
Sodium 180mg	**7%**
Total Carbohydrate less than 1g	**0%**
Dietary Fiber 0g	**0%**
Sugars 0g	
Protein 6g	

Vitamin A 4% • Vitamin C 0%
Calcium 15% • Iron 0%
*Percent Daily Values are based on a 2,000 calorie diet.

String cheese

FOCUS ON FITNESS

Model

Luis likes being outdoors. He participates in two activities that he enjoys—running and in-line skating. Luis also has physical education class two days each week. Below you can see a calendar of his activities for the past week. The description of each activity includes a list of the equipment he needs to stay safe.

Activity	Frequency	Time	Equipment
In-line skating	twice a week (Monday, Saturday)	Warm up (skate slowly), 10 minutes; skate, 20 minutes; cool down (skate slowly), 5 minutes	Helmet, knee pads, elbow pads, wrist guards, gloves
Baseball (physical education class in school)	twice a week (Tuesday, Thursday)	Warm up and stretch, 10 minutes; play, 30 minutes; cool down (walking), 5 minutes	Batting helmet, baseball glove
Running	once a week (Friday)	Warm up and stretch, 10 minutes; run, 20 minutes; cool down (jog slowly), 5 minutes	Running shoes

Practice

Grace's family belongs to the local YMCA, which offers a variety of activities. There is a basketball court, a track for running or walking, and several kinds of gym equipment. Grace enjoys all of these activities except running. In addition, she likes to ride her bike with her next-door neighbor, Haitsu.

On your own paper, set up an exercise program for Grace. Copy the fitness chart on the previous page and add the activities you suggest for her. Be sure to include a variety of activities she enjoys. Show how often and for how long she should do each activity. Also list ways for her to avoid injury. Be ready to explain how your choices benefit Grace.

Apply/Assess

Copy the fitness chart onto butcher paper or poster board, using colored markers. Then fill in your chart with the activities you would like to do. Include a warm-up, a cool-down, and activities that raise your heart rate. Remember to list the safety equipment you own or will need.

Share your finished chart with your classmates. Explain which activities you chose and why. Describe the equipment and other safety measures your activites require.

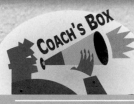
EXERCISE PROGRAM for GRACE

Activity	Frequency	Time	Equipment
Basketball			
Biking			
Walking on Treadmill			

SUMMARY

LESSON•1 Food contains nutrients, substances that your body needs. The six basic nutrient categories are carbohydrates, proteins, fats, vitamins, minerals, and water.

LESSON•2 The Food Guide Pyramid is a tool to help you plan healthy food choices. It explains how many servings you need to eat every day from each of the five basic food groups.

LESSON•3 A healthy eating plan includes a variety of foods. The food you eat provides your body with the calories it needs for energy.

LESSON•4 Physical activity improves your physical, mental/emotional, and social health. It helps build strength, endurance, and flexibility.

LESSON•5 The exercises you choose will depend on your personal fitness goals. To exercise safely, you should warm up first, work up to your target pulse rate, and cool down afterward.

Reviewing Vocabulary and Concepts

- calcium
- fat
- grains
- minerals
- nutrients
- sweets
- vegetable
- vitamins

On a sheet of paper, write the numbers 1–8. After each number, write the term from the list that best completes each statement.

Lesson 1

1. Carbohydrates, proteins, and fats are all types of _____.
2. _____ is a nutrient that provides energy, carries vitamins, and helps keep your skin healthy.
3. Nutrients that help regulate body functions are called _____.
4. Elements that help your body work properly are _____.

Lesson 2

5. You need to eat 3 to 5 servings each day from the _____ Group.

6. Foods in the Bread, Cereal, Rice, and Pasta Group are made from _____.
7. Foods in the Milk, Yogurt, and Cheese Group are a good source of the mineral _____.
8. It is best to eat small amounts of fats, oils, and _____.

On a sheet of paper, write the numbers 9–22. Write *True* or *False* for each statement below. If the statement is false, change the underlined word or phrase to make it true.

Lesson 3

9. <u>Sodium</u> is a mineral that helps your body build healthy teeth and bones.
10. Consuming too much saturated fat can increase your body's level of <u>calcium</u>.
11. The energy available in foods is measured in <u>calories</u>.

12. Eating less <u>saturated fat</u> is a good way to reduce the risk of heart disease.
13. People with the eating disorder <u>anorexia</u> eat large amounts of food and then purge by vomiting or using laxatives.

Lesson 4

14. Pushing or pulling against a force, such as gravity, builds <u>strength</u>.
15. You can build endurance by engaging in <u>anaerobic</u> exercise.
16. The ability to move body joints through a full range of motion is called <u>flexibility</u>.
17. You can become physically fit by doing <u>exercise</u>.
18. To stay healthy and fit, you should <u>increase</u> the amount of time you spend sitting still.

Lesson 5

19. A gentle activity that prepares the body for exercise is called a <u>cool-down</u>.
20. When exercising, you should always stretch <u>before</u> you warm up.
21. Your target pulse rate is <u>60 to 80 percent</u> of your heart's maximum rate.
22. It is best to wear <u>loose fitting</u> clothing when exercising.

Thinking Critically

Using complete sentences, answer the following questions on a sheet of paper.

23. **Analyze** How can a food label help you figure out how much a serving of food costs?
24. **Explain** Why does the Food Guide Pyramid recommend only small amounts from the Fats, Oils, and Sweets group?
25. **Predict** If you skipped breakfast every day for a week, how might it affect your schoolwork?
26. **Suggest** Why does choosing activities you enjoy make it easier to meet your fitness goals?

Career Corner

Dietetic Technician

Are you the one who helps plan family meals at your house? Are you concerned about people getting proper nutrition? Then you might enjoy a career as a dietetic technician. You just need a two-year associate degree and internship training to become licensed. Then you could be assisting a dietitian to help people plan balanced diets. You might volunteer for a community Meals on Wheels program to prepare for this career. Visit Career Corner at health.glencoe.com to find out more about this and other health careers.

Chapter 6

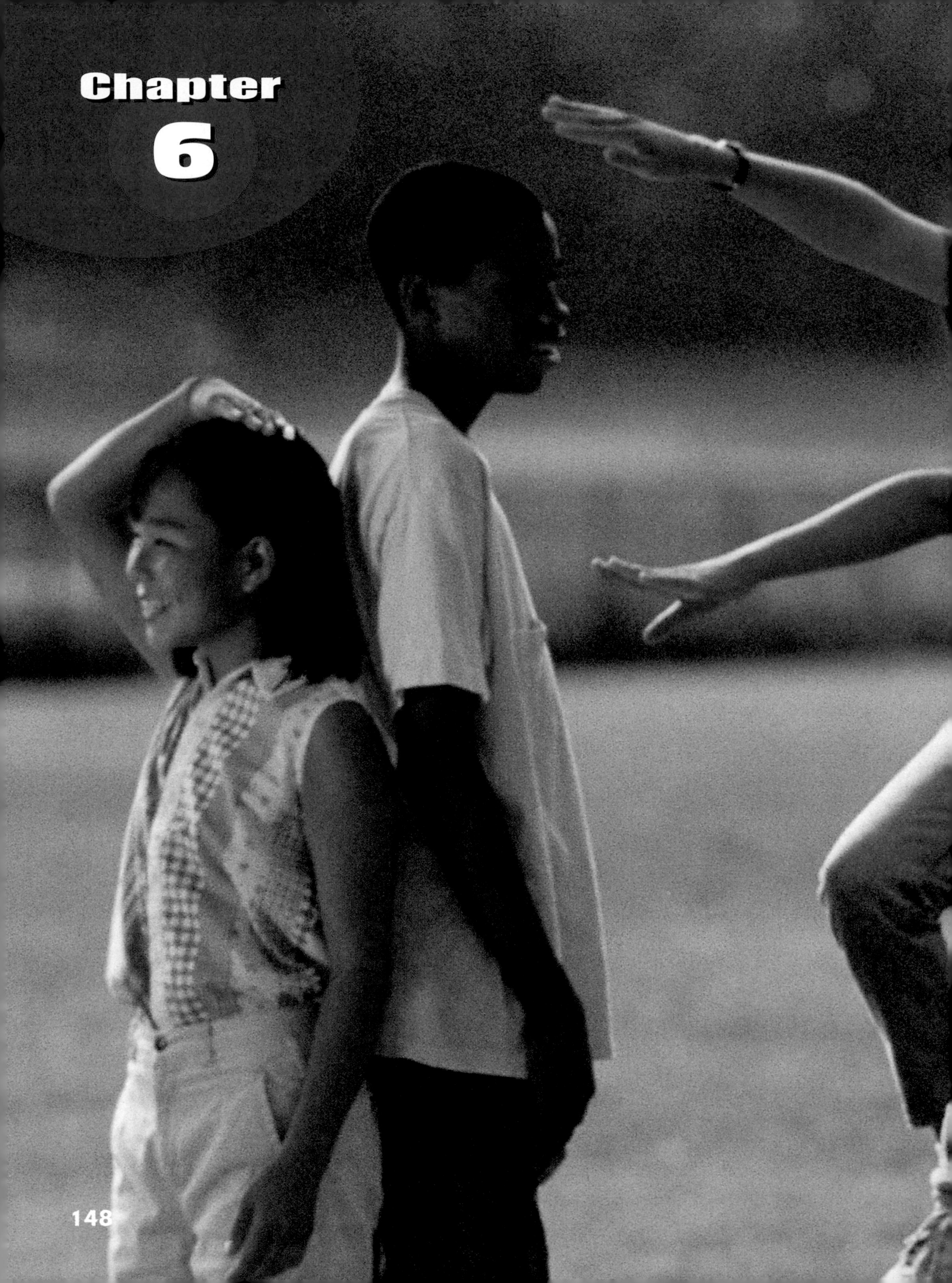

Growth and Development

Quick Write

Think about a few activities that you do every day, such as brushing your teeth, playing a sport, or talking with friends. How do your body and mind work together to perform these different actions?

Find out how well you take care of your body systems. Take the Health Inventory for Chapter 6 at health.glencoe.com.

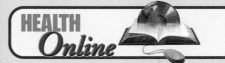

Reading Check

Is the following statement true or false? *Nerve cells carry messages from your brain to other parts of your body.* Explain your response.

From Cells to Body Systems

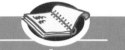

LEARN ABOUT...

- the relationship between cells, tissues, organs, and body systems.
- the names and functions of the major body systems.
- how body systems work together.

VOCABULARY

- cells
- tissues
- organ
- body system

Cells: The Building Blocks

Your entire body is made up of tiny units called cells. Your body contains many different kinds of cells, which vary in size and shape. Each type of cell does a special job. For example, nerve cells carry messages between your brain and other parts of your body. As **Figure 6.1** shows, nerve cells are long

FIGURE 6.1

FROM CELL TO SYSTEM

The body system shown here is the nervous system. Notice how the complex system begins with cells, the body's basic units.

B **Tissues** are *groups of similar cells that do the same kind of work.* The tissue shown here is made of clusters of nerve cells.

A **Cells** are *the basic building blocks of life.* Each cell in your body does a particular job. Nerve cells, like the ones shown here, carry messages to and from your brain.

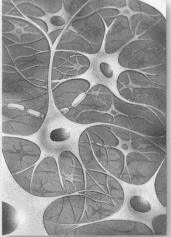

and narrow, like electrical wires, so they can carry messages. Skin cells, on the other hand, are flat and rectangular, so they can spread out to cover the surface of your body.

Systems: Parts of a Whole You

In many ways, your body is like a machine. The cells that make up your body combine to form larger structures called tissues, organs, and body systems. All of these parts work together to allow your body to function. **Figure 6.1** shows how cells combine to form the parts of a body system.

How Systems Are Organized

The parts of the body systems are organized by what they do, not by their location in your body. For example, the mouth and the small intestine are far apart, yet both are key parts of the digestive system. Some organs belong to more than one body system.

✓

Reading Check
Make a four-column chart. List the vocabulary words in the left column. Above the empty columns, write the headings *K* (Know), *W* (Want to Know), and *L* (Learned). Fill in columns *K* and *W*. As you read, fill in column *L*.

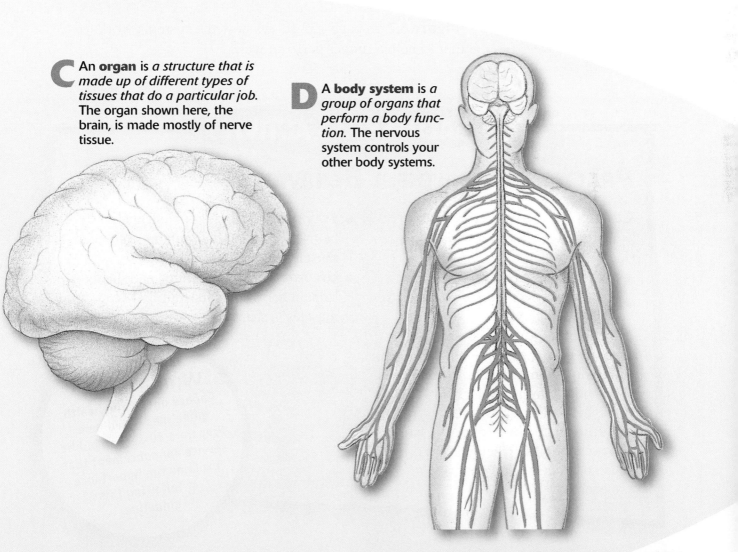

C An **organ** is *a structure that is made up of different types of tissues that do a particular job.* The organ shown here, the brain, is made mostly of nerve tissue.

D A **body system** is *a group of organs that perform a body function.* The nervous system controls your other body systems.

How Systems Work Together

Body systems are interrelated. This means that they work together and depend on one another to keep the body functioning well. The digestive and excretory systems work as a team to first break down food for energy (digestive), and then get rid of wastes (excretory). Some of the body systems and their functions within the body are listed below.

- **The skeletal and muscular systems** support and move the body and protect organs.
- **The circulatory system** brings food and oxygen to cells and takes wastes away.
- **The respiratory system** carries oxygen to blood and removes carbon dioxide.
- **The nervous system** controls all body systems, sends and receives messages, and helps you see, hear, taste, smell, and feel.
- **The digestive and excretory systems** break down food for energy and get rid of wastes.
- **The endocrine system** produces hormones that regulate body functions.

Figure 6.2 on page 153 shows how the systems work together to help a runner perform well.

HEALTH SKILLS ACTIVITY

PRACTICING HEALTHFUL BEHAVIORS

Caring for Your Body Systems

For good health, follow these guidelines.

- **GET PLENTY OF REST.** Rest helps muscles recover from physical activity and reduces mental stress.
- **EAT HEALTHFUL FOODS AND DRINK PLENTY OF WATER.** Good nutrition aids digestion and helps keep muscles and bones strong. Water feeds all cells and helps eliminate wastes.
- **AVOID ALCOHOL, TOBACCO, AND OTHER DRUGS.** Chemicals in drugs can damage all of your body's systems.
- **STAY ACTIVE.** Regular physical activity helps the heart and circulation and keeps muscles strong.
- **USE GOOD POSTURE.** Sitting and standing straight helps lungs function and keeps muscles in shape.

WITH A GROUP
Choose one of the health guidelines listed here. Prepare a 30-second public service announcement that explains the importance of following this guideline.

FIGURE 6.2

BODY SYSTEMS AT WORK

Each body system depends on the others to do its job effectively. *How many body systems are active when this teen runs?*

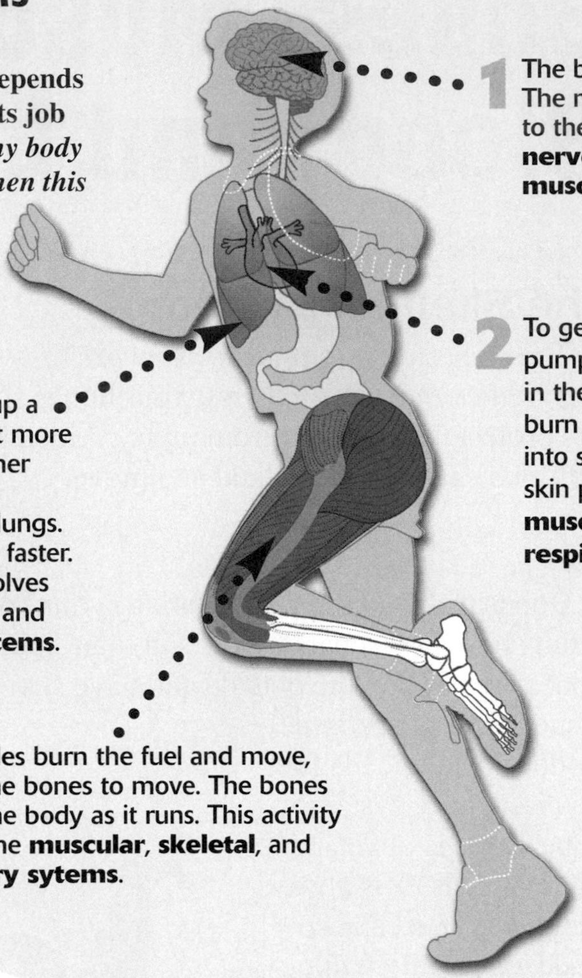

1 The brain sends out a message: Run! The message is carried through nerves to the muscles. This step involves the **nervous system** and the **muscular system**.

2 To get energy, muscles need blood that is pumped by the heart. Blood contains fuel in the form of sugar, as well as oxygen to burn that fuel. As blood flows, wastes pass into sweat glands that release them through skin pores. These processes involve the **muscular, circulatory, digestive, respiratory,** and **excretory systems**.

3 The muscles burn the fuel and move, causing the bones to move. The bones support the body as it runs. This activity involves the **muscular**, **skeletal**, and **circulatory sytems**.

4 Running burns up a lot of fuel. To get more oxygen, the runner gasps for breath provided by his lungs. His heart pumps faster. This process involves the **respiratory** and **circulatory systems**.

Lesson 1 Review

Using complete sentences, answer the following questions on a sheet of paper.

Reviewing Terms and Facts

1. **Vocabulary** Define the word *tissue* and explain how it is related to cells.
2. **Describe** How are the parts of a body system organized?
3. **Recall** Which body system carries food and oxygen to cells?

Thinking Critically

4. **Compare** Think about the different body systems identified in this lesson. Which do you seem to have control over? Which seem to work by themselves?
5. **Explain** Name a function of the body and tell why two or more systems sometimes need to work together to perform it.

Applying Health Skills

6. **Goal Setting** Review the guidelines in the Health Skills Activity for keeping your body systems functioning properly. Choose one guideline you think you could follow better than you do now. List some specific steps you could take every day to follow the guideline.

Bones, Muscles, Blood, and Lungs

The Skeletal System

The **skeletal system** is *a framework of bones and the tissues that connect those bones.* Your bones support your body and protect its soft parts from injury. Aided by your muscles, they also enable you to stand and move.

Bones

Bones make up the framework of your body. Adults have 206 separate bones in their bodies. Bones are hard on the outside and have spongy tissue inside. This tissue produces blood cells for the circulatory system. Bone tissue is alive and is made of cells. It is always being destroyed and re-made, especially while you are still growing.

Your skeletal system supports your body, allowing you to stand and walk. *Why might this gymnast be especially concerned about taking care of her bones and joints?*

Joints

Joints are *places where one bone meets another.* Different joints move in different ways. A pivot joint consists of the end of one bone rotating inside a ring formed by another. It can move up and down and from side to side. A hinge joint moves in only one direction, like a door hinge. Your knee is an example. A ball-and-socket joint, like your hip, consists of a round end of one bone moving inside the cup-shaped socket of another. It can move in all directions. See **Figure 6.3** for an illustration of important bones in your body and the three major types of joints.

Developing Good Character

Responsibility

Osteoporosis is a disease that weakens bones. To help prevent this disease, eat foods rich in calcium, such as milk, and strengthen bones with exercise.

FIGURE 6.3

THE SKELETAL SYSTEM

This skeleton shows some of the important bones found in your body and illustrates three major types of joints. *What type of joint is the hip joint?*

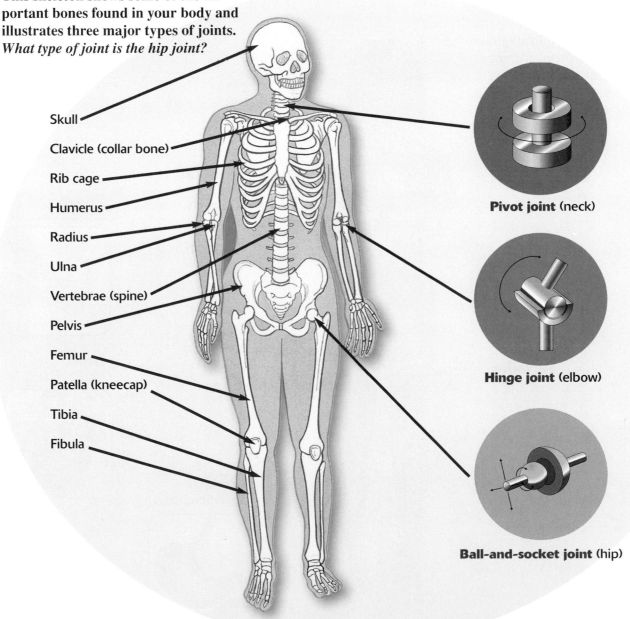

Skull

Clavicle (collar bone)

Rib cage

Humerus

Radius

Ulna

Vertebrae (spine)

Pelvis

Femur

Patella (kneecap)

Tibia

Fibula

Pivot joint (neck)

Hinge joint (elbow)

Ball-and-socket joint (hip)

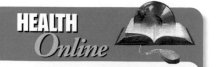
The Muscular System

The **muscular system** is made of *all the muscles in your body.* Muscles move bones, pump blood, and move food through the stomach and intestines, among other jobs. The three types of muscle are skeletal, cardiac, and smooth. The skeletal muscles are called voluntary muscles because you control them. They are located in places like your arms, face, abdomen, and back. Cardiac, or heart, muscles and smooth muscles, such as those in the stomach, are involuntary muscles—they work without your controlling them. See **Figure 6.4**.

FIGURE 6.4

THE MUSCULAR SYSTEM

Muscles move bones, pump blood, and move food through the digestive system. *What are the three major types of muscles?*

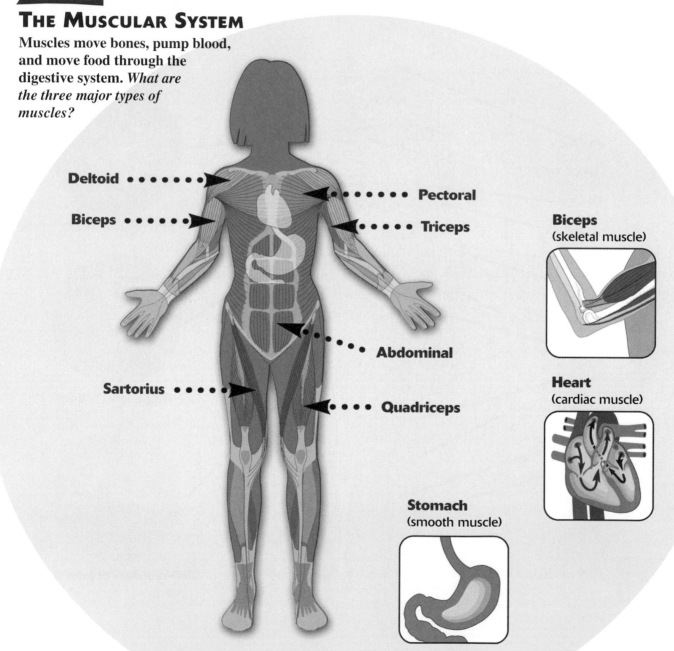

Deltoid

Biceps

Pectoral

Triceps

Abdominal

Sartorius

Quadriceps

Biceps (skeletal muscle)

Heart (cardiac muscle)

Stomach (smooth muscle)

The Circulatory System

The **circulatory system** *enables the body to transport, or move, materials from one place to another.* The blood moves to and from the tissues of the body, delivering oxygen, food, and other materials to cells and removing wastes. See **Figure 6.5**.

FIGURE 6.5

THE CIRCULATORY SYSTEM

The blood vessels shown in blue carry oxygen-poor blood away from the body and toward the heart and lungs. The red blood vessels carry oxygen-rich blood from the lungs to the heart and back to the rest of the body. *Why are the pulmonary arteries shown in blue?*

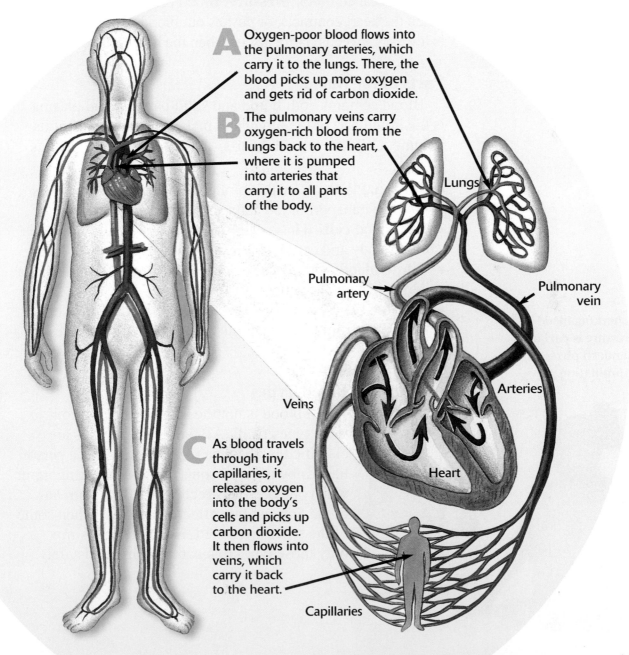

A Oxygen-poor blood flows into the pulmonary arteries, which carry it to the lungs. There, the blood picks up more oxygen and gets rid of carbon dioxide.

B The pulmonary veins carry oxygen-rich blood from the lungs back to the heart, where it is pumped into arteries that carry it to all parts of the body.

C As blood travels through tiny capillaries, it releases oxygen into the body's cells and picks up carbon dioxide. It then flows into veins, which carry it back to the heart.

Lungs

Pulmonary artery

Pulmonary vein

Arteries

Veins

Heart

Capillaries

Red blood cells, the smallest cells in the body, are continually being replaced. As you read this, your body is making red blood cells at the rate of about 2.4 million every second! *How many are made in 1 minute? In an hour? In a day?*

The Work of the Heart

The muscle that acts as the pump for the circulatory system is the **heart**. The heart pushes blood through the blood vessels, the tubes that carry blood throughout the body. The different types of blood vessels are arteries, veins, and capillaries. Arteries carry blood away from the heart. Veins return blood to the heart. The tiny blood vessels that connect arteries and veins are called capillaries. They provide blood directly to cells. **Figure 6.5** on page 157 shows how blood travels through the circulatory system.

Blood Pressure

The force of the blood pushing against the walls of the blood vessels is called **blood pressure**. Blood pressure is greatest when the heart contracts, or pushes out blood. Blood pressure is lowest between heartbeats, or when the heart relaxes.

Parts of the Blood

Blood contains both liquid and solid parts. Blood plasma is the liquid part of the blood and makes up about half of its volume. Cells are the solid parts. Each element of blood has a purpose:

- **Plasma.** Plasma is made up of about 92 percent water. Its job is to transport blood cells and dissolved food.
- **Red blood cells.** These cells carry oxygen to all other cells of the body and carry away some waste products.
- **White blood cells.** These cells help destroy disease-causing germs that enter the body.
- **Platelets.** These parts of cells help your blood clot. This keeps you from losing too much blood when you have a cut.

Checking blood pressure is part of a standard physical examination.

Blood Types

All blood is not the same. There are four main types: A, B, AB, and O. The types are classified by the type of red blood cells a person has. Knowing a person's blood type is important when one person is receiving blood from another. Serious side effects can result when some of the types are mixed. Health officials mix only those types that can be combined safely.

Blood may also contain something called an Rh factor. Blood is either Rh-positive or Rh-negative. People with Rh-positive blood can receive blood from people with either Rh-positive or Rh-negative blood. People with Rh-negative blood can receive blood only from people who are also Rh-negative.

The Respiratory System

Your **respiratory system** *enables you to breathe.* When you breathe in, or inhale, you take oxygen into your lungs. The **lungs** are *the main organs of the respiratory system.* When you breathe out, or exhale, the lungs get rid of carbon dioxide. See **Figure 6.6** for a closer look at the workings of the respiratory system.

FIGURE 6.6

THE RESPIRATORY SYSTEM

The respiratory system is divided into upper and lower sections, each of which performs different functions. *In which section are the alveoli located?*

Upper Respiratory System
Air comes into the body here, through the nose or mouth; it enters the trachea, or windpipe.

Lower Respiratory System
The trachea divides into two branches, called bronchi, that carry air to the lungs. The bronchi divide into smaller and smaller tubes, the smallest of which end in structures called alveoli (al·VEE·uh·ly).

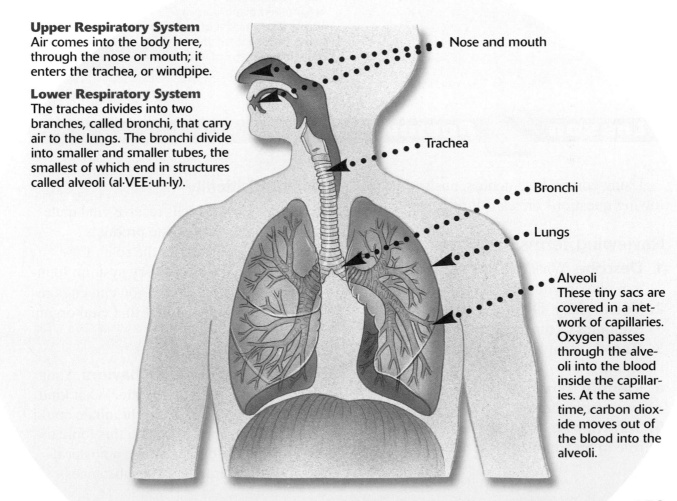

Nose and mouth

Trachea

Bronchi

Lungs

Alveoli
These tiny sacs are covered in a network of capillaries. Oxygen passes through the alveoli into the blood inside the capillaries. At the same time, carbon dioxide moves out of the blood into the alveoli.

How You Breathe

Breathing begins with the **diaphragm** (DY·uh·fram), *a large muscle at the bottom of the chest.* When you breathe in, the diaphragm contracts. When you breathe out, it expands. **Figure 6.7** shows how the breathing process works.

FIGURE 6.7

HOW YOUR LUNGS WORK

Notice what happens when you squeeze an empty plastic bottle. Your respiratory system works in a similar way. *What does the hand in this illustration represent?*

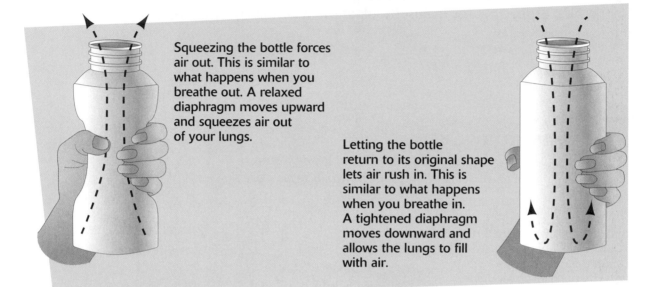

Squeezing the bottle forces air out. This is similar to what happens when you breathe out. A relaxed diaphragm moves upward and squeezes air out of your lungs.

Letting the bottle return to its original shape lets air rush in. This is similar to what happens when you breathe in. A tightened diaphragm moves downward and allows the lungs to fill with air.

Lesson 2 Review

Using complete sentences, answer the following questions on a sheet of paper.

Reviewing Terms and Facts

1. **Describe** What role does the skeletal system play in your body?
2. **Vocabulary** Define *joints* and give examples of three major types.
3. **Recall** What kind of muscles do you control?
4. **Identify** What blood vessels take blood away from the heart?
5. **Summarize** Explain the diaphragm's role in breathing.

Thinking Critically

6. **Explain** How do cells receive vital materials and get rid of waste products?
7. **Analyze** Think about the role of the heart within the circulatory system. Identify actions or behaviors you can engage in to protect the health of this vital organ.

Applying Health Skills

8. **Practicing Healthful Behaviors** Your respiratory system is delicate. What kind of things that a person might inhale could harm this system? Research this topic using reliable resources. Make a poster illustrating several harmful substances.

Nerves and Digestion

The Nervous System

The **nervous system** is *the control and communication system of the body.* Its command center is the **brain**, *the organ that controls your senses, thoughts, and actions.* The brain helps the body process and respond to the information it receives from the senses. It also processes thoughts.

The brain is made up of billions of neurons. **Neurons** (NOO·rahnz) are *cells that carry electrical messages,* the language of the nervous system. There are three types of neurons. Sensory neurons, such as the ones in your eyes, receive information from the outside world. Connecting neurons transmit messages between the sensory neurons and the motor neurons, which send messages to the muscles and glands.

Structure of the Nervous System

The nervous system has two main parts. The central nervous system consists of the brain and the **spinal cord**, *a tube of neurons that runs up the spine.* The largest part of the brain, the cerebrum (suh·REE·bruhm), is where thinking takes place.

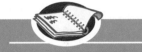

Quick Write

List all the body parts you know of that help you eat and digest food. After reading this lesson, check your list and add any other organs that you left out.

LEARN ABOUT...

- how your nervous system controls your body's functions.
- how the digestive and excretory systems process food.

VOCABULARY

- nervous system
- brain
- neurons
- spinal cord
- digestive system
- excretory system

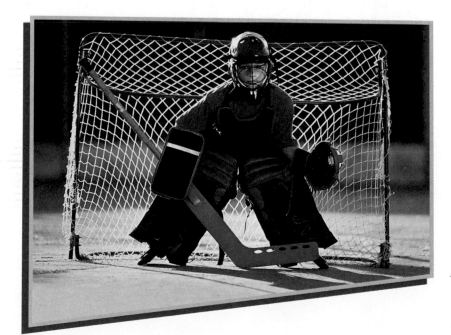

Your brain is one of your most vital organs. Wear the right equipment to protect it. *How is this teen protecting his brain from injury?*

The peripheral (puh·RIF·uh·ruhl) nervous system is made up of nerves that branch out from the spinal cord. It handles both your voluntary movements (the ones you control) and your involuntary movements (which you cannot control). The beating of your heart is an example of an involuntary movement. See **Figure 6.8** for a diagram of the nervous system.

Protecting Your Nervous System

The best way to keep your nervous system healthy is to protect yourself from head and spinal cord injuries. To do this, wear your safety belt whenever you ride in a car. When you skate or ride a bicycle, wear a helmet. Also, be careful when lifting heavy objects. Bend from the knees, not from the waist, and do not try to lift something that is too heavy for you.

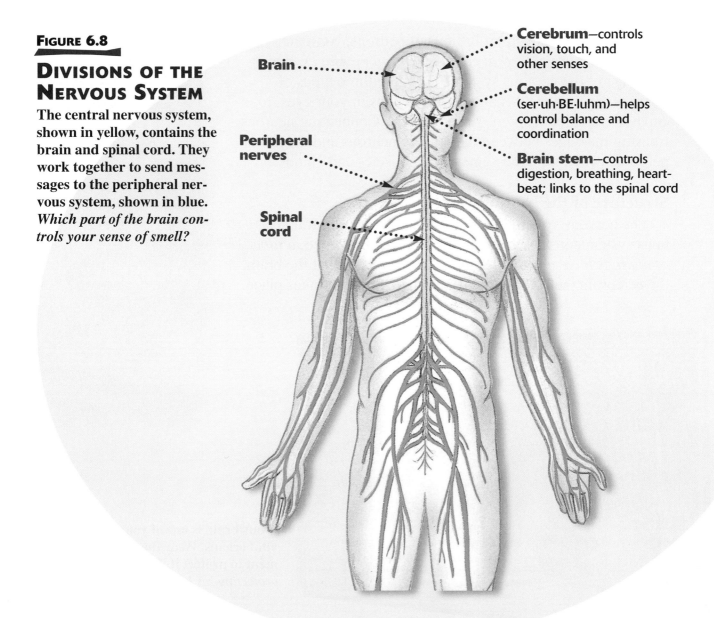

FIGURE 6.8

DIVISIONS OF THE NERVOUS SYSTEM

The central nervous system, shown in yellow, contains the brain and spinal cord. They work together to send messages to the peripheral nervous system, shown in blue. *Which part of the brain controls your sense of smell?*

Brain

Peripheral nerves

Spinal cord

Cerebrum—controls vision, touch, and other senses

Cerebellum (ser·uh·BE·luhm)—helps control balance and coordination

Brain stem—controls digestion, breathing, heartbeat; links to the spinal cord

FIGURE 6.9

THE DIGESTIVE SYSTEM

The digestive system involves many different body parts. *What other body systems can you name that help the process of digestion?*

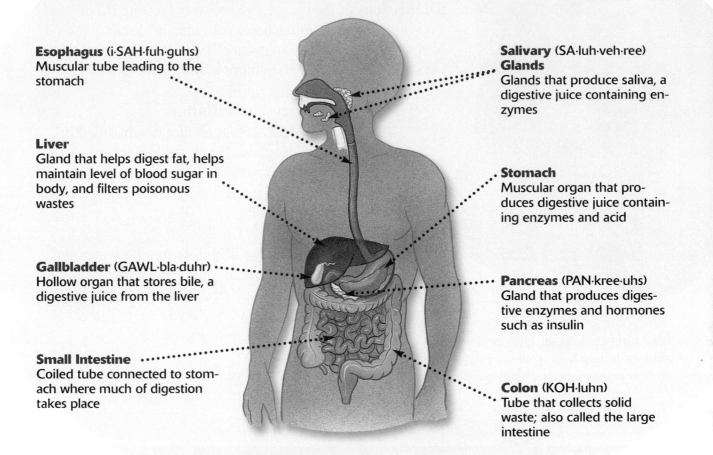

Esophagus (i·SAH·fuh·guhs)
Muscular tube leading to the stomach

Liver
Gland that helps digest fat, helps maintain level of blood sugar in body, and filters poisonous wastes

Gallbladder (GAWL·bla·duhr)
Hollow organ that stores bile, a digestive juice from the liver

Small Intestine
Coiled tube connected to stomach where much of digestion takes place

Salivary (SA·luh·veh·ree)
Glands
Glands that produce saliva, a digestive juice containing enzymes

Stomach
Muscular organ that produces digestive juice containing enzymes and acid

Pancreas (PAN·kree·uhs)
Gland that produces digestive enzymes and hormones such as insulin

Colon (KOH·luhn)
Tube that collects solid waste; also called the large intestine

The Digestive System

Your **digestive** (dy·JES·tiv) **system** *breaks down the food you eat into a form that your body cells can use as fuel.* This process, called digestion, turns food into nutrients.

Digestion begins with chewing, which crushes food into small pieces. Chemicals called enzymes (EN·zymz), found in your saliva (suh·LY·vuh), break down the food further. When you swallow, food enters the throat. Muscles contract and relax, pushing food along. Strong acid, enzymes, and churning muscles in your stomach break down food even further. The food particles move into the small intestine, where the nutrients are absorbed into the blood. The blood carries the digested food to all the body cells. **Figure 6.9** illustrates the digestive system.

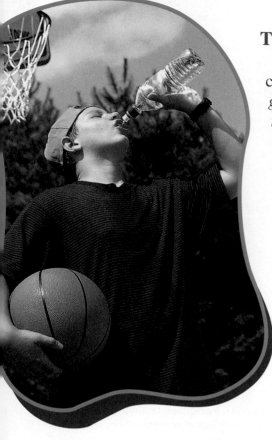

Drinking six to eight glasses of water a day will help keep your digestive and excretory systems healthy.

The Excretory System

Matter that cannot be absorbed through digestion becomes waste. Your **excretory** (EK·skruh·tohr·ee) **system** *gets rid of some of the wastes your body produces and maintains fluid balance.* The respiratory system performs some of the functions of the excretory system by getting rid of carbon dioxide when you exhale. Your skin also releases liquid wastes in the form of sweat. The major organs of this system, however, are the colon, kidneys, and bladder.

The Colon, Kidneys, and Bladder

The solid part of food that cannot be absorbed in the small intestine is passed to the colon, where water is removed. When the colon is full, a nerve sends a message for the colon to contract. This action removes solid waste from the body.

The kidneys filter the blood, removing water and waste substances and maintaining the body's fluid balance. The bladder is where liquid waste material, or urine, from the kidneys is stored. When the bladder is full, the urine is passed out of the body.

Lesson 3 Review

Using complete sentences, answer the following questions on a sheet of paper.

Reviewing Terms and Facts

1. **Vocabulary** Define *nervous system* and use it in an original sentence.
2. **Recall** What two body parts make up the central nervous system?
3. **List** What are the major organs of the excretory system?

Thinking Critically

4. **Analyze** Why does lifting heavy objects improperly present a risk of injury to the nervous system?

5. **Hypothesize** What do you think would happen if a person's kidneys were not working properly?

Applying Health Skills

6. **Practicing Healthful Behaviors**
   A healthy diet keeps your digestive and excretory systems working easily and efficiently—and that helps your whole body function well. Use what you know about nutrition and digestion to write a list of several things you can do to help your digestion and stay healthy.

Adolescence: A Time of Change

Changes During Adolescence

Adolescence (a·duhl·EH·suhns) is *the period between childhood and adulthood.* It is a time of rapid change in a person's life. During this period, you will develop the body of an adult. You will also grow mentally, emotionally, and socially.

Many of the changes of adolescence are caused by hormones, chemicals that control many body functions. The hormones your body produces during your teen years will help you develop. The glands that produce hormones are part of the endocrine system.

The Endocrine System

The **endocrine** (EN·duh·krin) **system** consists of *glands throughout the body that produce hormones.* Each hormone delivers instructions to the organs and tissues of your other body systems. Some hormones are responsible for growth and development. Others control the levels of different nutrients in your blood. **Figure 6.10** on the next page shows the glands of the endocrine system and the body functions they regulate.

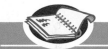

Quick Write

Think about the ways your body has changed in the past few years. Do you think your body will continue to change? List the other changes you think will take place.

LEARN ABOUT...

- how the endocrine system influences your growth.
- the physical, mental/ emotional, and social changes of adolescence.
- what factors influence your personality.

VOCABULARY

- adolescence
- endocrine system
- puberty
- personality
- behavior

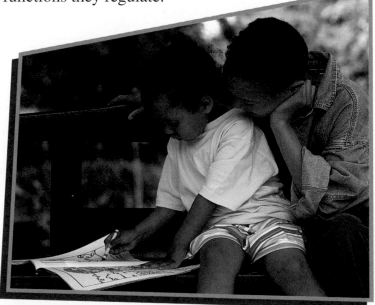

During adolescence, you will grow mentally and emotionally. *How can helping others be a good way to meet your emotional needs?*

FIGURE 6.10

THE ENDOCRINE SYSTEM

The glands of the endocrine system perform many different functions in your body. *Which glands are also part of the digestive system?*

The **pituitary** (pi·TOO·ih·tehr·ee) **gland** produces several hormones that control other glands and organs. It also regulates the body's growth and development.

The **thyroid** (THY·royd) **gland** produces a hormone that regulates the speed at which your body turns food into energy. It also helps regulate growth.

The **adrenal** (uh·DREE·nuhl) **glands** produce adrenaline, a hormone that controls the body's response to emergencies. They also play a role in digestion and help maintain a balance of salt and water in the body.

The **pancreas** produces insulin, which controls the ability of body cells to use sugar for energy.

The **ovaries** (OH·vuh·reez) and **testes** (TES-teez) produce hormones that control sexual development. Females have ovaries; males have testes.

Physical Development

Adolescence begins with puberty. **Puberty** (PYOO·ber·tee) is *the time when you develop certain physical traits of adults of your gender and become physically able to reproduce* (see **Figure 6.11**). Hormones cause the physical changes of puberty, which occur over several years. Puberty typically begins some time between the ages of 8 and 14 and ends between the ages of 16 and 20. However, puberty can occur earlier or later in some cases. Girls often enter puberty earlier than boys.

Mental and Emotional Development

During your teen years, you also develop mentally and emotionally. As you get older, you begin to think about things in new ways. You start to understand other people's points of view. You also learn that some problems do not have simple solutions. During this time, you learn about who you are and you develop many of the values you will hold throughout life.

During adolescence, you may experience powerful emotions that you do not always understand. You may have mood swings, feeling happy one minute and sad the next. These kinds of emotional changes are normal during your teen years. They are related to the changing levels of hormones in your body. Many hormones can affect your emotions.

Social Development

During adolescence, you begin to see yourself as separate from your parents. You learn to see them as human beings with needs and wants. At the same time, your parents begin to see that you are growing up. They may expect you to take on more responsibility.

FIGURE 6.11

PHYSICAL CHANGES OF ADOLESCENCE

Both boys and girls go through many physical changes during puberty.

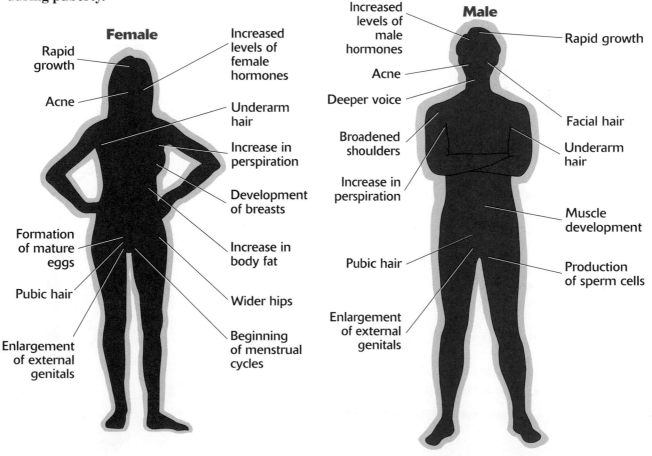

Female

Rapid growth

Acne

Formation of mature eggs

Pubic hair

Enlargement of external genitals

Increased levels of female hormones

Underarm hair

Increase in perspiration

Development of breasts

Increase in body fat

Wider hips

Beginning of menstrual cycles

Male

Increased levels of male hormones

Acne

Deeper voice

Broadened shoulders

Increase in perspiration

Pubic hair

Enlargement of external genitals

Rapid growth

Facial hair

Underarm hair

Muscle development

Production of sperm cells

Your friendships also become very important to you. In early adolescence, you may be strongly influenced by your friends. You may be part of a group that does everything together. Later on, you may break away from the group and form closer friendships with one or two individuals.

As you mature, you will worry less about your friends' approval and rely more on your own standards. By the end of your teens, you will be able to function on your own. You will have formed your own ideas about who you are and how you fit into the world. In short, you will be independent.

Hands-On Health

LOOKING AHEAD

Every day, you show in many ways how you are growing into a healthy, mature adult. This activity will help you recognize some of these changes in yourself.

WHAT YOU WILL NEED
- a pencil or pen
- a sheet of paper

WHAT YOU WILL DO
1. Number the paper 1–10.
2. Read through the list below. It describes many kinds of mature behavior. For each numbered item in the list, try to think of an example from your life.
3. Write down each of your examples on the line with the same number as the statement. Don't worry if you can't think of an example for every statement—just fill in as many as you can.

BECOMING AN ADULT
1. I think about the consequences before I act.
2. I do what I think is right, even when it is hard.
3. I feel comfortable with who I am; I don't try to be something I'm not.
4. I respect other people's ideas, even when they are different from mine.
5. I think about how my actions affect other people.
6. My parents and I show respect when we talk to each other.
7. I take time to listen to other people's problems.
8. I try to see situations from the viewpoint of my parents and other adults.
9. I think about how the choices I make now will affect my future.
10. I have a good idea of the kind of adult I would like to be.

IN CONCLUSION
1. Discuss your answers as a class. You do not have to share all of your answers unless you choose to.
2. With your classmates, brainstorm more examples of mature and responsible behavior.

YOUR FUTURE

Influences on Your Personality

Your **personality** is *the sum total of your feelings, actions, habits, and thoughts.* Like your fingerprints, your personality is unique. No one else is exactly like you.

Parts of your personality are inherited. Your personality is also shaped by your environment, the people and places that surround you. Your family is an important influence on your personality, especially early in your life. During your teen years, you may also be influenced by friends, teachers, and other role models. Finally, your personality includes your **behavior**, or *how you act in situations that occur in your life.* You cannot change your family or environment, but you do control what you do in any situation. If you act according to your values, you will grow up to be the kind of person you want to be.

Many people influence your personality during your lifetime. *Who do you think has the greatest influence on you at this time in your life?*

Lesson 4 Review

Using complete sentences, answer the following questions on a sheet of paper.

Reviewing Terms and Facts

1. **Vocabulary** Define the term *endocrine system.*
2. **Recall** At what age does puberty usually begin?
3. **List** Name five physical changes that occur during adolescence.
4. **Identify** Name three factors that affect your personality.

Thinking Critically

5. **Analyze** Explain the relationship between adolescence and puberty.

6. **Predict** In what ways do you think you will develop socially during your adolescence?

Applying Health Skills

7. **Communication Skills** Interview a classmate about his or her teen experience. Ask what your classmate likes best about being a young teen and what challenges he or she has faced as a teen. Demonstrate good listening skills as your classmate shares his or her responses. Then switch roles and have your classmate interview you. Use good speaking skills to relate your experiences to your classmate.

Heredity and Growth

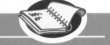
LEARN ABOUT...

- how traits are passed from parents to children.
- how a baby develops inside its mother's body.
- the stages in the life cycle.

VOCABULARY

- heredity
- chromosomes
- genes
- egg cell
- sperm cell
- fertilization
- uterus
- umbilical cord

Heredity

Heredity (huh·REHD·ih·tee) is *the process by which parents pass traits to their children*. These traits may include eye color, hair color, and body build. Children may also inherit musical or athletic ability. Sometimes children inherit diseases from their parents.

Parents pass down their traits through their **chromosomes** (KROH·muh·sohmz). These are *pairs of tiny, threadlike pieces of matter that carry the codes for inherited traits*. Each pair of chromosomes in your body contains one chromosome from your father and one from your mother.

Each chromosome is divided into small sections called genes. **Genes** (JEENZ) are *the basic units of heredity*. Each gene is related to a particular trait, such as height or eye color. Except for identical twins, who share 100 percent of their genes, each person has a unique arrangement of genes.

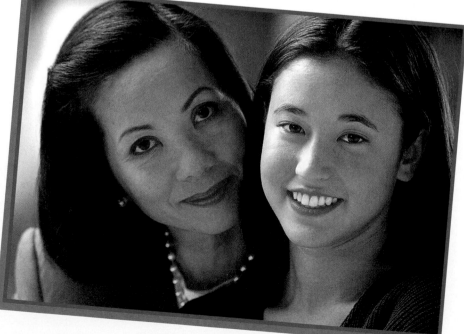

Parents and children often look alike because of heredity. *Do you resemble either of your parents?*

Combining Chromosomes

Almost every cell in your body contains 46 chromosomes—23 from each parent. The only human cells that do not have 46 chromosomes are reproductive cells, which can combine to produce a new person. The *reproductive cell in the female body* is an **egg cell**. The *reproductive cell in the male body* is a **sperm cell**. Egg cells and sperm cells have 23 chromosomes each. When they combine, their chromosomes pair up to produce a cell with 46 chromosomes.

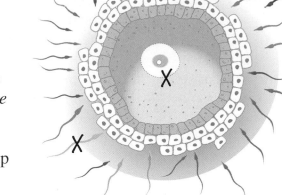

A girl has two X chromosomes. A boy has an X chromosome and a Y chromosome. *Why does every person have at least one X chromosome?*

The joining together of an egg cell and a sperm cell is called **fertilization**. Each person starts as a tiny fertilized egg cell—smaller than the period at the end of this sentence. During the development process, the cell divides millions of times.

X and Y Chromosomes

Special chromosomes in sperm cells determine whether a fertilized cell will develop into a male or a female. Each sperm cell contains either an X chromosome or a Y chromosome. Every egg cell contains only an X chromosome. If an X-carrying sperm combines with an egg, it will produce a girl. If the sperm cell has a Y chromosome, it will produce a boy.

HEALTH SKILLS ACTIVITY

ADVOCACY

The Health of Mother and Child

A mother can affect the health of her baby from the moment of fertilization. She needs to keep herself healthy to make sure the baby develops properly. Women can follow several steps to maintain good health during pregnancy:

- Have regular checkups with a health care professional who specializes in the care of pregnant women.
- Eat nutritious foods.
- Get enough rest.
- Follow an exercise plan that the health care professional recommends.
- Do not use alcohol or tobacco.
- Check with the doctor before taking any medicines.

ON YOUR OWN
Create a poster that encourages good health care during pregnancy. You can illustrate your poster with pictures showing good habits for pregnant women to follow.

Development Before Birth

The fertilized egg cell develops inside the mother's uterus. The **uterus** (YOO·tuh·ruhs) is *a pear-shaped organ that expands as a baby grows.* The baby gets its nourishment through the **umbilical** (uhm·BIL·i·kuhl) **cord**. This is *a tube that connects the lining of the uterus to the unborn baby.* It attaches to the place where the baby's navel, or belly button, will form. Blood from the mother carries food and oxygen through the cord to the baby. The cord also carries wastes away. **Figure 6.12** shows the stages the unborn baby goes through in the mother's uterus.

FIGURE 6.12

THE DEVELOPING BABY

After fertilization, it takes about nine months of growth and development before a baby is born. *Approximately how much does a baby weigh at birth?*

Time	Size	Features	Development
Fertilization	microscopic	single cell	undeveloped
3 months after fertilization	about 3 inches long; weighs about 1 ounce	arms, legs, fingers, toes, eyes, ears	heart is beating, nervous system is forming; cannot survive outside uterus
6 months after fertilization	about 14 inches long; weighs about 2 pounds	hair, eyebrows, fingernails, toenails	can move and kick, sucks thumb, can hear sounds; might survive outside uterus
9 months after fertilization	18–20 inches long; weighs 7–9 pounds	smooth skin, fully developed organs	eyes open and close, fingers can grasp, body organs and systems can now work on their own; ready for birth

The Life Cycle

During your life, you will go through many stages of growth and development. This series of stages is sometimes called the life cycle. It begins at birth and continues through childhood, adolescence, and adulthood.

- **Infancy.** Infancy is the first year of a baby's life. Infants grow, learn, and change at an astonishing rate. This growth and development continues throughout childhood.
- **Childhood.** Young children learn to walk and talk. They also develop other physical and mental skills that they will need throughout their lives. After they enter school, children grow mentally and socially. They learn about solving problems and getting along with others.

- **Adolescence.** Aside from infancy, adolescence is the time of most rapid change in a person's life. During this period, a person's body takes on its adult form. Adolescents also grow mentally, emotionally, and socially.
- **Early adulthood.** In early adulthood—from about age 19 to age 30—most people begin a career. They may move out of their parents' homes and begin to build their own homes and lives. Many young adults choose to marry and begin families at this stage of their lives.
- **Middle adulthood.** Adults over 30 may begin to look outward, toward their families and communities. Many focus their energy on raising children. Others try to contribute something to the world through their careers or other efforts, such as volunteer work or hobbies.
- **Late adulthood.** After age 60 or so, adults may begin to reflect on what they have accomplished in their lives. People who have fulfilled their goals and have lived according to their values can usually look back on their lives with satisfaction.

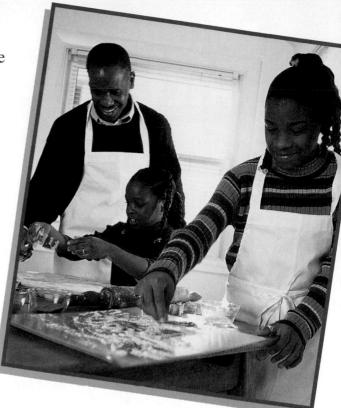

People go through many changes between childhood and adulthood. *What are some of the ways you have changed in the past three years?*

Lesson 5 Review

Using complete sentences, answer the following questions on a sheet of paper.

Reviewing Terms and Facts
1. **Vocabulary** Write a short paragraph explaining the meanings of *heredity, chromosomes,* and *genes.*
2. **Recall** Which cells in the human body do not have 46 chromosomes?
3. **Identify** In what part of the mother's body does a baby develop during pregnancy?

Thinking Critically
4. **Explain** What determines whether a baby will be male or female?

5. **Summarize** Describe the changes a person goes through over the course of the life cycle.

Applying Health Skills
6. **Analyzing Influences** How much does heredity influence you? Create a chart with three columns. Label them *Physical Traits, Mental/Emotional Traits,* and *Social Traits.* In each column, list parts of yourself that you think you have inherited from your parents or other relatives. How much of your appearance and personality appears to be inherited? How much do you think is due to other factors?

KEEPING BODY SYSTEMS HEALTHY

Model

Terry is a teen athlete. He knows that he needs to keep his body systems healthy to be able to stay in shape for his sports activities. This year, he is playing basketball and running track. Because these activities require strong lungs, he takes good care of his respiratory system. He always sits in the nonsmoking section of restaurants, and his parents do not allow guests to smoke in their house. He plans his outdoor activities for times when the air quality is good. Whenever he has a cough or cold, Terry rests and drinks plenty of fluids until he is well. These behaviors help him play better and also improve his total health.

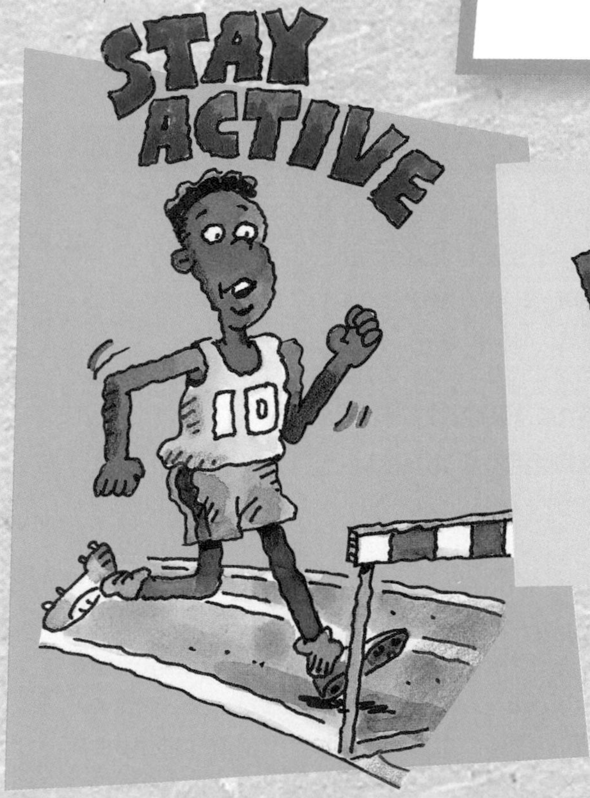

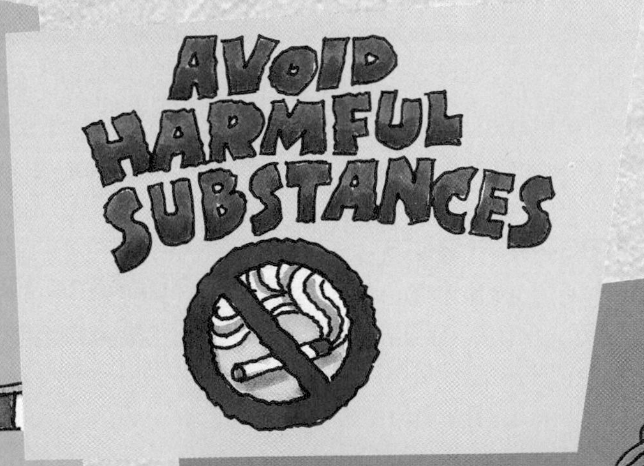

STAY ACTIVE

AVOID HARMFUL SUBSTANCES

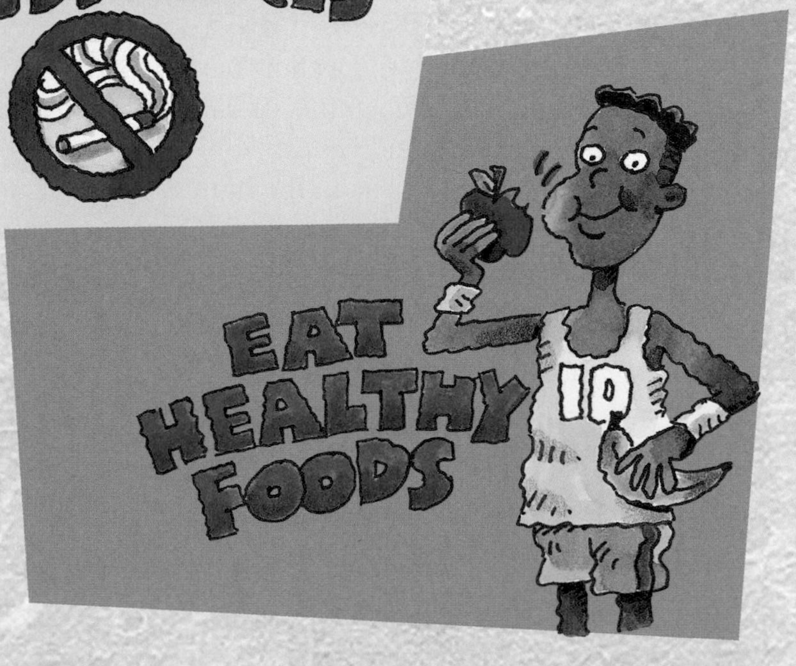

EAT HEALTHY FOODS

Practice

Form small groups. Choose one of the body systems you have learned about in this chapter. Write the name of that body system at the top of a sheet of paper. Then divide the paper into two columns labeled *Healthful Habits* and *Harmful Habits.* Use the first column to identify habits that can benefit your chosen body system. Use the second column to list habits that can harm that body system. At the bottom of the page, write a statement explaining why it is important to care for this body system.

Apply/Assess

Working with your group, create a news report about how to keep your body systems healthy. Your report should be three to five minutes long and should be in a style similar to a television news broadcast. In your report, describe at least three ways to care for all of your body systems. Include an explanation of how these three behaviors can benefit specific body systems. Present your report to the class.

COACH'S BOX

Practicing Healthful Behaviors

Caring for your body systems includes
- staying active.
- eating nutritious foods.
- avoiding harmful substances.
- taking care of illnesses.
- managing stress.

Self-√Check

- Is our report three to five minutes long?
- Did we describe at least three ways to care for body systems?
- Did we explain why these habits are healthy?

TAKE CARE OF ILLNESS

H₂O

MANAGE STRESS

HANDLING TEEN STRESS

Model

The changes of adolescence can be stressful. However, there are positive ways of dealing with the stress. Consider what Ben did when his skin started to break out a few months ago. At first, he worried a lot about his looks. He even started avoiding his friends because he was embarrassed. Then he realized that this was only adding to his stress. He decided to try a more positive approach. First, he talked to his parents. They took Ben to the doctor, who gave him some medication for his skin. At the same time, he started seeing his friends again. Being with them made Ben realize that they liked him for who he is.

By dealing with his problems positively, he reduced his stress and improved his self-esteem.

Practice

Read about Ruth, a sixth-grade student who had a very stressful day. Try to identify all the sources of stress she experienced and how she dealt with them. Which of her reactions were helpful? Which ones were harmful?

Ruth overslept because she had been up late working on a report for school. Because she was in a hurry, she didn't have time to shower or wash her hair, which made her feel self-conscious. When her friend Tyler started teasing her about her "wild" new hairstyle, Ruth got upset. Tyler realized that he had hurt her feelings and asked if she wanted to talk. After Ruth told Tyler about her stressful day, he apologized for teasing her.

COACH'S BOX

Stress Management

Stress-management strategies include
- identifying sources of stress.
- using positive coping strategies.
- building support systems.

Apply/Assess

What situations cause stress in your life? The cards below show examples of common causes of stress during adolescence and positive ways of dealing with them. Work with a small group. Have each group member take an index card and write down an example of a stressful situation a teen might face. You can use an experience of your own or invent a situation. Then work with your group to identify a positive response to each of the stressful situations you have listed. Write the response on the card. Include an explanation of how the response could produce helpful results. Then, as a group, make a list of people who can help teens deal with stressful situations.

Self-✓Check
- Did we name several sources of stress for adolescents?
- Did we list positive reactions to stress?
- Did we identify people who can provide support?

Cause of Stress: A friend teased me about being short for my age.

Positive Response: I talked to my friend about how the teasing made me feel.

How It Helps: I realized that my friend was only kidding, so I felt better. My friend realized that I'm sensitive about my height and agreed not to joke about it anymore.

Cause of Stress: My classes in school are a lot tougher than they used to be.

Positive Response: I asked my dad to help me with my homework.

How It Helps: I got a good grade and I understand the material a lot better now.

SUMMARY

LESSON·1 Your organs are grouped into body systems, which perform specific jobs in the body. All of your body systems work together to help you function.

LESSON·2 Your skeletal and muscular systems work together to support your body and help it move. Your circulatory system transports blood, which carries materials throughout your body. Your respiratory system takes in oxygen that your cells need and removes carbon dioxide.

LESSON·3 Your nervous system controls all your thoughts and body movements. Your digestive and excretory systems process food and eliminate wastes.

LESSON·4 During adolescence, you will change physically, mentally, emotionally, and socially as you prepare for adulthood. Hormones cause many of these changes.

LESSON·5 Parents pass traits down to their children through heredity. Every person develops from a fertilized egg cell that grows and changes inside its mother's uterus before birth. From birth on, people pass through the stages of the life cycle: infancy, childhood, adolescence, and adulthood.

- blood pressure
- body system
- circulatory
- digestive
- cells
- lungs
- muscular
- neurons
- organ
- peripheral

Reviewing Vocabulary and Concepts

On a sheet of paper, write the numbers 1–10. After each number, write the term from the list that best completes each sentence.

Lesson 1

1. Your entire body is made up of _____, the basic building blocks of life.
2. The brain is one very important _____ in your body.
3. A(n) _____ is a group of organs that performs a specific function in your body.

Lesson 2

4. The muscles of your body make up the _____ system.
5. The heart muscle pumps blood through the _____ system.
6. _____ is lowest between heartbeats, or when the heart relaxes.
7. The _____ are key organs in the respiratory system.

Lesson 3

8. The brain is made up of billions of _____, or cells that carry electrical messages.
9. The _____ nervous system is made up of nerves that branch out from the spinal cord.
10. The stomach, liver, and pancreas are all parts of the _____ system.

On a sheet of paper, write the numbers 11–18. Write *True* or *False* for each statement below. If the statement is false, change the underlined word or phrase to make it true.

Lesson 4

11. The <u>endocrine system</u> consists of glands throughout the body that produce hormones.

12. Your <u>behavior</u> is the sum total of your feelings, actions, habits, and thoughts.

13. <u>Puberty</u> is how you act in situations that occur in your life.

Lesson 5

14. <u>Genes</u> are tiny, threadlike pieces of matter that carry the codes for inherited traits.

15. An egg cell and a sperm cell join together in a process called <u>heredity</u>.

16. Aside from infancy, the period of greatest change in a person's life is <u>adolescence</u>.

17. The stages of growth and development are also known as the <u>life cycle</u>.

18. An unborn baby gets its nourishment through the <u>egg cell</u>.

Thinking Critically

Using complete sentences, answer the following questions on a sheet of paper.

19. Synthesize Explain how the exchange of oxygen for carbon dioxide in the lungs involves both the respiratory and the circulatory systems.

20. Contrast Explain the difference between the functions of the central nervous system and those of the peripheral nervous system.

21. Explain In what ways do relationships between parents and children change during adolescence?

22. Analyze Explain why adulthood, rather than adolescence, is the best time to have children.

Career Corner

Physician

Physicians are medical professionals who have completed many years of training. One of their goals is to help patients detect problems with their development. If a patient has one of these problems, the physician works to find the best way of treating it. Physicians can also help prevent these problems from occurring.

If you think you'd like to help people stay healthy, visit the Career Corner at health.glencoe.com.

SIGN IN

Preventing Diseases

Quick Write

Brainstorm a list of different diseases. Then write what you know about each disease. How do people get the disease? What can people do to protect themselves from the disease? After reading this chapter, go back to your list and see how much more you have learned about these diseases.

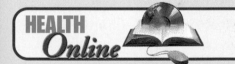
HEALTH Online

Visit health.glencoe.com and take the Chapter 7 Health Inventory to test what you know about HIV and AIDS.

✓ Reading Check

Discover what you already know about diseases. Listen to the statements provided by your teacher. For each statement, decide if you agree or disagree with it.

1

Causes of Diseases

Quick Write

Think about the last time you missed school because of an illness. Can you think of anything you could have done to avoid getting sick?

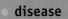

LEARN ABOUT...

- what makes you sick.
- how diseases can spread.
- how your body defends itself against disease.

VOCABULARY

- disease
- communicable disease
- noncommunicable disease
- pathogen
- infection
- immune system
- lymphocyte
- antibody
- immunity

Types of Diseases

A **disease** (dih·ZEEZ) is *an unhealthy condition of the body or mind.* Some diseases, such as cancer can be very dangerous or even deadly. Others, like colds, are far less serious.

There are two types of disease. A **communicable** (kuh·MYOO·ni·kuh·buhl) **disease** is *a disease that can be spread,* such as a cold. You can get a communicable disease from another person, an object, or an animal. A **noncommunicable disease** is *a disease that does not spread,* such as diabetes or cancer. You can't catch these diseases from another person.

With a microscope, a scientist can see disease-causing germs that are invisible to the unaided eye.

Germs That Cause Disease

Most communicable diseases are caused by germs, tiny organisms that can't be seen without a microscope. Lots of germs are present on your skin at all times, and most of them are harmless or even helpful. However, some germs are harmful. These *disease-causing germs* are called **pathogens**. **Figure 7.1** shows some common pathogens. *The result of pathogens invading the body, multiplying, and harming some of your body's cells,* is an **infection**. If your body cannot fight off the infection, you will get sick.

FIGURE 7.1

COMMON DISEASE-CAUSING GERMS

These photos show close-ups of four common disease-causing germs. *Have you had any of the diseases caused by these germs?*

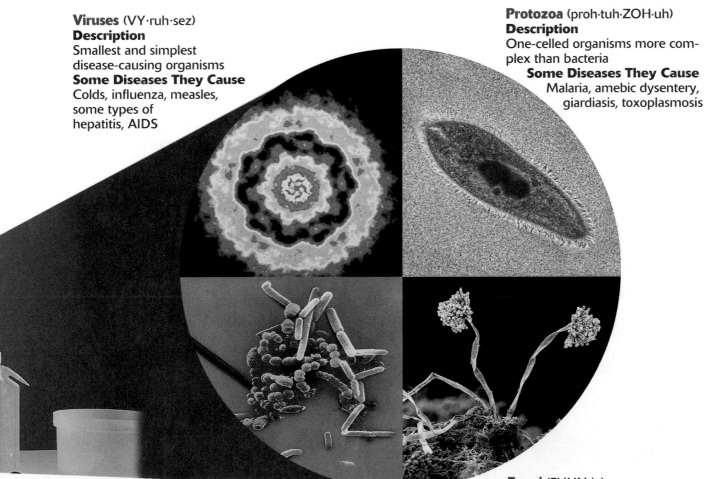

Viruses (VY·ruh·sez)
Description
Smallest and simplest disease-causing organisms
Some Diseases They Cause
Colds, influenza, measles, some types of hepatitis, AIDS

Protozoa (proh·tuh·ZOH·uh)
Description
One-celled organisms more complex than bacteria
Some Diseases They Cause
Malaria, amebic dysentery, giardiasis, toxoplasmosis

Bacteria (bak·TIR·ee·uh)
Description
One-celled organisms larger than viruses
Some Diseases They Cause
Strep throat, gonorrhea, tuberculosis, Lyme disease, whooping cough

Fungi (FUHN·jy)
Description
One- or many-celled primitive organisms such as molds and yeasts
Some Diseases They Cause
Athlete's foot, jock itch, ringworm, thrush, vaginal yeast infections

How Germs Spread

There are lots of different ways germs can enter your body. You may even be spreading them without knowing it. **Figure 7.2** shows the four most common ways that disease-causing germs are passed to people.

Your First Line of Defense

You are exposed to millions of disease-causing germs each day. So why aren't you sick all the time? The main reason is that a healthy body is in good fighting shape. If you keep yourself healthy and strong, your body will destroy many pathogens before they can hurt you. Some pathogens are destroyed before they enter your body. Your natural defenses find and wipe out many of those that do make their way in.

FIGURE 7.2

WAYS GERMS CAN SPREAD

This picture shows some ways germs can spread. *Try to think of one way you could block each of these routes into your body.*

Food or Water
You can get an infection by eating or drinking impure food or water. Bacteria that cause food poisoning can be spread this way.

Indirect Contact
Some germs can spread through the air. You can also pick up germs if you share cups, utensils, or other personal items with a sick person.

Contact with Animals or Insects
You can get an infection if an infected insect or animal bites you.

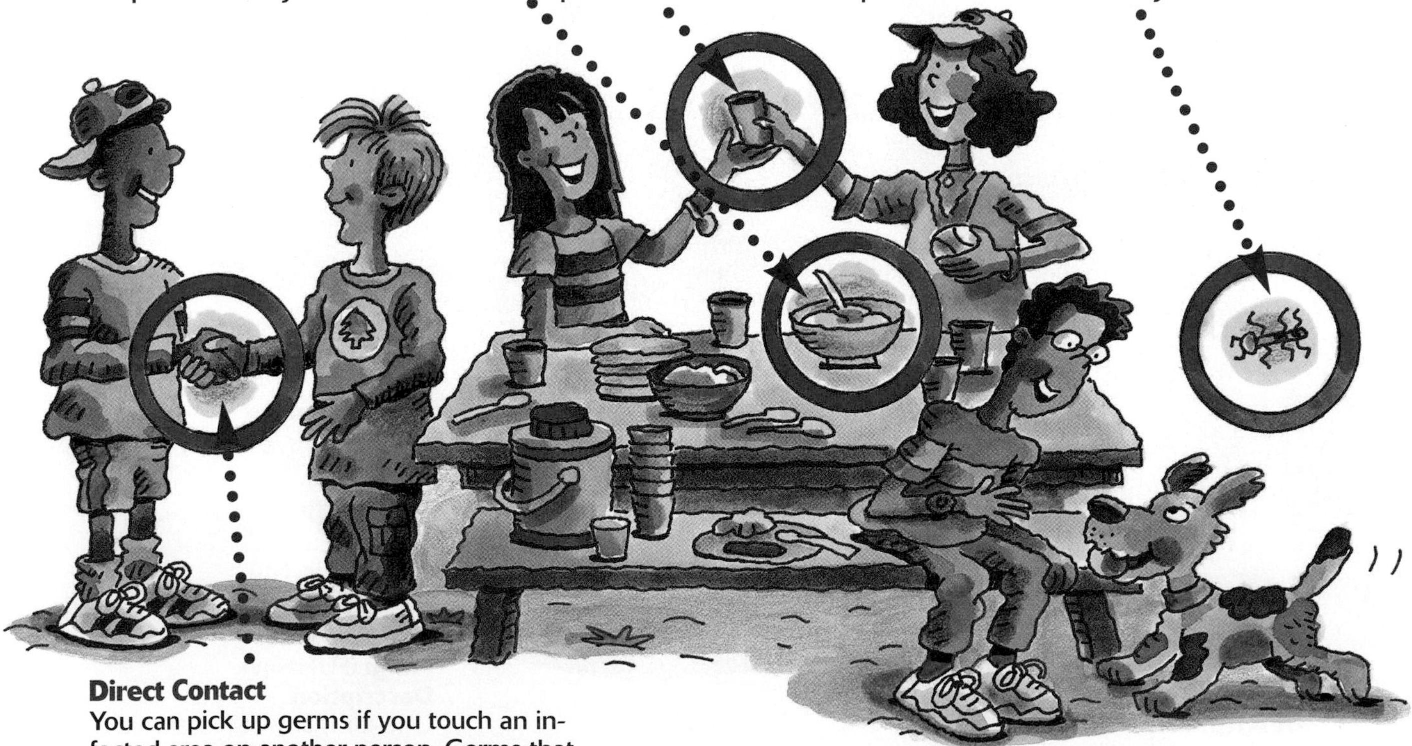

Direct Contact
You can pick up germs if you touch an infected area on another person. Germs that cause skin infections are spread this way. Some diseases, such as AIDS, are spread through direct sexual contact.

General Defenses

Your body has barriers to protect you from pathogens. These include your skin and mucous membranes, which line the inside of body parts such as your nose, mouth, and throat. Body fluids, such as tears and saliva are also barriers. They contain chemicals that destroy certain germs. If germs get past these barriers, your body responds with general reactions. They are called *general* because they are the same for all pathogens.

- Special blood cells surround pathogens and destroy them.
- A chemical is released to stop viruses from reproducing.
- Fever, or a rise in body temperature, kills some pathogens and makes it hard for others to reproduce.

Your Immune System

Your **immune** (i·MYOON) **system** is *a group of cells, tissues, and organs that fights disease.* One key part of the immune system is **lymphocytes** (LIM·fuh·syts), *white blood cells that attack pathogens.* Some lymphocytes attack germs directly. Others produce **antibodies**, *chemicals produced specifically to fight a particular invading substance* (see **Figure 7.3**). If the same germ enters your body again, existing antibodies will attack and destroy it. This *resistance to infection* is called **immunity**.

FIGURE 7.3

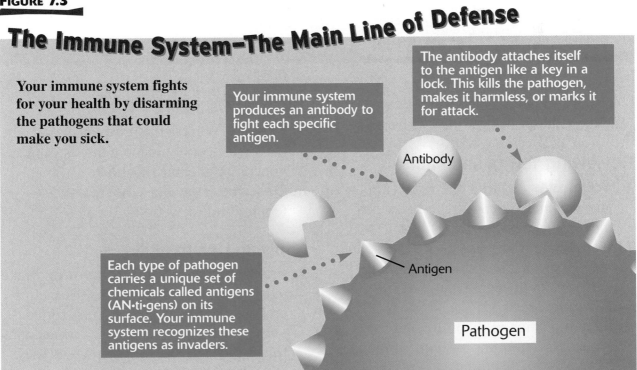

The Immune System–The Main Line of Defense

Your immune system fights for your health by disarming the pathogens that could make you sick.

Your immune system produces an antibody to fight each specific antigen.

The antibody attaches itself to the antigen like a key in a lock. This kills the pathogen, makes it harmless, or marks it for attack.

Antibody

Each type of pathogen carries a unique set of chemicals called antigens (AN·ti·gens) on its surface. Your immune system recognizes these antigens as invaders.

Antigen

Pathogen

LEARNING HOW GERMS SPREAD

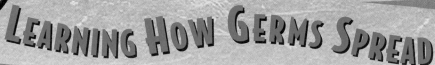

People's hands can spread germs easily. This activity shows how.

WHAT YOU WILL NEED
- cotton balls
- peppermint or lemon extract flavoring

WHAT YOU WILL DO
1. Form groups of 5 or more. Place a few drops of flavoring on a cotton ball. Have one member of each group rub the cotton over the palm of his or her hand and wait for the liquid to dry.
2. Have the person who applied the food flavoring shake hands with two other people in the group. Those people, in turn, should shake hands with the rest of the people in the group.
3. Smell your hand to determine whether the flavoring was transferred to you.

IN CONCLUSION
1. If the food flavoring had been a group of cold viruses, how many people in the group would have picked up the germs on their hands?
2. What might they have done later to allow the viruses to enter their bodies?
3. How does frequent handwashing help prevent the spread of germs?

Lesson 1 Review

Using complete sentences, answer the following questions on a sheet of paper.

Reviewing Terms and Facts

1. **Vocabulary** Define the words *infection* and *immune system*. Write a sentence that includes both terms.
2. **List** Name four ways germs can spread.
3. **Identify** What barriers and general reactions help keep pathogens from infecting your body?
4. **Recall** Which in the following list are parts of the immune system: antibodies, lymphocytes, bacteria?

Thinking Critically

5. **Explain** What is the difference between a communicable disease and a noncommunicable disease?
6. **Describe** How does the immune system fight off infection?

Applying Health Skills

7. **Practicing Healthful Behaviors** Make a list of healthful behaviors that could prevent disease-causing germs from entering your body. Make sure you account for each of the four ways in which they can enter your body.

Communicable Diseases

Common Communicable Diseases

The most common communicable disease is the common cold. It is responsible for more school absences than any other illness. More than 200 different viruses can cause colds. Symptoms include mild fever, runny nose, itchy eyes, sneezing, coughing, sore throat, and headache. If you have these symptoms, you should stay at home for the first 24 hours after they appear. During this period, your cold is most **contagious** (cuhn·TA·jus). This means that it is *able to spread to others by direct or indirect contact.*

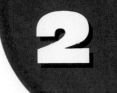

Quick Write

What do you usually do when you catch a cold? Describe your favorite cold treatment and explain why you think it is effective.

LEARN ABOUT...

- the most common communicable diseases.
- how you can keep from getting sick so often.
- what vaccines you need.

VOCABULARY

- contagious
- vaccine

It is important to stay home and rest when you have a cold. Also drink plenty of water.

Other communicable diseases include influenza (known as "the flu"), mononucleosis, hepatitis (types A, B, and C), strep throat, and tuberculosis. **Figure 7.4** describes these five diseases. Some of these diseases can be prevented with **vaccines** (vak·SEENZ), *preparations of killed or weakened germs.* Vaccines cause your immune system to produce antibodies, protecting you against the disease.

FIGURE 7.4

COMMON COMMUNICABLE DISEASES

Disease	Common Symptoms	How It Spreads	Treatment	Prevention/Reducing Risk
Common cold	Congestion, sore throat, cough	Infected droplets in the air from coughs/sneezes; direct or indirect contact with infected people	Rest, liquids, over-the-counter medicines	Handwashing; avoiding contact with infected people and objects they have touched
Influenza (in·floo·EN·zuh), or flu	High fever, fatigue, muscle and joint aches, cough	Infected droplets in the air from coughs/sneezes; direct contact with infected people	Rest, liquids, steam inhalations, pain relievers, antiviral medicine for serious cases	Handwashing; avoiding contact with infected people and objects they have touched; annual vaccine for adults
Mononucleosis (MAH·noh·noo·klee·OH·sis), or mono	Swollen glands (in neck, underarms, groin), headaches, sore muscles, sore throat, fever, fatigue	Infected droplets in the air from coughs/sneezes; direct contact with an infected person's saliva (kissing, sharing utensils)	Pain relievers, rest, liquids	Avoiding contact with infected person
Hepatitis (he·puh·TY·tis)	Weakness, fatigue, nausea, vomiting, fever, yellowing of eyes, abdominal pain, dark urine	Type A: Consuming food or water containing viruses Types B & C: Usually through direct contact with infected person's blood or other body fluids	Rest, healthful food choices Types B & C: medication	Type A: cleaning food carefully; vaccination for those at high risk Type B: vaccination Type C: avoiding sexual contact and drug use
Tuberculosis (tuh·ber·kyoo·LOH·sis), or TB	Cough, fatigue, persistent fever, night sweats, weight loss	Infected droplets in the air from coughs/sneezes	Antibiotics taken over a long period of time	Antibiotics for those in close contact with infected person; vaccine
Strep throat	Sore throat, fever, chills, body aches, loss of appetite, nausea, vomiting, swollen tonsils or glands	Infected droplets in the air from coughs/sneezes	Antibiotics, soft food, liquids, gargling with salt water	Handwashing; avoiding contact with infected person

Preventing Communicable Diseases

You can avoid germs by staying away from people who are sick. You can also remove germs by washing your hands properly, as shown in **Figure 7.5**. Finally, you can increase your body's ability to fight germs by practicing healthful behaviors, such as eating right and staying active. If you do catch a cold, take care of yourself. Rest and drink lots of liquids. Medicine can help you feel better, but time is the best cure for a cold.

Vaccines

Vaccines can protect you from many communicable diseases. When you receive a vaccine, you don't get sick because the disease-causing germs are dead or weakened. The antibodies you produce, however, make you immune to the disease. **Figure 7.6** on page 190 lists some common vaccines.

FIGURE 7.5

HANDWASHING FOR HEALTH

Washing your hands removes germs that can cause colds, flu, and more serious diseases.

Scrub your hands for at least 15 seconds with soap and warm or hot running water. Rub your hands together vigorously as you wash.

Rinse all traces of soap away with warm water.

Wash well around fingernails and creases in your hands, where germs accumulate. A nail brush will help you remove germs from under your fingernails.

Dry with a clean towel, a paper towel, or an air dryer.

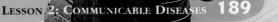

FIGURE 7.6

VACCINES GIVEN AT DIFFERENT AGES

Vaccine and the Diseases It Protects Against	Typical Vaccination Schedule
Hep B: hepatitis B	Birth–2 months, 1–4 months, 6–18 months
DTaP: diphtheria, tetanus, pertussis (whooping cough)	2, 4, 6, and 15–18 months, 4–6 years, Td (tetanus and diphtheria toxoid) boosters at 11–12 years and every 10 years thereafter
Hib: diseases caused by *Hemophilus influenza* type B (Hib) bacteria	2, 4, 6, and 12–15 months
IPV: poliomyelitis	2, 4, and 6–18 months 4-6 years
PCV: diseases caused by *Streptococcus pneumoniae* bacteria	2, 4, 6, and 12–15 months
MMR: measles, mumps, rubella (German measles)	12–15 months 4–6 years, or any time before 12 years
Varicella: chicken pox	12–18 months
Hep A: hepatitis A	2 doses at least 6 months apart, any time between 2 and 18 years; used only in high-risk areas or for high-risk groups

Source: Table based on immunization schedule recommended by the Centers for Disease Control and Prevention, the American Academy of Pediatrics, and the American Academy of Family Physicians

Lesson 2 Review

Using complete sentences, answer the following questions on a sheet of paper.

Reviewing Terms and Facts

1. **Vocabulary** Define the word *contagious* and use it in a sentence.
2. **Describe** List the symptoms of a common communicable disease. Explain what a person with that disease could do to get rid of it or feel better.
3. **List** Name five diseases that can be prevented with vaccines.

Thinking Critically

4. **Explain** What steps can you take to keep yourself and others around you germ free?
5. **Infer** How does getting a vaccine help protect both your health and the health of people around you?

Applying Health Skills

6. **Practicing Healthful Behaviors** Create a poster explaining what people can do to keep themselves and others healthy during the "cold season," or winter months. Display your poster in the school hallway.

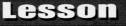
Understanding STIs

Sexually Transmitted Infections

Sexually transmitted infections (STIs) are *communicable diseases that are passed from one person to another through sexual contact.* Anyone who is sexually active runs the risk of becoming infected with one of these diseases. STIs are different from other communicable diseases in several ways.

- STIs can damage the reproductive system and cause sterility.
- Most STIs are spread only through sexual contact.
- There are no vaccines for STIs.
- Someone who has an STI may have no visible symptoms, or have symptoms that come and go, but still be contagious.
- Having an STI once doesn't make you immune.
- Many STIs can cause death if left untreated.
- To get rid of an STI, a person *must* see a doctor.

Some other communicable diseases, such as hepatitis, can also spread through sexual contact. They are not called STIs because they can also be transmitted in other ways. **Figure 7.7** on page 192 lists the symptoms of five common STIs.

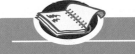

Quick Write

You probably know that HIV, the virus that causes AIDS, sickens and kills many people. Make a list of the ways you think HIV is spread.

LEARN ABOUT...

- what sexually transmitted infections are.
- how HIV and other STIs are spread.
- what you can do to protect yourself from sexually transmitted infections.
- why it is important to seek help in dealing with STIs.

VOCABULARY

- sexually transmitted infections (STIs)
- HIV
- AIDS

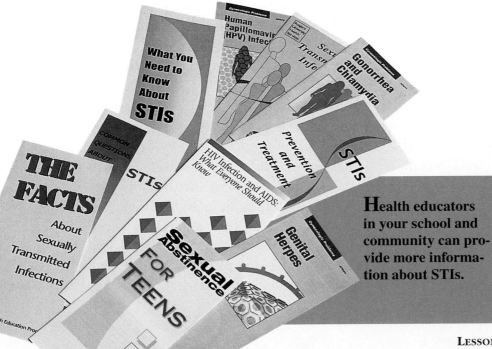

Health educators in your school and community can provide more information about STIs.

FIGURE 7.7

COMMON STIs

People under 24 are the age group most likely to get STIs. *Which of these five common STIs cannot be cured?*

STI	Causes	Common Symptoms	Treatment
Chlamydia (kluh·MIH·dee·uh)	Bacteria	Pain or burning feeling during urination, unusual discharge from penis or vagina; often has no symptoms (especially in females), but can still be spread	Cured with antibiotics
Gonorrhea (gah·nuh·REE·uh)	Bacteria	Pain or burning feeling during urination, unusual discharge from penis or vagina, abdominal pain; sometimes has no symptoms (especially in females), but can still be spread	Cured with antibiotics
Genital herpes (HER·peez)	Herpes simplex virus (HSV)	Itching or pain followed by painful, itchy sores in genital area; symptoms come and go, but virus is still present and able to be spread	Antiviral medication relieves symptoms when sores appear; no cure
Syphilis (SI·fuh·lis)	Bacteria	Red, wet, painless sores at place where virus enters body, followed by rash and flu-like symptoms; can lead to brain damage and other serious health problems, especially in infants	Cured with antibiotics
Genital warts	Human papilloma virus (HPV)	Small pink or red bumps in genital area; can increase risk of certain cancers in women	Warts can be removed by a doctor, but may return because virus remains present in the body

HIV and AIDS

HIV, or human immunodeficiency virus, is *the virus that causes AIDS*. HIV attacks a person's immune system, decreasing its ability to fight infection. **Figure 7.8** shows how HIV attacks the immune system.

People can be infected with HIV for 10 years or longer before any symptoms appear. However, eventually they will develop AIDS, or acquired immunodeficiency syndrome. **AIDS** is *an HIV infection combined with severe immune system problems*. When AIDS weakens the immune system, other infections set in. Symptoms can include fatigue, frequent long-lasting fevers, sweating heavily at night, and a chronic cough. Drugs can delay the onset of AIDS and help fight the symptoms, but there is no cure. People with AIDS eventually die from diseases that a healthy immune system could easily have resisted.

How HIV Spreads

HIV is carried in the body fluids of people infected with the disease. Significant amounts of the virus—enough to transmit HIV to other people—may be found in

- semen.
- vaginal fluid.
- blood.
- breast milk.

When these infected fluids enter another person's body, HIV infection may occur. HIV spreads mostly through sexual contact and sharing needles. A woman with HIV can also pass the virus to her baby during pregnancy or while breast-feeding. Before 1985, HIV was sometimes spread when people infected with HIV donated blood. Today, all donated blood in the United States is tested for HIV, and infected blood is discarded. It is safe to donate and receive blood in this country.

Reading Check

Identify main ideas and important details. Summarize what you have read in this lesson. What information about AIDS would you add to Figure 7.7?

FIGURE 7.8

HOW HIV ATTACKS THE IMMUNE SYSTEM

HIV keeps the immune system from doing its job. A person with AIDS will have trouble resisting certain infections.

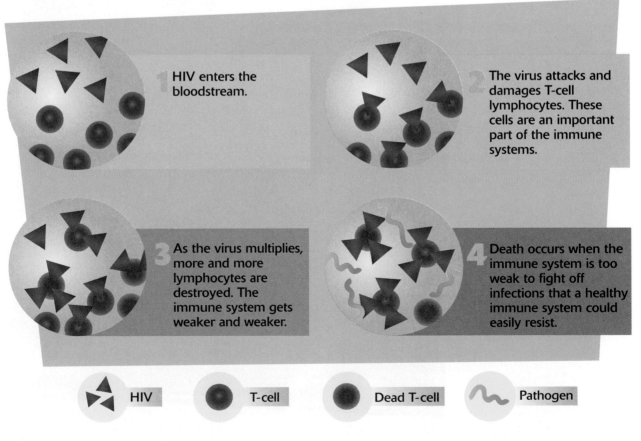

1 HIV enters the bloodstream.

2 The virus attacks and damages T-cell lymphocytes. These cells are an important part of the immune systems.

3 As the virus multiplies, more and more lymphocytes are destroyed. The immune system gets weaker and weaker.

4 Death occurs when the immune system is too weak to fight off infections that a healthy immune system could easily resist.

HIV   T-cell   Dead T-cell   Pathogen

The AIDS Memorial Quilt contains more than 44,000 panels, contributed by people all over the world. Each panel is a tribute to one or more people who have died from AIDS. The money people pay to view the quilt goes to help people living with the disease. So far, the quilt has raised over $3 million.

It is important to realize that HIV spreads only through contact with infected body fluids. You *cannot* get HIV from

- the air.
- sweat and tears.
- mosquito bites.
- donating blood.
- touching, such as shaking hands or hugging.
- contact with objects, such as eating utensils or toilet seats.

Detecting HIV

Many people infected with HIV show no symptoms for a long time. They can still pass on the virus, however. Laboratories perform tests to find out if a person is infected with HIV. These tests show the presence of antibodies to the virus. If a blood test is negative, it should be repeated in six months. A person recently infected with the virus may not have had time to develop antibodies.

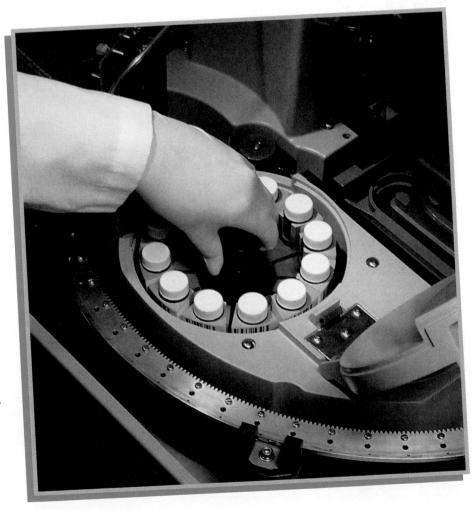

Blood samples are carefully tested to determine if they are infected with HIV.

Preventing STIs and HIV

STIs can cause serious health problems and even death. To avoid these risks, you must avoid contact with other people's body fluids, including blood, semen, and vaginal fluid. Specifically, you should avoid

- having sexual contact. Abstinence from sexual activity is the only sure way to prevent STIs. Go out with groups of friends to avoid being pressured to be sexually active.
- sharing needles or other objects that break the skin. Sharing a needle with an HIV-infected person exposes you to HIV-infected blood. If you get your ears pierced, have it done professionally by someone who uses sterilized equipment.
- using alcohol or drugs. People are more likely to engage in risky behaviors when under the influence of alcohol or drugs.

Getting Help

Many people, and especially teens, do not seek help when they think they have an STI. Getting help can be embarrassing, so they just wait and hope the disease will go away. This is the worst thing a person can do. If left untreated, STIs can cause serious damage.

Teens who suspect that they have an STI should talk to a parent or trusted adult. At first, it may feel uncomfortable. However it is the first step toward getting the needed treatment. It is also a necessary step in preventing permanent damage to the reproductive system.

Lesson 3 Review

Using complete sentences, answer the following questions on a sheet of paper.

Reviewing Terms and Facts

1. **Vocabulary** Define the term *sexually transmitted infection* (STI) and use it in an original sentence.
2. **List** Name five common STIs.
3. **Recall** Explain the relationship between HIV and AIDS.

Thinking Critically

4. **Compare and Contrast** How are STIs similar to and different from other communicable diseases?
5. **Hypothesize** Why might teens be reluctant to seek help for STIs?

Applying Health Skills

6. **Practicing Healthful Behaviors** Write a letter to an imaginary teen explaining why practicing abstinence is the best way to avoid STIs.

Noncommunicable Diseases

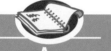
What Are Noncommunicable Diseases?

Heart disease, cancer, diabetes, allergies, and asthma are noncommunicable diseases. Some people are born with these diseases, while others develop them later in life (see **Figure 7.9**). For example, you may get sick because of your lifestyle or because of substances around you. Also, some communicable diseases can damage your body in ways that put you at risk for developing a noncommunicable disease. Many noncommunicable diseases are **chronic** (KRAH·nik), or *long-lasting.*

FIGURE 7.9

CAUSES OF NONCOMMUNICABLE DISEASES

People can get noncommunicable diseases in any of these three ways. Sometimes, more than one factor is present. *What can you do to protect yourself from lifestyle diseases?*

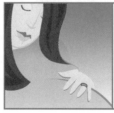

Diseases Present at Birth
Some people are born with noncommunicable diseases. Sometimes problems occur during the development or birth of a baby. Other times, heredity is the cause.

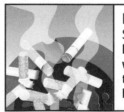

Lifestyle Diseases
Some noncommunicable diseases are caused by unhealthy habits. For example, having an unhealthy weight and being physically inactive may contribute to heart disease or diabetes. Tobacco use may lead to heart disease or cancer.

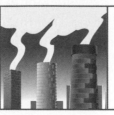

Environmental Diseases
Poisons in the enviroment may contribute to lung cancer, asthma, and other noncommunicable diseases. Pollution is a factor that can cause disease.

Heart Disease

Heart disease includes several problems of the heart and blood vessels. **Figure 7.10** describes the major types of heart disease and shows how each type can lead to others.

Heart disease is the number one cause of death in the United States. You can lessen your chances of developing heart disease later in life by adopting healthy habits now.

- **Stay active.** Aerobic activity can strengthen your heart and blood vessels and lower blood pressure.
- **Maintain a healthy weight.** Having less body fat reduces the strain on the heart and blood vessels.
- **Eat nutritious foods.** Choose foods that are high in fiber and low in salt, fat, and cholesterol.
- **Learn to manage stress.** Reducing or managing stress can help lower blood pressure and decrease the risk of heart disease.
- **Avoid tobacco products.** Avoiding tobacco can lower your risk of stroke and heart attack (and other diseases, too).

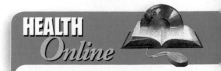

HEALTH *Online*

Get facts about heart disease from the Web Link to the American Heart Association at health.glencoe.com.

FIGURE 7.10

TYPES OF HEART DISEASE

There are several types of heart disease. The arrows in this illustration show how one type of disorder can lead to another. *Can you explain why arteriosclerosis might lead to high blood pressure?*

Arteriosclerosis
(ahr•tir•ee•oh•skluh•ROH•sis)
a group of conditions in which artery walls thicken, harden, and do not stretch as easily, decreasing blood flow; sometimes called "hardening of the arteries"

Atherosclerosis
(a•thuh•roh•skluh•ROH•sis)
a type of arteriosclerosis in which fatty deposits called plaque, made up mostly of cholesterol, build up on the inside of arteries, causing blockages

Stroke
the destruction of brain tissue caused by lack of blood flow to the brain, often leading to disability or death

Heart attack
the death of heart tissue caused by lack of blood flow to the heart, often leading to disability or death

High blood pressure
a condition in which the blood exerts an unusually high force on the walls of the arteries for a long period of time; also called hypertension

✓

Reading Check

Sort the following words into categories: *sunscreen, chewing tobacco, oatmeal, doctors, sunburns, cigarettes, radiation.* Label each category and add more words that would fit in each group.

Treating Heart Disease

It is better to prevent heart disease now than to treat it later. However, there are many treatments available.

- Medication can dissolve blood clots, enlarge blood vessels, lower blood pressure, and control a person's heartbeat.
- Surgical procedures can open up blocked arteries or insert devices to regulate the heartbeat. Advanced surgical techniques even allow a new heart to be transplanted into a person's body.
- Changes in lifestyle can help lower blood pressure and prevent more heart damage. These changes include regular physical activity, healthy eating and avoiding tobacco.

Cancer

Cancer is *a disease caused by abnormal cells that grow out of control.* It is the second most common cause of death in the United States. Many cancers start out as **tumors**, or *masses of abnormal cells,* in one tissue or organ. Some tumors are noncancerous, or benign (bi·NYN). This means they do not spread to other parts of the body. Tumors that are cancerous, or malignant (muh·LIG·nuhnt), invade surrounding tissue. Eventually, cancerous cells from the tumor may spread throughout the body.

What causes cancer? A history of cancer in a family increases risk. The most important factor, however, seems to be exposure to cancer-causing substances. For skin cancer—the most common type—sun exposure is the main risk. However, the single biggest cancer threat is tobacco use. Cigarette smoking accounts for at least 30 percent of all cancer deaths. You can lower your cancer risk by avoiding tobacco, protecting yourself from the sun, and eating more low-fat, high-fiber foods.

Skin cancer is the most common of all cancers. Over 1 million new cases are diagnosed each year. *What habits help you lower your risk of skin cancer?*

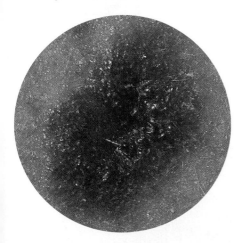

Treating Cancer

To be treated successfully, cancer must be discovered early. People who detect one of these seven warning signs should see a doctor right away:

- **C** hange in bowel or bladder habits
- **A** sore that does not heal
- **U** nusual bleeding or discharge
- **T** hickening or lump in the breast or elsewhere
- **I** ndigestion or difficulty swallowing
- **O** bvious change in a wart or mole
- **N** agging cough or hoarseness

Thanks to advances in treatment, more than half of all cancers can be completely cured. Three common treatments for cancer are surgery, radiation, and chemotherapy. Surgery is used to remove tumors and repair damaged organs. Radiation (ray·dee·AY·shuhn) destroys cancer cells with X-rays or other types of radiation. Surgery and radiation are more effective when the cancer has not yet spread.

Chemotherapy (kee·moh·THEHR·uh·pee) destroys cancer cells with powerful drugs. Chemotherapy can be used to fight cancers that have already spread throughout the body.

Allergies

An **allergy** is *the body's sensitivity to certain substances*. A *substance that causes an allergic reaction* is called an **allergen** (AL·er·juhn). When you have allergies, your immune system reacts to allergens as if they were germs entering your body.

If you feel sick when you are around certain things, see your doctor. He or she can perform simple tests to determine the source of your allergy. Though there is no cure for an allergy, certain medicines can relieve the symptoms. You can also try to avoid the allergen. Keeping your home clean can help, especially if you have dust allergies.

MEDIA WATCH

OVERCOMING THE ODDS

Cyclist Lance Armstrong survived an advanced case of testicular cancer and went on to win the Tour de France several years in a row. *Can you name some other famous cancer survivors?*

HEALTH SKILLS ACTIVITY

ACCESSING INFORMATION

Learning More About Noncommunicable Diseases

If you develop healthy habits now, you can reduce your risk of getting many non-communicable diseases, including cancer, heart disease, and diabetes. Here are some examples of healthy habits that can prevent disease.

- Do not use tobacco products.
- Stay active. Get some physical activity every day.
- Eat nutritious foods, including plenty of fiber. Avoid fat, especially saturated fat, and large amounts of salt.
- Protect yourself from exposure to the sun.
- Maintain a healthy weight.
- Manage your stress.

WITH A GROUP
Form groups of 3 or 4. Using library resources and the Internet, each group should research a different noncommunicable disease. Identify behaviors that can reduce your chances of getting the disease. Share your results with the class.

Asthma

Asthma (AZ·muh) is *a chronic breathing disease caused by allergies, physical exertion, air pollution, or other factors.* Untreated, it can lead to lung infections and permanent lung damage. Most people develop it during elementary school, but sometimes symptoms may also appear later in life.

People with asthma experience asthma attacks, illustrated in **Figure 7.11**. Many factors can trigger an attack, including common allergens like pollen or mold, animal dander, or certain foods. Smoke, physical activity, or a cold virus can also bring on an attack. To avoid an attack, it's best to avoid any known allergens or take preventive medicine as prescribed. Medication helps people with asthma to lead normal lives.

FIGURE 7.11

AN ASTHMA ATTACK

This figure illustrates how the airways become narrowed during an asthma attack. *Why does a person have difficulty breathing during an asthma attack?*

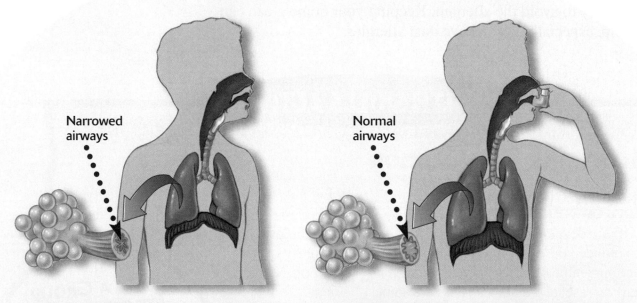

Narrowed airways

Normal airways

During an asthma attack, the airways in the lungs become swollen and clogged with mucus. Since the airways are narrower, less air can enter the lungs. Symptoms of an attack can include wheezing (a whistling sound), tightness in the chest, and a dry cough. The person may panic because breathing is so difficult. Without medication, attacks can last several hours or more.

Medication can help open up the air passages in the lungs. An inhaler is a small hand-held device that dispenses the exact amount of medication needed. Some people have to take this medicine every day. All people with asthma should carry it with them at all times in case of an asthma attack.

Diabetes

Diabetes (dy·uh·BEE·teez) is *a disease that prevents the body from using the sugars and starches in food for energy.* It is caused by problems with **insulin**, *a hormone produced by the pancreas* that normally moves sugars into cells. In type 1 diabetes, the body does not produce insulin. Type 2 diabetes prevents the body from using insulin effectively. Being overweight or inactive can contribute to type 2 diabetes. **Figure 7.12** lists the symptoms and treatment of diabetes.

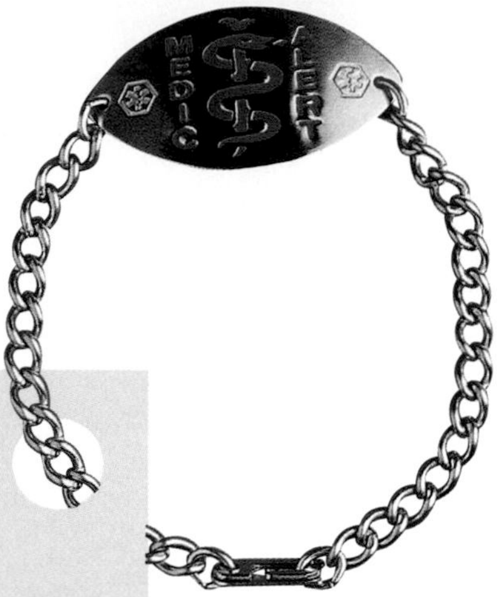

FIGURE 7.12

DIABETES SYMPTOMS AND TREATMENT

Diabetes cannot be cured, but it can be controlled. *Why might wearing a medical alert bracelet be a good idea for people with diabetes?*

Symptoms

- excess production of urine
- increased hunger and thirst
- weight loss
- lack of energy
- blurred vision

Treatment

- regular checks of blood sugar level
- regulating food choices
- controlling weight
- oral medication
- insulin injections

Lesson 4 Review

Using complete sentences, answer the following questions on a sheet of paper.

Reviewing Terms and Facts

1. **Vocabulary** What is a *chronic* disease?
2. **List** Name the seven warning signs of cancer.
3. **Identify** Which of these noncommunicable diseases can be triggered by exposure to allergens: diabetes, allergies, heart disease?
4. **Vocabulary** Define the term *insulin*.

Thinking Critically

5. **Compose** Choose one of the diseases discussed in this lesson. Write a paragraph about how the disease is treated.
6. **Synthesize** Name two healthy lifestyle choices that help prevent more than one noncommunicable disease.

Applying Health Skills

7. **Goal Setting** Being overweight and inactive can increase a person's chances of getting type 2 diabetes. Name some healthy habits that can lower this risk.

PROTECTING YOUR HEALTH

Model

Jenny has set a goal to become more physically active. This goal has ongoing rewards. By increasing her activity level, Jenny will reduce her lifelong risk of developing certain diseases, such as diabetes and heart disease. She will also be able to maintain a healthy weight, which further reduces her disease risk. As a final reward, she will have more energy for the activities she enjoys, such as hiking with her family. Here are the steps Jenny is using to reach her goal.

1. SET A SPECIFIC GOAL.
"I plan to be physically active for 60 minutes each day."

2. LIST THE STEPS TO REACH YOUR GOAL.
"I will add more daily physical activity by walking the dog every morning. I will ride my bicycle to school when the weather is good. I will increase my activity level gradually until I am active for a full hour each day."

3. GET HELP FROM OTHERS.
"I will ask my parents to join me on weekends for walks and bike rides. I will ask my doctor for advice about other ways to increase my activity level. When I am with my friends, I will suggest physical activities like playing ball instead of going to the movies."

4. EVALUATE YOUR PROGRESS.
"I will start an activity calendar to keep track of how much time I spend being physically active each day."

Practice

Max and Scott are meeting at Scott's house for an after-school snack. Read their conversation and use what you know about disease prevention to answer the questions below.

SCOTT: I'm starving! Let's make a sandwich.
MAX: Hold on a minute—time out to wash my hands.
SCOTT: But I'm starving now!
MAX: Me too, but I'm trying to avoid getting a cold this winter. Part of the plan is to wash my hands a lot more often, especially before I eat. I also want to get enough sleep—my mom is helping me with that.
SCOTT: So is your plan working?
MAX: So far, it's been two months, and I'm feeling great.
SCOTT: Hey, that makes a lot of sense. Pass the soap!

1. What is Max's goal?
2. What actions will he take to achieve his goal?
3. How does Scott's willingness to share Max's goal help Max?

COACH'S BOX

Goal Setting

1. Set a specific goal.
2. List the steps to reach your goal.
3. Get help from others.
4. Evaluate your progress.
5. Reward yourself.

Apply/Assess

Choose one of the diseases discussed in this chapter. Set a goal to prevent the disease or, if you already have the disease, to control it. List the steps you will take to reach your goal.

Find other students who chose the same disease. As a group, create a brochure that illustrates the steps for preventing or controlling this disease. Illustrate your brochure with drawings, magazine pictures, or computer graphics. Share your brochure with the class.

Self-√ Check

- Did we set a clear, realistic goal?
- Does our brochure show a plan for reaching the goal?
- Does our brochure contain accurate information about our chosen disease?

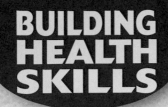
ADVOCATING FOR HEALTH

Model

An advocate is a person who speaks or writes in support of something. You are an advocate for health when you persuade others to make healthy choices. Read how Parker became an advocate for his grandfather's health.

When Parker learned about heart disease, he became concerned about his grandfather. After a heart attack, Parker's grandfather quit smoking. However, he did not change his eating habits or increase his activity level. Parker decided to write his grandfather a letter to tell him about his concerns.

Dear Grandpa,

I am writing this letter to tell you some important things I learned about heart disease. First of all, I learned that stopping smoking was one of the best things you can do for your heart. I was really proud of you when you quit smoking. It made me feel like I was more important than those cigarettes. I'm so glad you quit.

I've learned some other things about heart disease, too. Staying physically active can make your heart stronger and lower your blood pressure. It can also help you control your weight, and that's good for your heart. I was thinking that we could walk together every day and that would help both our hearts. I also learned that what we eat is important. We need to include more fruits and vegetables so we get the fiber and nutrients our bodies need. Maybe we could work together on this too.

Most of all, I want your heart to stay healthy so we can keep going fishing and watching hockey games together. I want you to be around a long, long time.

Love,
Parker

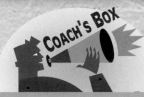

Practice

As you have learned, abstinence from sexual activity is the best protection against STIs. Practice your advocacy skills by pretending to be an advice columnist. Read this teen's letter and write a response that promotes abstinence from sexual activity before marriage.

> *Dear Dr. Leslie,*
>
> *I am a student at Webster Middle School. Today in health class, we talked about abstinence from sexual activity. My teacher said that abstinence is the best choice for teens. But movies and TV shows never even talk about it. How should I interpret these mixed messages?*
>
> *Wondering at Webster*

Share your letter with others in your class. How is your response similar to or different from theirs?

Advocacy

Using the skill of advocacy asks you to
- take a clear stand on an issue.
- persuade others to make healthy choices.
- be convincing.

Apply/Assess

See if you can get right to the point by developing a bumper sticker that contains an abstinence message. Your challenge will be to get a message across in just a few words.

Create a bumper sticker that makes a clear stand for abstinence. Draw your bumper sticker on a strip of butcher paper or poster board. You may use art, borders, or graphics to illustrate your work. Be prepared to explain why abstinence is the best choice for teens.

Self-√Check

- Did I take a clear stand?
- Is my bumper sticker persuasive to teens?
- Did I give reasons why abstinence is the best choice?

The SAFEST SEX is NO SEX!

Abstinence ♥ Makes the HEART grow fonder

I'm WAITING . . . . because I'm WORTH IT!

SUMMARY

LESSON·1 Communicable diseases are caused by germs that are spread from person to person. The body's natural defenses work to keep out or destroy pathogens. They also protect the body from becoming infected by the same kinds of pathogens again.

LESSON·2 Healthy behaviors help a person's body fight off infection and keep infections from spreading. Vaccines can give a person immunity to several communicable diseases.

LESSON·3 Sexually transmitted infections (STIs) are communicable diseases that are spread through sexual contact. Practicing abstinence protects you against STIs.

LESSON·4 Noncommunicable diseases can be present at birth or can be caused by unhealthy habits or environmental hazards. Common noncommunicable diseases are heart disease, cancer, allergies, asthma, and diabetes.

- antibodies
- disease
- handwashing
- hepatitis
- immunity
- lymphocytes
- noncommunicable diseases
- pathogens
- vaccine

Reviewing Vocabulary and Concepts

On a sheet of paper, write the numbers 1–9. After each number, write the term from the list that best completes each sentence.

Lesson 1

1. A(n) _____ is an unhealthy condition of the body or mind.
2. You can't catch _____ from another person.
3. Germs that cause disease are known as _____.
4. White blood cells that attack pathogens are called _____.
5. Your immune system produces chemicals called _____ specifically to fight a particular invading substance.

6. If your body is resistant to a particular infection, you have a(n) _____ to it.

Lesson 2

7. _____ is a good way to prevent the spread of germs.
8. Nausea, weakness, and yellowing of the eyes are common symptoms of _____.
9. One way to protect yourself from certain communicable diseases is to have a(n) _____, a preparation of killed or weakened germs.

On a sheet of paper, write the numbers 10–20. Write *True* or *False* for each statement. If the statement is false, change the underlined word or phrase to make it true.

Lesson 3

10. People who have no visible symptoms <u>cannot</u> spread STIs to others.

11. Gonorrhea, chlamydia, and <u>the common cold</u> are all types of sexually transmitted infections.

12. The virus that causes AIDS is called <u>HIV</u>.

13. HIV <u>can</u> be spread through casual contact, such as shaking hands or hugging.

14. By practicing sexual <u>abstinence</u> you will avoid the dangers of STIs.

Lesson 4

15. Most cancers start as <u>infections,</u> or masses of abnormal cells in an organ or tissue.

16. Radiation and chemotherapy are two ways of treating <u>heart disease</u>.

17. Foods and pollen are common <u>allergens</u>, or causes of allergies.

18. A person who has sudden difficulty breathing and tightness in the chest during exercise may have <u>asthma</u>.

19. Asthma is a chronic, or <u>short-lasting</u>, disease.

20. Being overweight or inactive can contribute to <u>type 1</u> diabetes.

Thinking Critically

Using complete sentences, answer the following questions on a sheet of paper.

21. Describe Explain how your immune system works to prevent disease. What are the other ways your body guards itself against germs?

22. Analyze Why would people whose parents or grandparents had heart disease be more likely to get it later in life? What could you do to "stop the cycle"?

23. Infer Why do you think arteriosclerosis can lead to a heart attack?

24. Analyze Explain which of the seven warning signs of cancer could be a sign of skin cancer and why.

25. Suggest You can have asthma and still lead a normal life. What actions can lessen the chances of having an asthma attack?

Career Corner

Medical Technologist

Do you like looking at things under a microscope? Do you enjoy doing science experiments? If so, you might think about a career as a medical technologist. These professionals work in hospitals and laboratories. Their job is to test patients' blood and other tissues. This helps doctors diagnose and treat diseases. To do this job, you will need a four-year degree in medical technology or life sciences. Visit Career Corner at health.glencoe.com to learn more about this and other careers.

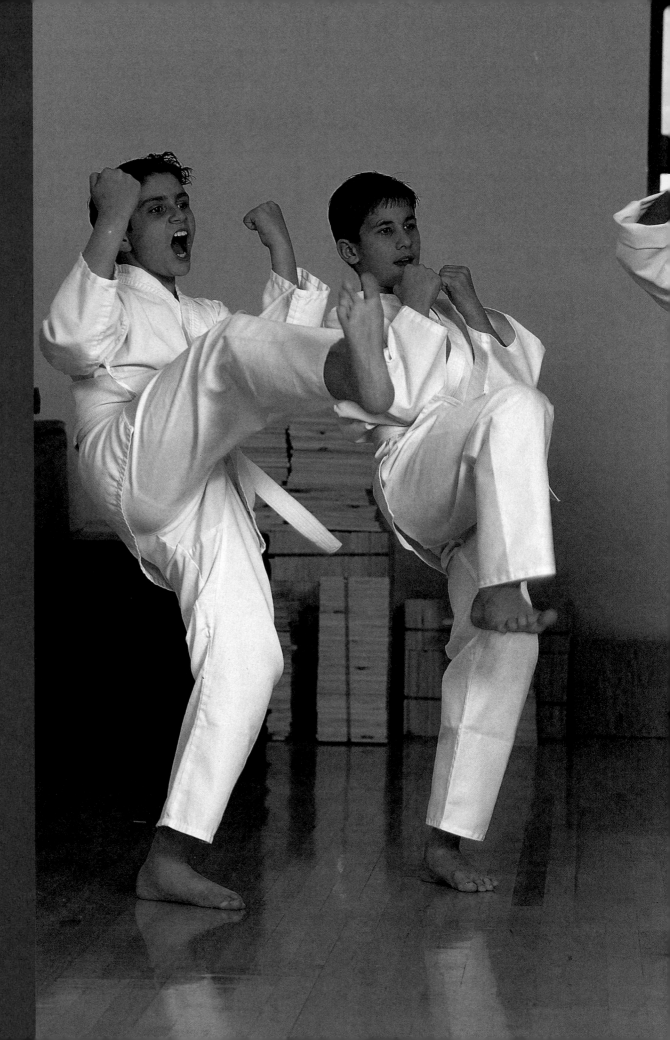

Protecting Your Health

Technology Project

Presentation Software
Get your health message out to others by creating an exciting, colorful slide show to demonstrate the benefits of practicing healthful behaviors.
- Log on to health.glencoe.com.
- Click on Technology Projects and find the "Presentation Software" activity.
- Include pictures, sounds, and animations to make an effective presentation.

In Your Home and Community

Refusal Skills
Interview one or two adult members of your family, or choose other adults you feel comfortable questioning. Ask them to share with you some successful ways they found to say no to people when they did not want to do something that might harm their health.

Tobacco

Quick Write

Using tobacco is a health risk. List at least two reasons people might start smoking when they know the health risks involved. Share your responses with classmates.

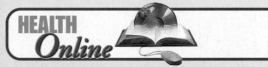

Go to health.glencoe.com and take the Health Inventory for Chapter 8. In the activity, you will rate your commitment to staying tobacco free.

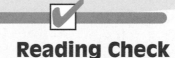

Reading Check

Brainstorm as many different words as possible that relate to tobacco.

Why Tobacco Is Harmful

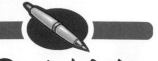

Quick Write

Write a paragraph about the reasons many people choose to remain tobacco free.

LEARN ABOUT...

- how using tobacco products damages your health.
- why tobacco use leads to addiction.
- the harmful effects of smokeless tobacco.
- the dangers of secondhand smoke.

VOCABULARY

- nicotine
- tar
- carbon monoxide
- addiction
- emphysema
- snuff
- secondhand smoke

Tobacco Use: The Inside Story

Tobacco products include cigarettes, clove cigarettes, bidis (hand-rolled, flavored cigarette), cigars, pipes, and smokeless tobacco. All of them contain dangerous substances. Tobacco smoke contains more than 4,000 chemicals, and least 43 of them cause cancer. Harmful substances in tobacco include:

- **Nicotine** (NI·kuh·teen), *a drug that speeds up the heartbeat and affects the central nervous system.* Nicotine, which is only found in tobacco, narrows blood vessels and contributes to heart disease. People who use tobacco regularly develop a physical need for nicotine.
- **Tar**, *a thick, oily, dark liquid that forms when tobacco burns.* Tar coats the inside of the lungs. Over time, chemicals in tar can cause cancer and lung diseases.
- **Carbon monoxide** (KAR·buhn·muh·NAHK·syd), *a poisonous, odorless gas produced when tobacco burns.* When inhaled, it reduces the amount of oxygen in the blood.

Avoiding the harmful chemicals in tobacco offers lifelong benefits. *Why is avoiding tobacco smoke an important choice for this teen?*

Tobacco: An Addictive Drug

Nicotine, which is found in all tobacco products, can cause addiction. **Addiction** is *the body's physical or mental need for a drug or other substance.* The need for a substance is also called dependence. There are two kinds of dependence.

- Psychological, or mental, dependence means that users believe they need the substance to feel good.
- Physical dependence means the body needs the substance to function. When people stop using the substance, they experience painful symptoms. These symptoms may include shakiness, headache, nervousness, and sleeping problems.

Nicotine is a highly addictive drug. Most tobacco users admit that it is hard to quit. **Figure 8.1** shows how people become addicted to tobacco. Addiction leads to heavier use, which can harm the whole body. **Figure 8.2** on page 214 shows how tobacco use harms many different body parts.

✓ **Reading Check**
Find pairs of phrases in the following list that have a cause-and-effect relationship: *nicotine, reduced oxygen, tar, carbon monoxide, faster heartbeat, addiction, black lungs, can't quit.*

FIGURE 8.1

STAGES OF TOBACCO ADDICTION

Addiction can start with the first use, or it can be a slow process, taking many years. *When do you think most adult smokers began smoking?*

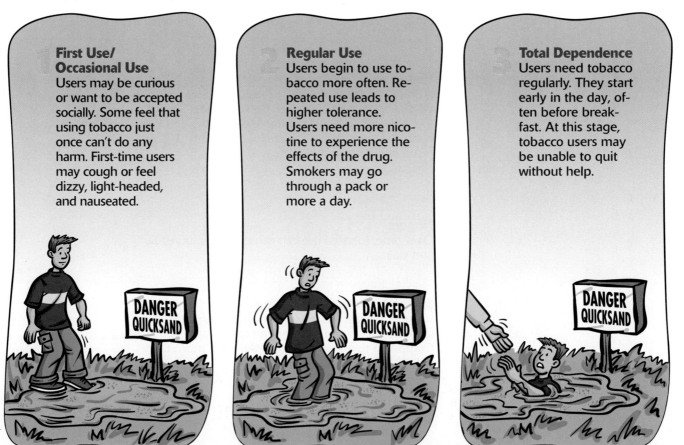

First Use/ Occasional Use
Users may be curious or want to be accepted socially. Some feel that using tobacco just once can't do any harm. First-time users may cough or feel dizzy, light-headed, and nauseated.

Regular Use
Users begin to use tobacco more often. Repeated use leads to higher tolerance. Users need more nicotine to experience the effects of the drug. Smokers may go through a pack or more a day.

Total Dependence
Users need tobacco regularly. They start early in the day, often before breakfast. At this stage, tobacco users may be unable to quit without help.

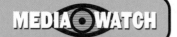

FIGURE 8.2

THE HARMFUL EFFECTS OF TOBACCO

The chemicals in tobacco harm many parts of the body. *What is the harmful effect on the blood vessels?*

Skin
Smoking ages the skin, causing it to wrinkle earlier than a nonsmoker's skin.

Mouth, Teeth, and Throat
Cigarette smoke and smokeless tobacco lead to bad breath and stained teeth. Chemicals in tobacco cause mouth and throat cancers. Smokeless tobacco can cause leukoplakia—white sores in the mouth that can lead to cancer—as well as bone loss around the teeth. It also wears away tooth enamel.

Throat

Lungs
The tar in cigarette smoke coats the inside of the lungs so they cannot work efficiently. Exposure to tar is one cause of **emphysema** (em·fuh·SEE·muh), *a disease that occurs when the tiny air sacs in the lungs lose their elasticity, or ability to stretch.* Chemicals in tobacco smoke can also contribute to lung cancer. Smoking causes nearly 87 percent of lung cancers.

Heart
Nicotine increases the heart rate and causes blood vessels to become narrower. Narrow vessels make the heart pump harder to move blood through the body. This extra effort raises blood pressure and can result in heart attack or stroke.

Fingers
Over time, tobacco use can cause fingers to yellow and stain.

Stomach, Bladder, and Colon
Harmful substances in tobacco smoke can lead to stomach ulcers and bladder and colon cancers. Compared to nonsmokers, smokers are more than twice as likely to get bladder cancer.

Brain

Nicotine is carried from the lungs to the brain within seven seconds. It releases chemicals in the brain that cause tobacco users to want more nicotine. Nicotine also interferes with the flow of information between nerve cells.

Blood Vessels

Carbon monoxide from tobacco smoke reduces the amount of oxygen carried in the blood. This means that body organs receive less oxygen from the blood. Physical activity is more difficult. Athletes are not able to perform as well.

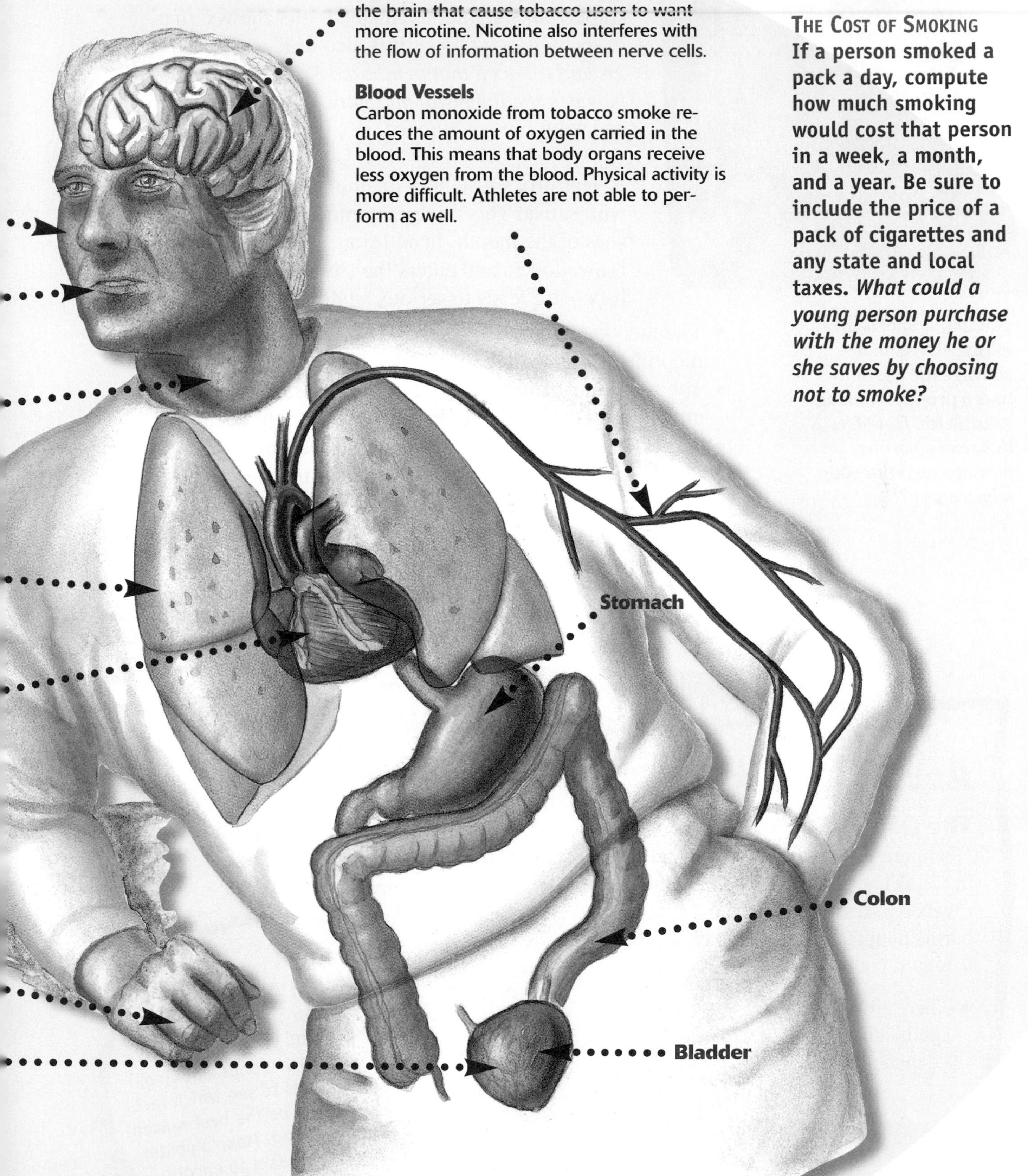

Stomach

Colon

Bladder

THE COST OF SMOKING
If a person smoked a pack a day, compute how much smoking would cost that person in a week, a month, and a year. Be sure to include the price of a pack of cigarettes and any state and local taxes. *What could a young person purchase with the money he or she saves by choosing not to smoke?*

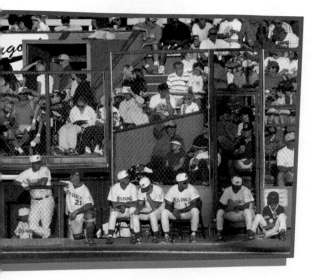

All major sports are taking efforts to discourage the use of tobacco products among its athletes. *How does this send a positive message about staying tobacco free?*

Smokeless Tobacco

As its name indicates, smokeless tobacco is not smoked like cigarettes. Instead, it is chewed in a coarsely ground form. It is also used as **snuff**, *finely ground tobacco that is inhaled or held in the mouth between the lower lip and gum.* Chewing tobacco and snuff are not smoked, so are they safe? No.

Harmful substances in smokeless tobacco mix with saliva. This mixture contacts the sensitive tissues of the mouth. In addition, some of this mixture is swallowed and enters the stomach. Smokeless tobacco use leads to serious health problems.

- The nicotine in smokeless tobacco is just as addictive as the nicotine in smoked tobacco.
- Tobacco juice can cause white spots to form on the gums and inside the cheeks. These spots can turn into cancer.
- Swallowed tobacco can cause sores in the stomach.
- People who use smokeless tobacco tend to lose their senses of taste and smell.
- Smokeless tobacco causes bad breath and stains the teeth.
- Grit and sugar in tobacco can cause cavities and red, inflamed gums (gingivitis). This can lead to an advanced stage of gum disease that causes tooth decay and tooth loss.

HEALTH SKILLS ACTIVITY

ADVOCACY

The Dangers of Smoking

Cigarette ads often show smokers having fun. They never show the dangers of tobacco use. By showing how tobacco harms people, you can help teens decide to stay tobacco free.

- There are at least 43 cancer-causing chemicals in tobacco and tobacco smoke.
- Smoking at an early age increases the risk of lung cancer.
- Cigarettes kill more than 400,000 Americans every year. That is more than 1,000 per day.

WITH A GROUP
Use library resources, the Internet, and your textbook to find more facts about smoking. Poll classmates to see which fact they believe to be the best reason to avoid smoking. Make a poster that uses this fact to encourage teens to avoid tobacco.

Secondhand Smoke

Secondhand smoke is *tobacco smoke that stays in the air.* Nonsmokers who breathe secondhand smoke can develop some of the same health problems as smokers. Secondhand smoke kills more than 40,000 nonsmokers each year. About 3,000 of them die of lung cancer. The remaining deaths are from heart disease and other cancers.

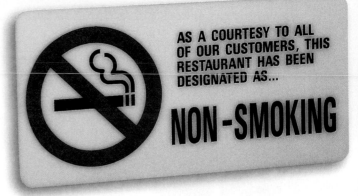

Secondhand smoke causes other health problems. In children under 18 months old, it can cause pneumonia, bronchitis, and other lower respiratory tract infections. Each year, 150,000 to 300,000 children develop these diseases as a result of secondhand smoke. Between 7,500 and 15,000 of these children are hospitalized. Many children with asthma have more frequent and more severe attacks when secondhand smoke is present.

Because of the health risks of secondhand smoke, smoking has been banned in many public buildings. *Name some buildings in your community that are officially smoke free.*

Many offices, factories, restaurants, and other places have banned smoking due to the health risks to nonsmokers. Some towns and cities have even banned smoking outside, in places such as beaches, building entrances, outdoor dining areas, children's play areas, and public gardens.

Lesson 1 Review

Using complete sentences, answer the following questions on a sheet of paper.

Reviewing Terms and Facts

1. **List** Name three harmful substances found in tobacco smoke and describe each one.
2. **Recall** Identify the three stages of tobacco addiction.
3. **Identify** What are two forms of smokeless tobacco?
4. **Vocabulary** Define the term *secondhand smoke.* Use it in an original sentence.

Thinking Critically

5. **Relate** Identify one of the diseases associated with tobacco use. Explain how developing this disease could affect a person's lifelong health.
6. **Explain** Why can smoking be considered a social problem as well as a health problem? Why should communities be concerned about smoking?

Applying Health Skills

7. **Advocacy** Create a radio advertisement against tobacco use. The ad might mention the many health problems caused by tobacco use. You might read your ad in front of the class or over the school's public address system.

Quick Write

Think about your favorite television show. Do any of the characters smoke? Write a short paragraph describing how the other characters reacted to this character's smoking.

LEARN ABOUT...

- why people start using tobacco.
- how you can stay tobacco free.

VOCABULARY

- media

Staying Tobacco Free

The Reality of Teens and Tobacco Use

Most teens don't risk their health by using tobacco. Those who do use it may be unaware of the realities of tobacco use.

- Some teens think tobacco will help them fit in. In reality, as **Figure 8.3** shows, less than 15 percent of teens ages 12 to 17 smoke.
- Teens may think that using tobacco makes them seem more grown-up. However, the number of adult smokers has dropped drastically. Many former smokers quit to improve their health and the health of their families.
- Teens may believe that tobacco won't hurt their health for many years. In fact, some of tobacco's harmful effects—such as increased heart rate—start with the first use.
- Teens may try tobacco to look "cool." However, tobacco actually harms the user's appearance. It can cause bad breath, stained teeth, and wrinkled skin.

FIGURE 8.3

NONSMOKERS IN DIFFERENT AGE GROUPS

This graph shows the percentage of nonsmokers in three different age groups. *Why do you think most teens choose not to smoke?*

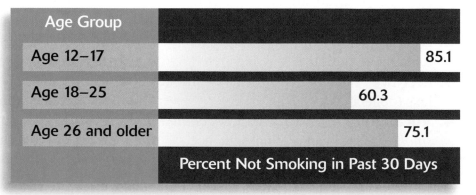

Age Group	Percent Not Smoking in Past 30 Days
Age 12–17	85.1
Age 18–25	60.3
Age 26 and older	75.1

Source: U.S. Substance Abuse and Mental Heath Services Administration, *National Household Survey on Drug Abuse,* 1999.

Pressures You May Face

If tobacco is so harmful, why do some teens start using it? There is no one answer. They may be influenced by factors such as the media, friends, and family.

- **Pressure from the media.** Many teens use tobacco because of the images they see and hear in the media. The media are *the various methods of communicating information, including newspapers, magazines, radio, television, movies, and the Internet.* In some movies, for example, characters may express their personality by smoking. In addition, tobacco companies spend billions of dollars each year on advertising. Studies have shown that tobacco companies target teens, especially through magazines.

- **Pressure from peers.** Peer pressure is a major factor in teen tobacco use. If a teen's friends use tobacco, then he or she is more likely to try it. By choosing friends who are tobacco free, teens can avoid this pressure.

- **Pressure from family.** Family influence is another large factor in teen tobacco use. Teens are more likely to use tobacco if parents or siblings use it. If parents don't use tobacco, teens are much less likely to use it.

- **Other pressures.** Teens may think that tobacco use will help them cope with stress. Others think it will help control their weight. However, tobacco use can actually add to stress because smokers experience discomfort if they do not have nicotine regularly. Tobacco users may also find it harder to participate in physical activity, a key to healthy weight control.

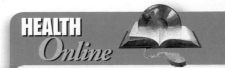

HEALTH *Online*

Do you know the facts about the dangers of using tobacco? Test your knowledge in Web Links at health.glencoe.com.

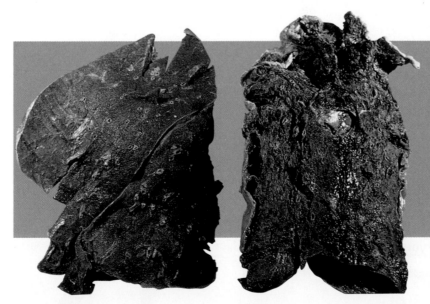

Compare the condition of the smoker's lung on the right with the healthy lung shown on the left. *How might these pictures influence teens who are thinking about using tobacco?*

Reasons to Say No

There are many reasons to say no to tobacco. Tobacco use damages nearly all of your body systems and increases the risk of developing cancer and other serious diseases. It exposes others to dangerous secondhand smoke. Tobacco products are also very expensive. They make your breath, clothing, skin, and hair smell bad. **Figure 8.4** gives more reasons to say no.

Here is one more reason. In many states, it is illegal to possess tobacco if you are younger than 18. In some states, teens can go to jail for possessing tobacco.

Hands-On Health

STRAW BREATHING

Smoking can damage the lungs and cause emphysema, a disease that damages the tiny sacs in the lungs called alveoli. People with emphysema struggle to get air into and out of their lungs. How do you think this disease would affect your ability to do physical activities? Find out by performing this simple experiment.

WHAT YOU WILL NEED
- a small drinking straw
- paper and pencil or pen
- a stopwatch, clock with a second hand, or other timer

WHAT YOU WILL DO
1. Stand up and do an exercise, such as running in place or jumping jacks, for one minute. Have someone time you.
2. After doing a minute of exercise, write down how you feel. How tired are you? How easily can you breathe?
3. Put a small straw in your mouth. Then hold your nose closed and breathe only through the straw. Do this for one minute.
4. Continue to breathe through the straw as you stand up and perform a minute of exercise. Have someone time you.
5. After you finish your exercise, write down how it felt this time. Was it much harder than the first time?

IN CONCLUSION
1. How did you feel when your breathing was restricted?
2. How do you think it would affect your life if you felt that way all the time?
3. Do you think this experiment is a convincing argument against smoking?

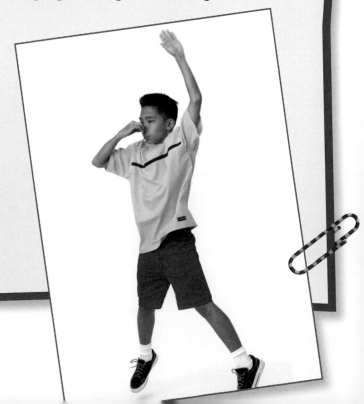

FIGURE 8.4

SAYING NO TO TOBACCO

If someone offers you tobacco, you should be well armed with different ways to say no. *Can you think of any other ways to refuse tobacco?*

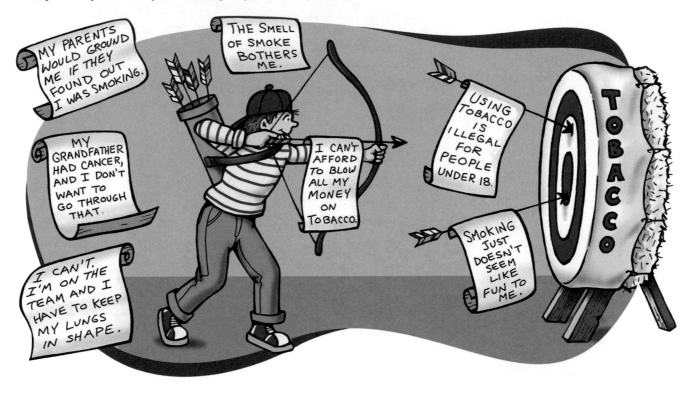

Lesson 2 Review

Using complete sentences, answer the following questions on a sheet of paper.

Reviewing Terms and Facts

1. **Vocabulary** Define the term *media.* Explain how the media can influence teens' decisions about tobacco use.
2. **Recall** Identify three pressures teens face to start using tobacco.
3. **List** Give three ways to say no to tobacco.

Thinking Critically

4. **Justify** If you were a health insurance company, would you have tobacco users pay a higher insurance rate? Explain.

5. **Hypothesize** Why do you think many state governments have placed such strict controls on the sale of tobacco to minors and possession by minors?

Applying Health Skills

6. **Analyzing Influences** In a journal, keep track of pressures to use tobacco that you see and hear in one day. Write down if people use tobacco around you, if you see advertisements for tobacco products, or if you see someone using tobacco on television. Which of these do you think affects you the most? How do you remain tobacco free around these influences?

STAND FIRM AGAINST TOBACCO

Model

Saying no to tobacco isn't always easy, but remember—practice makes you better at it. Read about a teen named Tasha, shown below. She's at a party with her friends. Her friend Betty takes out a cigarette, lights it, and passes it to Tasha. Tasha has already decided not to smoke. Here are some ways she uses refusal skills. Would you be able to do as well?

SAY NO IN A FIRM VOICE.
"No thanks, I don't smoke."

TELL WHY.
"I just don't want to do something that isn't good for me."

OFFER OTHER OPTIONS.
"No, I don't want one. Why don't we go to a movie instead?"

PROMPTLY LEAVE THE SITUATION.
When Betty and the other girls keep pressuring her, Tasha calls her mother and leaves the party.

Practice

Imagine the following scene. Then answer the questions at the end.

It's the end of the school day. Michael and Jeremy are at their lockers. Michael pulls out a can of smokeless tobacco and offers Jeremy a dip. Jeremy has already decided he doesn't want to use tobacco in any form.

JEREMY: No thanks, I don't want any.
MICHAEL: Don't be a baby. I'll bet you've never tried it.
JEREMY: No, I've already made my decision. Besides, we could get caught and kicked out of school.
MICHAEL: Hey, a vacation would be nice. Anyway, there aren't any teachers around.
JEREMY: Look, I'm just not interested. I have to meet some friends for a basketball game. I'll see you later.

1. Which refusal skills did Jeremy use?
2. Do you think this conversation was realistic?
3. Which refusal skills would be comfortable for you?

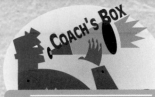

Apply/Assess

Read the following three situations. Choose one situation and write your own conversation. Use the skills you have learned to refuse tobacco in your conversation. You might role-play your conversation with another student in front of your class. Ask the class to identify the refusal skills you use.

While Marcus is camping out in his backyard, his neighbor Tyrone enters the tent. Tyrone is a couple of years older than Marcus. After making himself comfortable, Tyrone reaches in his pocket and pulls out a pack of cigarettes. He lights one up and offers the pack to Marcus.

Marshall and Zack are best friends. They go to the same school and are on the baseball team. One day after practice, Zack surprises Marshall by reaching into his backpack and pulling out a pouch of chewing tobacco. Zack holds the pouch out to Marshall.

Anna is at the grocery store picking up some things for her mother. In the parking lot, she sees Matt, the cutest guy in her science class. Anna waves and Matt comes over to talk. As they are talking, he offers her a cigarette.

FIND THE HIDDEN MESSAGES

Model

Every day, you are exposed to advertisements. Because teens have a lot of purchasing power, advertisers spend large amounts of money trying to convince you to purchase their products. However, some of these products, like tobacco, can harm your health. Study the ads below. They show messages that advertisers use to sell tobacco. Notice that none of the messages reveal the dangers or risks of tobacco use. Why do you think tobacco advertisers avoid the truth?

What the ad suggests:
Everyone else is using tobacco.

The truth:
Most teens don't use tobacco.

Join the Crowd!

What the ad suggests:
You will have fun and lots of friends if you use tobacco.

The truth:
Using tobacco makes you sick and less able to enjoy life.

FUN AND FLAVOR!

FREE COOL STUFF

KOFF

Taste the Good Life

What the ad suggests:
Tobacco companies will give you great stuff for nothing.

The truth:
Wearing a tobacco company's logo gives the company free advertising.

What the ad suggests:
Using tobacco will make you rich and famous.

The truth:
Using tobacco will cost you money.

Practice

Form small groups. Look through magazines and newspapers for tobacco advertisements. Locate and cut out three advertisements for cigarettes, cigars, or chewing tobacco. Glue or tape the ads on a sheet of poster board. Under each ad, write the hidden message it tries to send about tobacco. Share your ads with your classmates. Do they agree with your descriptions? Which ads would influence someone your age? Why?

Apply/Assess

Develop your own antitobacco advertisement. Use one or more of the techniques you have seen in tobacco ads to influence teens to stay tobacco free. You can also include other messages, such as information about how tobacco is harmful. Share your advertisements with the class. Which advertisements would have the most influence on teens? Explain why.

Analyzing Influences

Advertisements try to appeal to our basic needs and desires, such as:
- curiosity
- friendship
- success
- fun
- independence

Self-√Check
- Does my ad take a strong stand against tobacco?
- Did my ad use advertising techniques?
- Would my ad influence teens to be tobacco free?
- Did my ad provide information about the harmful effects of tobacco?

What the ad suggests:
Using tobacco will make you attractive, glamorous, or cool.

The truth:
Using tobacco damages your skin, stains your teeth, and makes your breath smell bad.

Sophisticated TASTE

Come to the Great Outdoors

What the ad suggests:
Using tobacco will bring you closer to nature.

The truth:
Smoking pollutes the air.

SUMMARY

LESSON·1 Tobacco is an addictive drug that can cause cancer and other health and social problems. Several substances in tobacco are harmful to health. Nicotine contributes to heart disease. Tar coats the inside of the lungs and leads to cancer and lung diseases. Carbon monoxide is a gas that reduces the amount of oxygen in the blood. Smokeless tobacco has many of the same health risks as smoked tobacco. Secondhand smoke can cause the same health problems for non-smokers.

LESSON·2 Most teens do not use tobacco, though it may seem otherwise. Teens' attitudes about tobacco use are influenced by several sources. The media pressure teens with advertisements and images of tobacco use. Peers and families serve as positive examples when they do not use tobacco. Some teens wrongly think that tobacco use will help them deal with stress or lose weight. There are many ways and reasons to say no to tobacco.

Reviewing Vocabulary and Concepts

On a sheet of paper, write the numbers 1–11. After each number, write the term from the list that best completes each sentence.

- addiction
- carbon monoxide
- chemicals
- emphysema
- nicotine
- psychological
- physical
- secondhand smoke
- smokeless tobacco
- snuff
- tar

Lesson 1

1. Tobacco smoke contains over 4,000 _____.
2. A thick, oily, dark liquid that forms when tobacco burns is _____.
3. _____ is a poisonous, odorless gas that reduces the amount of oxygen in the blood when inhaled.
4. The addictive chemical found in tobacco is called _____.
5. You have formed a(n) _____ when you physically or mentally depend on a substance.

6. A person whose body cannot function without a drug has a _____ dependence.
7. A _____ dependence is a person's belief that he or she needs a particular substance to feel good.
8. Smoking can cause _____, a disease that damages the tiny air sacs in the lungs.
9. _____ is finely ground tobacco that is inhaled or held in the mouth between the lower lip and the gum.
10. Using _____ stains the teeth and causes bad breath.
11. Many children with asthma experience more severe reactions when they breathe _____.

Lesson 2

On a sheet of paper, write the numbers 12–15. After each number, write the letter of the answer that best completes each statement.

12. People may begin using tobacco because
   a. their family members use tobacco.
   b. they think it will make them look more grown-up.
   c. they think it will make them fit in with peers.
   d. All of the above.

13. A form of media that might pressure you to use tobacco is
   a. your family.
   b. your peers.
   c. magazines.
   d. stress.

14. It is illegal in many states for people under the age of 18 to
   a. listen to tobacco advertisements.
   b. possess tobacco products.
   c. breathe tobacco smoke.
   d. advocate for a smoke-free environment.

15. Smoking is not a healthy way to manage stress because
   a. stress doesn't need to be managed.
   b. the craving for nicotine actually increases stress levels.
   c. the substances in tobacco are completely harmless.
   d. most people do not have any stress.

Thinking Critically

Using complete sentences, answer the following questions on a sheet of paper.

16. Explain How does a person who begins to use tobacco become addicted? Describe the stages of addiction he or she experiences.

17. Analyze Why might an adult smoker with a family want to quit the tobacco habit?

18. Interpret Why would an office building ban smoking at its entrances?

19. Infer Why do you think teens whose parents smoke are more likely to smoke themselves?

20. Suggest Imagine that one of your friends wants to start smoking. How would you convince him or her not to smoke?

Career Corner

Anesthesiologist

When people have surgery or certain other medical treatments, they may need to use drugs to prevent pain. These drugs are called anesthetics. The physician who gives them is called an anesthesiologist. Like other doctors, these health professionals need at least four years of medical school. After that, they go through a residency. This is a period of advanced training in a medical specialty. Find out more about this and other health careers by clicking on Career Corner at **health.glencoe.com.**

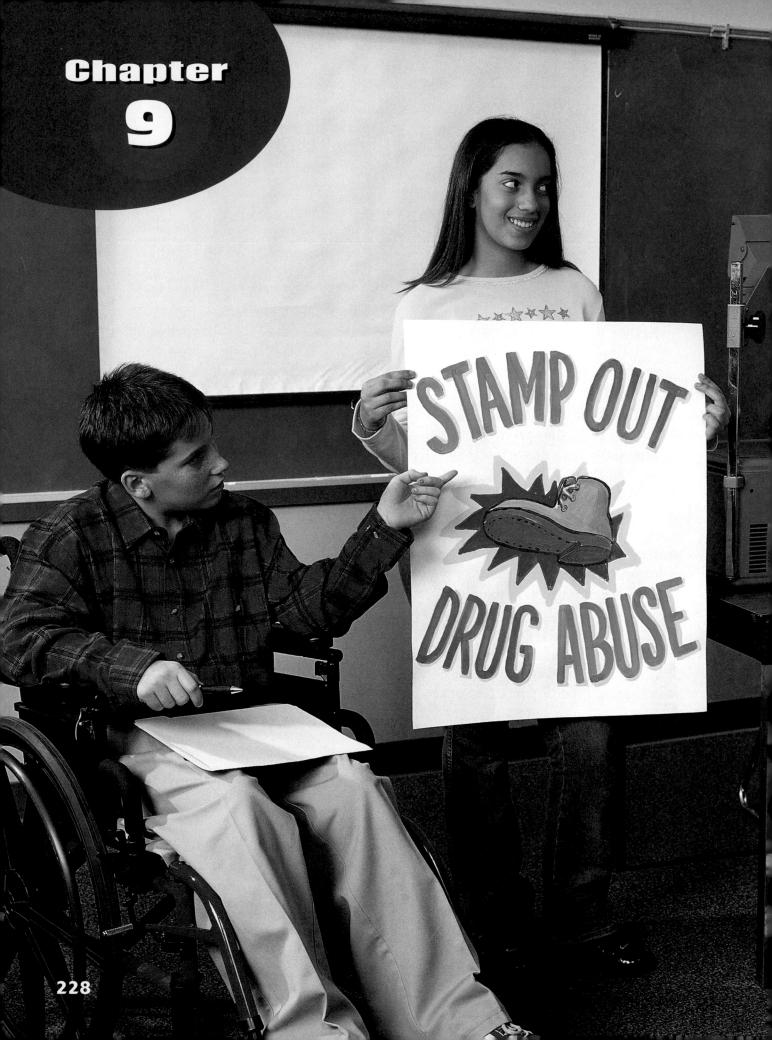

Alcohol and Other Drugs

Quick Write

How much do you know about the harmful effects of alcohol and other drugs? Begin a list of your responses. After you finish the chapter, expand your list using the new information you have learned.

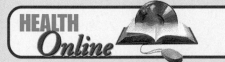

Rate your commitment to being alcohol and drug free. Go to health.glencoe.com and take the Chapter 9 Health Inventory.

✔ Reading Check

Write your own definition for the word *drug*. When you have finished reading the chapter, change or add to your definition if necessary.

Why Alcohol Is Harmful

Quick Write

Alcohol causes the brain and other parts of the body to work more slowly. List five ways in which drinking alcohol might affect a person's behavior.

LEARN ABOUT...

- how alcohol affects a person's physical and mental health.
- the short-term and long-term risks of using alcohol.
- why pregnant women should not drink alcohol.

VOCABULARY

- alcohol
- drug
- cirrhosis
- alcoholism
- fetal alcohol syndrome (FAS)

What Is Alcohol?

Alcohol (AL·kuh·hawl) is *a substance that is produced by a chemical reaction in some foods*. Alcohol is also a drug. A **drug** is *any substance that changes the structure or function of the body or mind*.

When a person drinks alcohol, it passes through the stomach and small intestine and moves into the bloodstream. When alcohol reaches the brain, it slows down the body's functions and reactions. See **Figure 9.1**.

Why Do Some Young People Drink?

In the United States, it is illegal for anyone under 21 years old to drink alcohol. Some teens break this law because they want to fit in with friends or family members who drink. They may think that drinking will make them seem more grown-up. Teens may also think drinking will help them escape their problems. However, drinking cannot solve problems—it creates new ones.

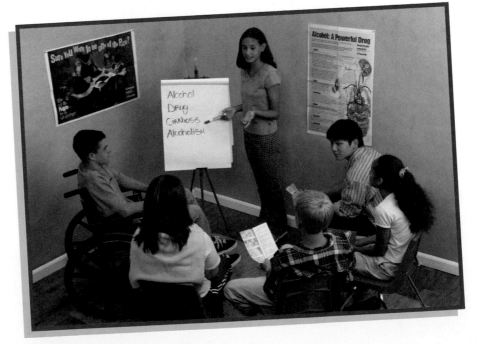

These teens are discussing the dangers of drinking. *Why is it important to stay alcohol free?*

FIGURE 9.1

HARMFUL EFFECTS OF ALCOHOL ON THE BODY

Alcohol affects many parts of the body.

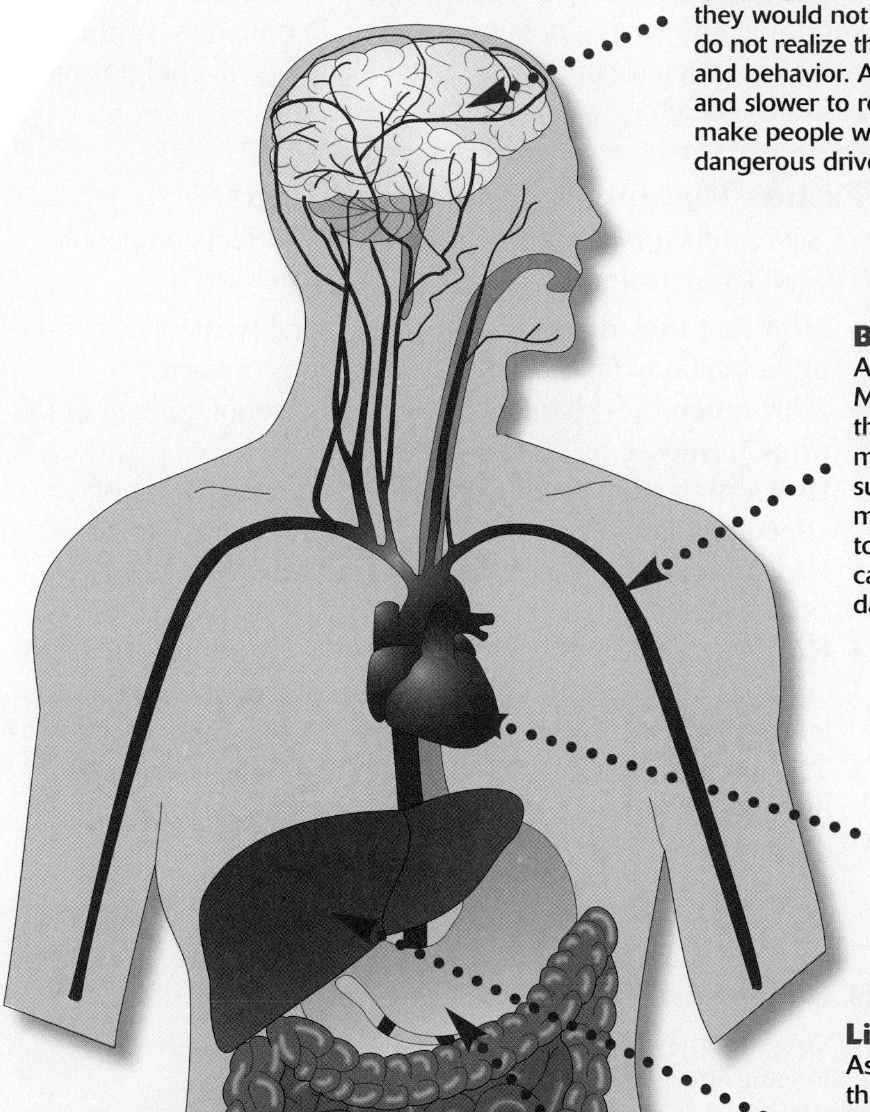

Brain
Alcohol slows down the way the brain works. When people drink, they have trouble thinking, speaking, and moving. They may say or do things they would not normally say or do. Drinkers often do not realize that alcohol has affected their thinking and behavior. Alcohol also makes a person clumsy and slower to react in an emergency. These effects make people who have been drinking very dangerous drivers.

Blood vessels
Alcohol expands the blood vessels. More blood passes through, making the drinker feel warmer. However, as more blood flows close to the body surface, the body loses heat. This may lead a person to stay outdoors too long in very cold weather, causing body temperature to fall dangerously low.

Heart
Heavy drinking can lead to high blood pressure and may damage the heart muscle.

Liver
As blood passes through the liver, this organ slowly breaks down any alcohol that is in the blood. Heavy drinking over a long period can damage the liver. It can cause hepatitis, liver cancer, or **cirrhosis** (suh·ROH·sis), which is *destruction and scarring of liver tissue*. Cirrhosis can lead to death.

Stomach
Heavy drinking can damage the lining of the stomach. Eventually, it can cause sores called ulcers.

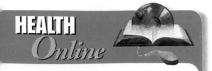
Alcohol's Short-Term and Long-Term Effects

Alcohol begins to affect the body soon after it is swallowed. The blood vessels expand and the heart rate increases. The drinker's reactions, behavior, and judgment are also affected. Drinking large amounts of alcohol in a short time can cause a condition known as alcohol poisoning. People may vomit, become unconscious, or have trouble breathing. Alcohol poisoning can cause death.

Factors That Influence Alcohol's Effects

Several factors can influence alcohol's effects on people. These factors include:

- **How fast they drink.** When drunk quickly, alcohol builds up in the body faster than the liver can process it.
- **How much they drink.** The size and alcohol content of the drink influence its effects. See **Figure 9.2**.
- **How much they weigh.** The same amount of alcohol affects a small person more than a larger one.
- **How much they have eaten.** Having an empty stomach causes alcohol to pass into the bloodstream more quickly.
- **How they feel.** A person's mood before drinking affects his or her mood after drinking. For example, depression may increase after drinking.
- **The use of other drugs.** Even medicines like aspirin may increase the effect of alcohol. Mixing alcohol with some drugs can be fatal.

FIGURE 9.2

ALCOHOL CONTENT IN DIFFERENT DRINKS

The three drinks here are different sizes, but they contain the same amount of alcohol and have the same effect on the brain and body. *How many ounces of beer would produce the same effect as 6 ounces of wine?*

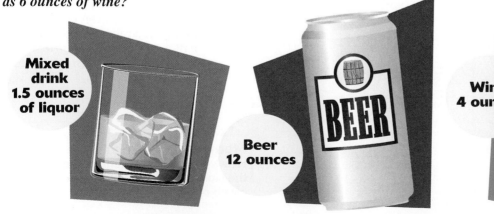
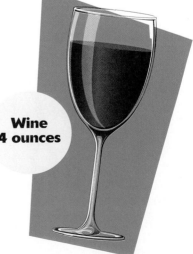

Mixed drink
1.5 ounces of liquor

Beer
12 ounces

Wine
4 ounces

Addiction and Alcoholism

Alcohol also has serious long-term effects. Not only does it damage the body, but it can lead to addiction. *The physical and mental need for alcohol* is a disease called **alcoholism**. People who have this illness are called alcoholics. Alcoholism cannot be cured, but it can be treated. The alcoholic must go through a process to remove the effects of alcohol from his or her body. Once that has happened, the alcoholic must never drink alcohol again.

Pregnancy and Alcohol

When a pregnant woman drinks, alcohol passes from her body into the bloodstream of her developing baby. This can lead to **fetal** (FEE·tuhl) **alcohol syndrome**, or **FAS**, *a group of permanent physical and mental problems caused by alcohol.* Babies with FAS often weigh less than average. They may suffer from birth defects and mental retardation. To make sure their babies do not develop FAS, women should avoid alcohol completely during pregnancy.

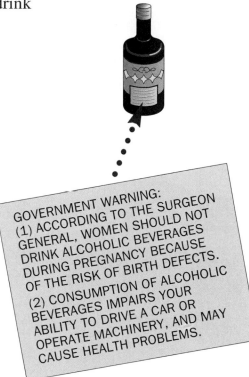

All alcoholic beverages must carry a label warning about the dangers of alcohol. *What does this label say about alcohol's short-term and long-term effects?*

GOVERNMENT WARNING: (1) ACCORDING TO THE SURGEON GENERAL, WOMEN SHOULD NOT DRINK ALCOHOLIC BEVERAGES DURING PREGNANCY BECAUSE OF THE RISK OF BIRTH DEFECTS. (2) CONSUMPTION OF ALCOHOLIC BEVERAGES IMPAIRS YOUR ABILITY TO DRIVE A CAR OR OPERATE MACHINERY, AND MAY CAUSE HEALTH PROBLEMS.

Lesson 1 Review

Using complete sentences, answer the following questions on a sheet of paper.

Reviewing Terms and Facts

1. **Vocabulary** Define the word *alcohol* and use it in an original sentence.
2. **Summarize** How does alcohol affect the brain, blood vessels, heart, liver, and stomach?
3. **List** Name four factors that influence the effect alcohol has on the body.
4. **Explain** Why is it unwise for pregnant women to drink alcohol?

Thinking Critically

5. **Explain** Why might a person who has been drinking think that the alcohol has not affected his or her ability to drive?
6. **Infer** In what ways might drinking affect a person's relationships?

Applying Health Skills

7. **Advocacy** Work with a partner to think of a slogan that would persuade young people not to drink. Put your slogan on a button or poster.

Quick Write

Write down a list of medicines you see advertised in television commercials. What symptoms or diseases do they treat?

LEARN ABOUT...

- how medicines help you when you're sick.
- why medicines have warning labels.
- how to use medicines safely.

VOCABULARY

- medicine
- prescription medicine
- over-the-counter (OTC) medicine
- antibiotic
- side effect
- tolerance
- drug misuse
- drug abuse

Using Medicines Responsibly

How Medicines Help Your Body

Medicines are *drugs that are used to cure or prevent diseases or other conditions.* There are two types of medicines. **Prescription** (pri·SKRIP·shuhn) **medicines** can be *sold only with a written order from a doctor.* **Over-the-counter (OTC) medicines** are *medicines available without a written order from a doctor.* Prescription medicines generally require a doctor's supervision because they have more risks than OTC medicines. However, this does not mean that OTC medicines are risk free. It is important to follow the directions on the medicine label. You should also pay attention to any warnings about when and how to use them.

Some medicines prevent disease. Others cure disease or relieve the symptoms of disease or injury. Still others are used to treat chronic conditions, such as heart disease or asthma. Some of the most widely used medicines are described below.

- Vaccines are medicines that protect you from certain diseases. You probably received vaccines for polio, measles, and other diseases during your infancy and childhood. Vaccines are also required before traveling to many foreign countries.

Vaccines are medicines that help to prevent disease. *What immunizations did you receive in the past year?*

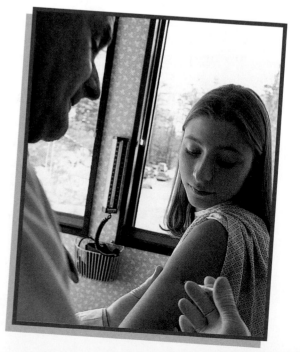

- **Antibiotics** (an·ti·by·AH·tiks) are *medicines that kill or stop the growth of certain germs.* Antibiotics can treat infections caused by bacteria, such as strep throat. However, they cannot cure illnesses caused by viruses, such as colds or the flu.
- Some medicines help control heartbeat, reduce high blood pressure, and open blocked blood vessels.
- Some medicines reduce pain, such as that from a headache, sore muscles, or a broken bone. Aspirin is one example.

How Medicines Affect the Body

All medicines can have powerful effects on your body and mind. Your reaction to a medicine depends on these factors:

- The type and amount of the medicine
- The way the medicine enters the body (see **Figure 9.3** on page 236)
- Your age, weight, and general health
- Other medicines you are taking
- Any allergies you have

Negative Reactions to Medicines

You may experience a reaction to some types of medicines. A **side effect** is *any reaction to a medicine other than the one intended.* Common side effects are drowsiness, dizziness, stomach upset, or a rash. Taking more than one medicine at a time can cause more dangerous side effects. It may greatly increase or decrease the effects of one or both medicines. It can also cause unexpected reactions. Always tell your doctor about all the medicines you are taking, including over-the-counter medicines.

If you take a medicine for a long time, you may develop a tolerance. **Tolerance** (TAHL·er·ence) is *a condition in which the body becomes used to the effects of a medicine and needs greater amounts to get the same effect.* If a medicine seems to have stopped working for you, ask your doctor or pharmacist about your options.

Read the label carefully when taking any type of medicine. *Why is it important to check the side effects of a medicine?*

FIGURE 9.3

HOW MEDICINES ENTER THE BODY

Common ways of taking medicines include direct application to the affected area, swallowing, inhaling, and injection. *Give examples of medicines that are used in each of these four ways.*

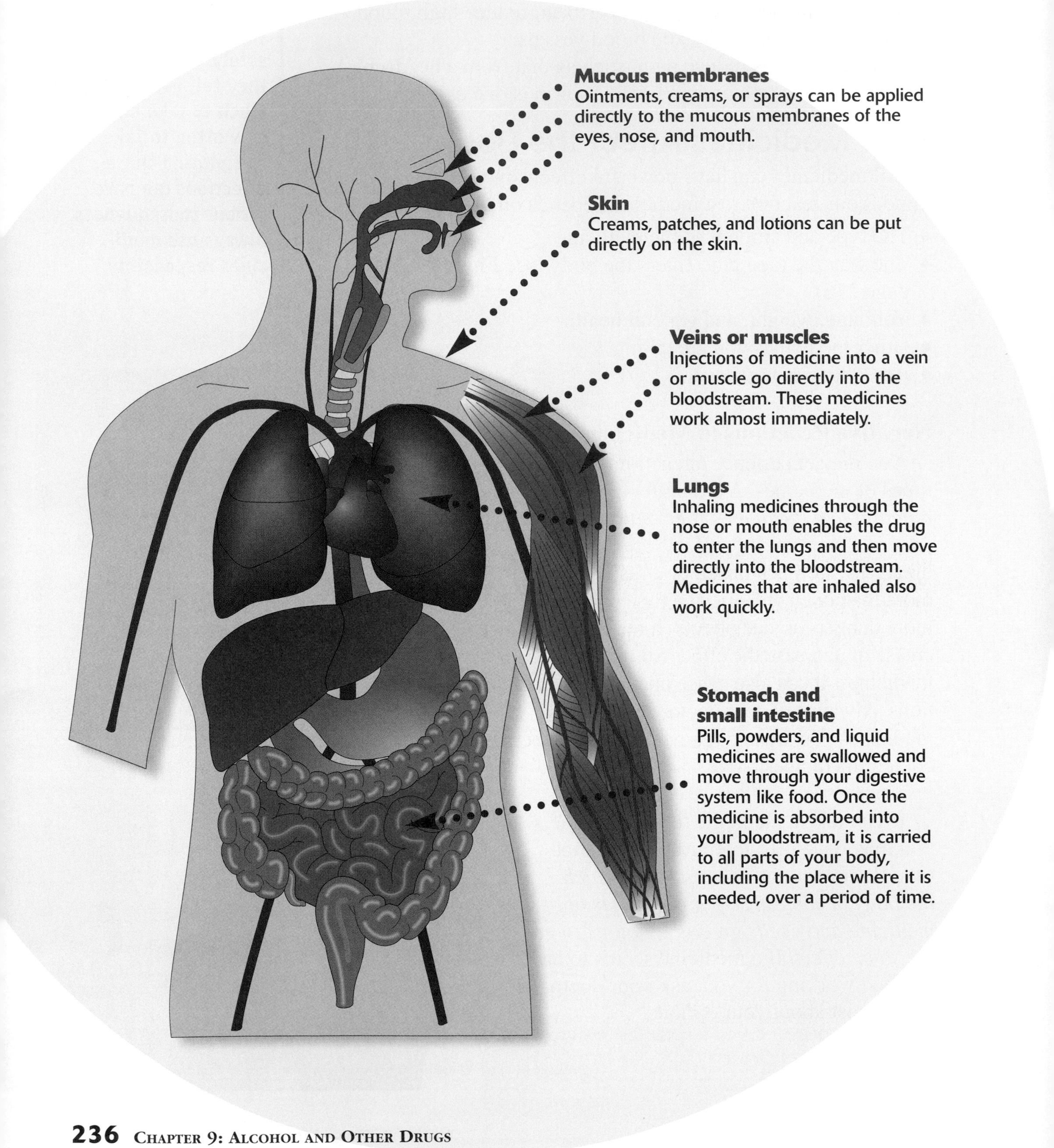

Mucous membranes
Ointments, creams, or sprays can be applied directly to the mucous membranes of the eyes, nose, and mouth.

Skin
Creams, patches, and lotions can be put directly on the skin.

Veins or muscles
Injections of medicine into a vein or muscle go directly into the bloodstream. These medicines work almost immediately.

Lungs
Inhaling medicines through the nose or mouth enables the drug to enter the lungs and then move directly into the bloodstream. Medicines that are inhaled also work quickly.

Stomach and small intestine
Pills, powders, and liquid medicines are swallowed and move through your digestive system like food. Once the medicine is absorbed into your bloodstream, it is carried to all parts of your body, including the place where it is needed, over a period of time.

Drug Safety

The Food and Drug Administration (FDA) is a government agency that reviews all medicines sold in the United States to make sure they are safe. It can often take several years to determine a medicine's long-term effects. The FDA then decides whether a medicine must be sold with a prescription or if it can be sold over the counter. Even medicines sold over the counter, however, are only safe when used as directed.

Reading Medicine Labels

The FDA requires drug manufacturers to put certain information on medicine labels. The label must tell how and when to take the medicine, how much to take, and special instructions for taking it. **Figure 9.4** is an example of a prescription label. **Figure 9.5** on page 238 is an example of a label on OTC medicine.

FIGURE 9.4

LABEL ON A PRESCRIPTION MEDICINE

Prescription medicine labels usually show the name of the doctor who prescribed the medicine. *Why is this information important to include on the label?*

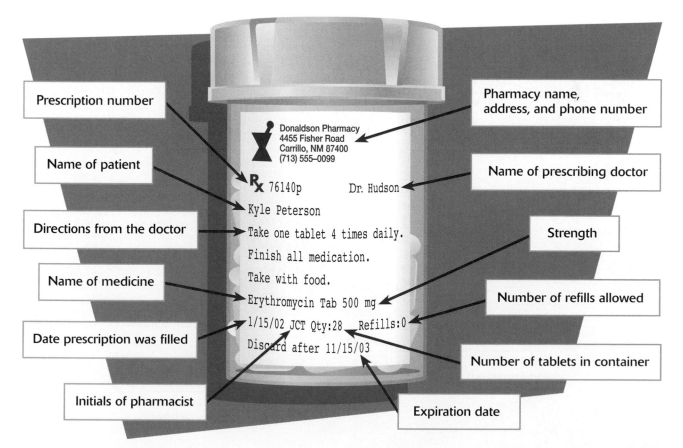

Prescription number

Name of patient

Directions from the doctor

Name of medicine

Date prescription was filled

Initials of pharmacist

Pharmacy name, address, and phone number

Name of prescribing doctor

Strength

Number of refills allowed

Number of tablets in container

Expiration date

Donaldson Pharmacy
4455 Fisher Road
Carrillo, NM 87400
(713) 555-0099

Rx 76140p   Dr. Hudson

Kyle Peterson

Take one tablet 4 times daily.

Finish all medication.

Take with food.

Erythromycin Tab 500 mg

1/15/02 JCT Qty:28   Refills:0

Discard after 11/15/03

Using Medicines Safely

Any drug that can do some good can also do some harm. For that reason, all medicines should be used with caution. To stay safe, follow these guidelines when taking any kind of medicine.

- Ask your doctor or pharmacist if you are not sure which OTC medicine to buy or how to use it.
- Take medicines only as directed on the label or as instructed by your doctor or pharmacist.
- Take medicines only for their intended purpose.
- If the medicine does not help you, talk with a parent or another adult. You may need to call your doctor.
- Parents should keep medicines in child-resistant containers and place them out of the reach of young children.
- Throw away all medicines after they pass their expiration dates.
- Finish all of the medicine prescribed by the doctor for bacterial infections.

FIGURE 9.5

LABEL ON AN OVER-THE-COUNTER MEDICINE

Labels on OTC medicines usually include instructions on how to take the drug safely. *Name three types of people who should not take the drug shown here.*

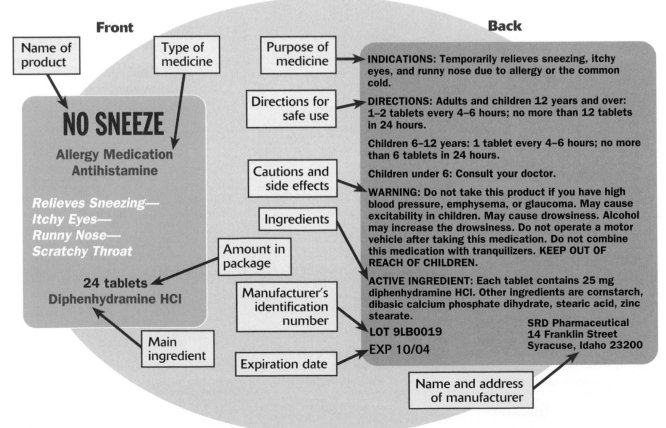

Front

Name of product

Type of medicine

NO SNEEZE

Allergy Medication
Antihistamine

*Relieves Sneezing—
Itchy Eyes—
Runny Nose—
Scratchy Throat*

24 tablets
Diphenhydramine HCl

Amount in package

Main ingredient

Back

Purpose of medicine

Directions for safe use

Cautions and side effects

Ingredients

Manufacturer's identification number

Expiration date

Name and address of manufacturer

INDICATIONS: Temporarily relieves sneezing, itchy eyes, and runny nose due to allergy or the common cold.

DIRECTIONS: Adults and children 12 years and over: 1–2 tablets every 4–6 hours; no more than 12 tablets in 24 hours.

Children 6–12 years: 1 tablet every 4–6 hours; no more than 6 tablets in 24 hours.

Children under 6: Consult your doctor.

WARNING: Do not take this product if you have high blood pressure, emphysema, or glaucoma. May cause excitability in children. May cause drowsiness. Alcohol may increase the drowsiness. Do not operate a motor vehicle after taking this medication. Do not combine this medication with tranquilizers. **KEEP OUT OF REACH OF CHILDREN.**

ACTIVE INGREDIENT: Each tablet contains 25 mg diphenhydramine HCl. Other ingredients are cornstarch, dibasic calcium phosphate dihydrate, stearic acid, zinc stearate.

LOT 9LB0019

EXP 10/04

**SRD Pharmaceutical
14 Franklin Street
Syracuse, Idaho 23200**

The Misuse and Abuse of Drugs

People can harm themselves if they misuse or abuse drugs. **Drug misuse** means *taking medicine in a way that is not intended*. Taking more or less medicine than the doctor instructed is an example of drug misuse. So is taking medication that was prescribed for someone else. **Drug abuse** (uh·BYOOS) means *using drugs in ways that are unhealthy or illegal*. See **Figure 9.6**.

FIGURE 9.6

EXAMPLES OF DRUG MISUSE AND ABUSE

All drugs can cause harm if misused or abused. Whom should you consult if you are not sure how to use a medicine?

Drug Misuse

- Taking a medicine for a shorter or longer time than prescribed
- Changing the amount of medicine taken without a doctor's approval
- Taking more than one medicine without approval from your doctor
- Using medicine that was prescribed for an earlier illness without a doctor's approval
- Using medicine prescribed for someone else

Drug Abuse

- Using a drug that is illegal
- Using a medicine for nonmedical purposes
- Swallowing or breathing a substance that was not meant to enter the body
- Using a drug in any way that is physically, mentally, or socially harmful

Lesson 2 Review

Using complete sentences, answer the following questions on a sheet of paper.

Reviewing Terms and Facts

1. **Vocabulary** Define *side effect* and use the term in an original sentence.
2. **List** What are five ways that medicines can enter the body?
3. **Recall** Which U.S. government agency helps ensure that medicines are safe?
4. **Contrast** What is the difference between misuse and abuse of drugs?

Thinking Critically

5. **Infer** Why might a doctor prescribe different medicines for two people with the same illness?

6. **Explain** Why might it take a long time for the FDA to approve a new medicine?

Applying Health Skills

7. **Accessing Information** Choose an over-the-counter medicine to research. Find out as much as you can about the medicine, including what it does, how it is taken, and what side effects it can have. Share your information with the class, and be prepared to explain why your sources are reliable.

What Are Illegal Drugs?

Quick Write

Write a list of physical, mental/emotional, and social problems that people might develop from using illegal drugs.

LEARN ABOUT...

- the dangers of illegal drugs.
- the main types of illegal drugs.

VOCABULARY

- withdrawal
- stimulant
- depressant
- narcotic
- hallucinogen
- inhalant
- marijuana
- anabolic steroids

The Dangers of Drug Abuse

Any use of illegal drugs, as well as the abuse of legal medicines, can seriously harm the user and even cause death. Sometimes these effects occur the first time the drug is used. Drug abuse damages relationships and harms performance in school or at work. People who use illegal drugs may also get into trouble with the law, ruining their future plans.

Drug abuse often leads to addiction. Addicts have a psychological and physical need, or dependence, for the substance they are abusing. Ending a drug dependence is a difficult and painful process. The user must remove all traces of the drug from the body. This causes **withdrawal**, *a series of mental and physical symptoms that occur when a person stops using an addictive substance.* These symptoms may include headaches, chills, vomiting, memory loss, hallucinations, and severe anxiety. Because withdrawal can be dangerous, this process should be medically supervised. After the drug has been removed from their bodies, users must deal with their psychological dependence by learning to control their cravings.

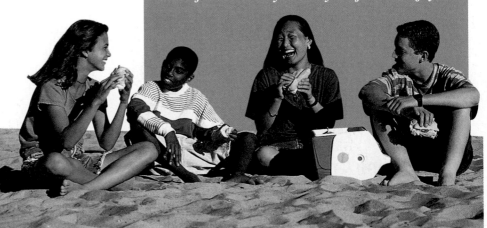

Teens who value their health avoid tobacco, alcohol, and other drugs. *What are some healthful activities you and your friends enjoy?*

Stimulants

Stimulants (STIM·yuh·luhnts) are *drugs that speed up the body's functions*. They cause blood pressure to rise, the heart to beat faster, breathing rate to increase, and the pupils of the eyes to dilate. Stimulants may be swallowed, smoked, inhaled, or injected. Amphetamines (am·FE·tuh·meenz) and cocaine (koh·KAYN) are two types of stimulants. Both are highly addictive and very dangerous.

Amphetamines

Amphetamines are sometimes called *uppers* or *speed*. Doctors may prescribe them to treat obesity, sleep disorders, or attention disorders in children. All other uses are illegal.

Any use of amphetamines can have dangerous side effects. These include

- headaches.
- blurred vision.
- dizziness.
- restlessness.
- anxiety.

At high doses, the drugs can cause more severe side effects, such as

- loss of coordination.
- irregular or rapid heartbeat.
- physical collapse.
- heart failure.

Long-term use of amphetamines can lead to severe mental problems. Injecting or inhaling amphetamines can cause blood pressure to rise quickly, leading to seizure and death.

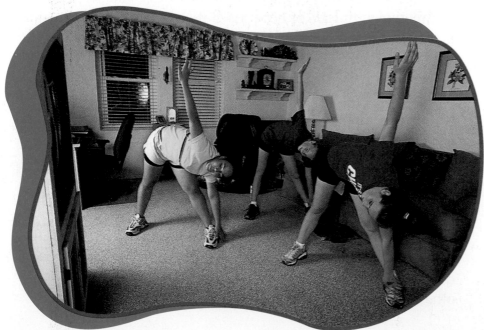

Responsible teens know that using illegal drugs is not a solution to the stress of everyday life. *How are these teens managing stress in a healthy way?*

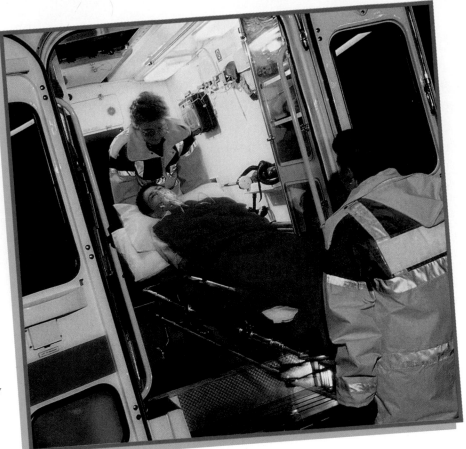

Cocaine and crack are very dangerous drugs. *Why is it risky to try these illegal drugs even once?*

Cocaine and Crack

Cocaine is an illegal stimulant drug that is highly addictive. Its effects are unpredictable and very dangerous. Even the first use of the drug can cause the user's blood pressure and heart rate to soar to levels that result in a fatal seizure or heart attack. Other dangers of cocaine use include

- sleeplessness, loss of appetite, nervousness, and suspicion.
- infection with HIV or hepatitis B if cocaine is injected.
- serious or fatal burns from preparing crack or freebase, a form of cocaine that is smoked.

Depressants

Depressants are *drugs that slow down the body's functions and reactions.* They cause heart rate and blood pressure to drop. Breathing and brain activity also slow down. Alcohol is an example of a depressant. The two other main types of depressants are barbiturates and tranquilizers. A doctor may prescribe them to reduce anxiety and help people sleep. However, they are highly addictive. The dangers of depressant use include lack of coordination, slurred speech, drowsiness, poor judgment, confusion, and addiction. When combined with alcohol or other drugs, they can be deadly.

Narcotics

Narcotics (nar·KAH·tics) are *certain drugs that relieve pain.* They include morphine, codeine, and heroin. Doctors may prescribe morphine to reduce severe pain. For example, it may be used after surgery or serious injury. Some prescription cough syrups and painkillers contain codeine. Legal narcotics are strongly addictive and must be used very carefully.

Heroin is very dangerous and has no legal uses. Heroin users risk unconsciousness or death. People who inject heroin also risk HIV infection from shared needles.

Hallucinogens

Hallucinogens (huh·LOO·suhn·uh·jenz) are *illegal drugs that cause the user's brain to distort images and to see and hear things that aren't real.* In other words, these drugs cause hallucinations. Users often behave strangely or violently. PCP (angel dust) and LSD (acid) are two very dangerous hallucinogens.

People who use PCP or LSD often think they have super strength. They may try dangerous acts that can lead to death. People who use these drugs sometimes have delayed effects, called flashbacks, long after they stop using the drugs. The person has no control over when a flashback could occur.

Another hallucinogen, called MDMA or Ecstasy, is also a stimulant. Users may experience confusion, depression, and nausea. Continued use can result in permanent brain damage.

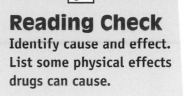

Reading Check
Identify cause and effect. List some physical effects drugs can cause.

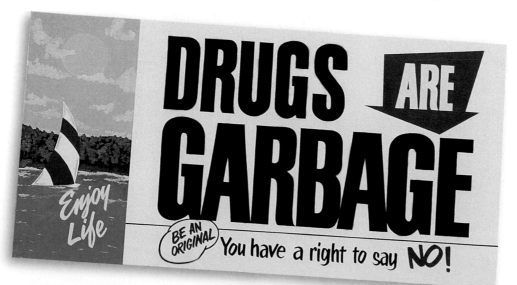

This antidrug ad appeared on the back of a garbage truck. *Do you think the ad is effective?*

Inhalants

Inhalants (in·HAY·luhnts) are *substances whose fumes are inhaled to produce hallucinations.* Most inhalants are common household products not meant to be taken into the body. If swallowed, these would commonly cause death. When inhaled, they can fill the lungs and suffocate the user. They also kill brain cells, causing permanent brain damage or a comatose condition. This can happen with the *first* usage.

Marijuana

Marijuana (mar·uh·WAHN·uh) is *an illegal drug that comes from the hemp plant.* Marijuana is also known as pot or grass. It increases heart rate and may cause panic attacks. It also interferes with concentration and memory. People who use marijuana may lack energy. They often lose interest in activities they once enjoyed. Users lack coordination, injure themselves more often, and are unable to react well in emergencies. Long-term use may cause lasting damage to the brain. People who use marijuana may be more likely to try other, more dangerous drugs.

Hands-On Health

"SAY NO TO DRUGS" SKIT

What's the best way to refuse drugs? In this activity, you and your classmates will practice your refusal skills.

WHAT YOU WILL NEED
- one friend or classmate
- pencil and paper

WHAT YOU WILL DO
1. With your partner, list ways someone might try to persuade you to use a drug.
2. On a second sheet of paper, list ways to use your refusal skills with the items on your first list.
3. Review your lists. Select the three most persuasive reasons that you might encounter and your three best refusals.
4. Use these statements to create a skit to perform for your classmates. Ask them to evaluate your presentation.

IN CONCLUSION
1. Did your classmates find your refusal statements convincing?
2. If not, how could they be strengthened?

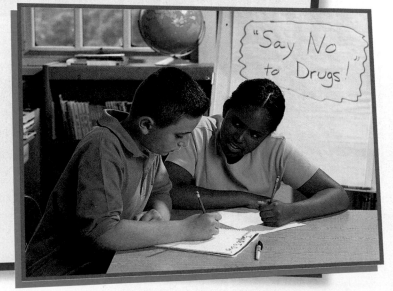

Anabolic Steroids

Anabolic steroids (a·nuh·BAH·lik STIR·oydz) are *synthetic drugs based on a male hormone.* Doctors sometimes prescribe steroids to treat certain medical conditions. Some athletes use steroids illegally to increase their body weight and strength. Steroids should never be used for this purpose. Users may become violent, aggressive, and deeply depressed. Steroids also cause severe acne, sexual underdevelopment in both males and females, liver and brain cancer, and heart attacks.

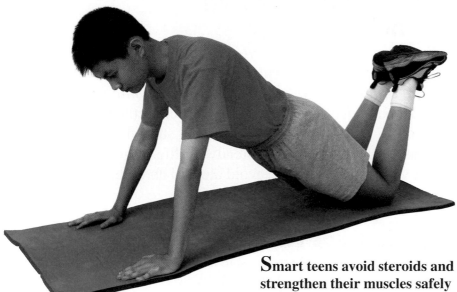

Smart teens avoid steroids and strengthen their muscles safely with strength-building exercises such as push-ups.

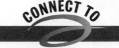

CONNECT TO
Social Studies

TESTING ATHLETES WORLDWIDE
To stop drug use among athletes, several countries have established independent agencies to manage the testing of athletes. The United States Anti-Doping Agency (USADA) and the Australian Sports Drug Agency (ASDA) are two such organizations. The World Anti-Doping Agency (WADA) coordinates antidrug programs on the international level. WADA's motto is "Think positive, test negative."

Lesson 3 Review

Using complete sentences, answer the following questions on a sheet of paper.

Reviewing Terms and Facts

1. **Explain** How are the terms dependence and withdrawal related?
2. **Recall** Which of the following drugs is not a stimulant: amphetamines, crack, or barbiturates?
3. **List** How can the use of inhalants cause injury or death?
4. **Identify** What are the harmful side effects of anabolic steroids?

Thinking Critically

5. **Apply** How would you reply if someone told you that using cocaine only once is harmless? Explain your answer.
6. **Predict** What do you think could happen to the schoolwork of someone who uses marijuana? Give reasons for your answer.

Applying Health Skills

7. **Advocacy** Create a TV commercial that highlights the dangers of one of the drugs discussed in this lesson. Be sure that your commercial provides information that persuades people to avoid the drug. Share your finished work with classmates.

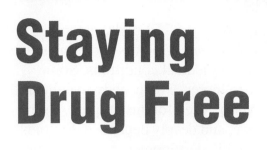

Staying Drug Free

Quick Write

What are the activities that you enjoy most? Write a paragraph explaining how the use of alcohol and other drugs could interfere with your favorite activities.

LEARN ABOUT...

- ways to avoid using alcohol and drugs.
- the laws about substance abuse.
- how families of substance abusers can find help.

VOCABULARY

- substance abuse
- alternative

Why You Should Avoid Alcohol and Drugs

Feeling good and looking your best during your teenage years means saying no to **substance abuse**—*use of illegal or harmful drugs, including any use of alcohol while under the legal drinking age.* Most young people across the nation are drug free . . . and proud of it! By staying substance free, you and they will stay healthy and ready for life. **Figure 9.7** shows you many reasons to avoid alcohol and other drugs.

FIGURE 9.7

REFUSAL MADE EASY

There are many good reasons to avoid alcohol and other drugs. *What other reasons can you add to the ones listed here?*

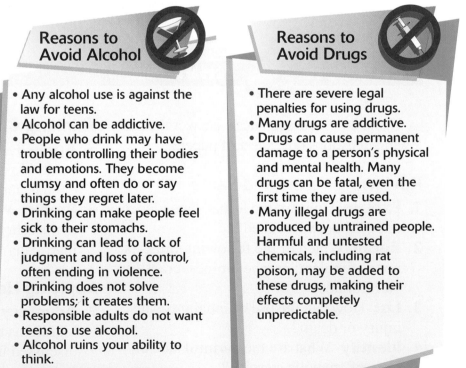

Reasons to Avoid Alcohol

- Any alcohol use is against the law for teens.
- Alcohol can be addictive.
- People who drink may have trouble controlling their bodies and emotions. They become clumsy and often do or say things they regret later.
- Drinking can make people feel sick to their stomachs.
- Drinking can lead to lack of judgment and loss of control, often ending in violence.
- Drinking does not solve problems; it creates them.
- Responsible adults do not want teens to use alcohol.
- Alcohol ruins your ability to think.
- You can have fun without consuming alcohol.

Reasons to Avoid Drugs

- There are severe legal penalties for using drugs.
- Many drugs are addictive.
- Drugs can cause permanent damage to a person's physical and mental health. Many drugs can be fatal, even the first time they are used.
- Many illegal drugs are produced by untrained people. Harmful and untested chemicals, including rat poison, may be added to these drugs, making their effects completely unpredictable.

The Law Is on Your Side

In all states, a person must be 21 years old to legally possess or purchase alcohol. In addition, many laws ban the use of dangerous drugs. Some drugs, such as morphine and codeine, are illegal except for certain medical uses. Drugs such as heroin, LSD, and crack are always illegal. Selling any of these drugs on the street or near schools is a crime with serious penalties.

Like other dangerous drugs, marijuana is illegal. The penalties for use and possession vary from state to state. Depending on where a person is caught and how much marijuana he or she has, a person can pay a large fine and serve lengthy jail time.

Ways to Stay Substance Free

Pressure to use alcohol and drugs may come from many sources. Advertisements and some peers may try to convince you that drinking and using drugs is cool. Pressure can also come from within. Some young people might think that they will fit in better if they drink or use drugs. Others might try alcohol or drugs to prove they are not afraid to do it.

The best way to refuse these harmful—and illegal— substances is to state your decision to yourself and others with confidence. You can also choose friends who are substance free. If someone persists in trying to persuade you to have a drink or use a drug, use one of the responses in **Figure 9.8**.

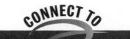

FIGURE 9.8

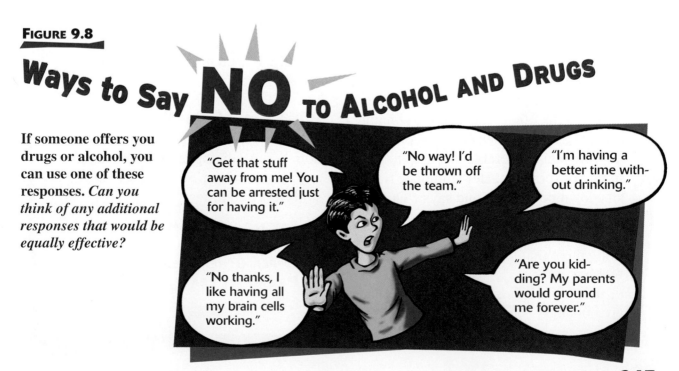

Ways to Say NO to Alcohol and Drugs

If someone offers you drugs or alcohol, you can use one of these responses. *Can you think of any additional responses that would be equally effective?*

"Get that stuff away from me! You can be arrested just for having it."

"No way! I'd be thrown off the team."

"I'm having a better time without drinking."

"No thanks, I like having all my brain cells working."

"Are you kidding? My parents would ground me forever."

Reading Check

Explore memory aids. How does S.T.O.P. help you remember the steps to the refusal process?

Alternatives to Drug and Alcohol Use

When you refuse drugs or alcohol, you may want to suggest a positive alternative. An **alternative** (ahl·TER·nuh·tihv) is *another way of thinking or acting*. If the person you are with wants to sneak a beer, you might suggest playing video games instead. Other healthy alternatives include the following:

- **Have fun at drug-free and alcohol-free events.** Asking questions about an event ahead of time can help you avoid situations where alcohol or other drugs are present.
- **Improve your talents.** Choose an activity you like and practice it until you become an expert. Become a great skateboarder, a computer whiz, or the best artist at school.
- **Be part of a group.** Join a sports team, a club, or a community group. A network of substance-free friends with a common interest will help you feel confident and supported.
- **Start your own business.** Let friends and neighbors know that you are available for baby-sitting, yard work, or other odd jobs. Post a sign advertising your business at the local supermarket or community center.

HEALTH SKILLS ACTIVITY

REFUSAL SKILLS

Say No and Mean It

Tammy loves soccer. She is thrilled to be a member of the school team this year. In her first game, she is too excited to concentrate. She loses control of the ball, and the other team scores, winning the game in the last seconds of play. Tammy feels miserable and tries to hide in the locker room. Her teammate Sara sits down next to her and says, "Don't worry about it. Why don't you come over to my house tonight? We'll have something there that's guaranteed to make you feel better."

Tammy is relieved that her teammates are not angry—until she arrives at Sara's house. Sara offers her a pill, saying, "Try it—you'll feel great." Tammy wants to be part of the team, but she doesn't want to use drugs.

What Would You Do?

Apply refusal skills to Tammy's situation. Write a dialogue between Tammy and Sara in which Tammy uses refusal skills to avoid drugs.

SAY NO IN A FIRM VOICE.
TELL WHY NOT.
OFFER OTHER IDEAS.
PROMPTLY LEAVE.

Help for Families of Substance Abusers

Drug and alcohol abuse doesn't just harm users. It also affects their friends and family. Several organizations provide help and support for people whose lives are affected by a loved one's addiction to alcohol or drugs. Local phone books can help people find these organizations. They include hospitals, substance abuse treatment centers, and special groups.

- Alateen helps children of alcoholic parents learn how to cope with problems at home.
- Al-Anon helps family members and friends of alcoholics learn more about the disease. They also discuss how to meet their own needs.
- Nar-Anon, similar to Al-Anon, holds meetings for families of drug addicts.

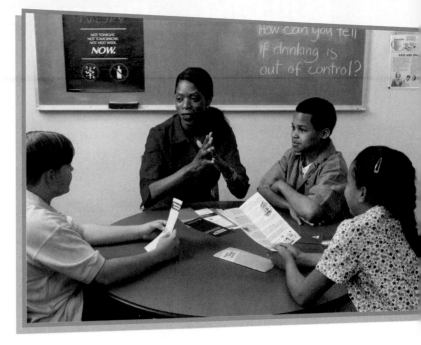

Many organizations can help families and friends of substance abusers. *Do you know where you would go for help if you needed it?*

Lesson 4 Review

Using complete sentences, answer the following questions on a sheet of paper.

Reviewing Terms and Facts

1. **Vocabulary** Define the term *substance abuse*. Use it in an original sentence.
2. **List** Name five reasons to avoid drug and alcohol use.
3. **Give examples** Describe one healthy alternative to using alcohol or other drugs.
4. **List** Name two organizations that help the families and friends of alcoholics and drug addicts.

Thinking Critically

5. **Analyze** Why do teens who are substance free have more fun than those who use alcohol and drugs?

6. **Apply** What would you say to a friend who is being pressured to use drugs?

Applying Health Skills

7. **Communication Skills** Work with a partner to write a skit about a teen who is worried about a family member's drinking problem. How would the teen express concern and persuade the family member to get help? Make sure you include effective communication skills in your skit. Perform your skit for the class.

HOW TO AVOID ALCOHOL

Model

Knowing about alcohol's negative effects on physical and mental health can help you decide to say no to alcohol. Read about a teen named Debra and her cousin Lisa.

Lisa's older sister, Tanya, and Tanya's boyfriend have taken the two girls to the beach. When lunchtime comes, Tanya and her boyfriend open up the picnic basket. It contains a six-pack of beer, but nothing else to drink. Debra is concerned and looks at Lisa, who also appears troubled.

1. STATE THE SITUATION.
"There's nothing here to drink but beer."

2. LIST THE OPTIONS.
"We could drink the beer, we could drink nothing until we get home, or we could walk down the beach and find a water fountain or a snack stand."

3. WEIGH THE POSSIBLE OUTCOMES.
"I don't like the smell of beer, and it could make me sick. If we walk down the beach, we will get tired and hot, and we still might not find anything else to drink. If we don't drink anything, we will get very thirsty and maybe get sick."

4. CONSIDER YOUR VALUES.
"It's not right for us to drink beer. It's against the law."

5. MAKE A DECISION AND ACT.
"Let's walk down the beach."

Practice

Read the following paragraph. What would you do in John's situation? Use your own paper to write the steps John could take to make a decision.

Nick used to be the star of the football team. This season, however, he is struggling—both on the football field and in the classroom. Last week, his friend John overheard some classmates saying that Nick had been drinking with some of the older kids in the neighborhood. When John asked Nick if that was true, Nick became angry and said he could handle his drinking.

Apply/Assess

As a class, brainstorm a list of ways a teen might be affected by someone else's use of alcohol. With a small group, choose one of these ideas and write a scenario about a teen who is in that situation. In the scenario, show how the teen uses the steps of the decision-making process to handle the situation.

COACH'S BOX

Decision Making

1. State the situation.
2. List the options.
3. Weigh the possible outcomes.
4. Consider your values.
5. Make a decision and act.
6. Evaluate the decision.

6. EVALUATE THE DECISION. "We found a snack stand and bought some bottled water. I feel good about our decision because we did the right thing and protected our health."

Self ✓ Check

- Did we state the situation clearly?
- Did the teen in our story use the steps for decision making?

GO FOR THE GOAL

Model

As a teen, you probably have many goals for your future. Using drugs and alcohol can ruin your ability to reach your goals. As you read the conversation below, ask yourself what goal these three teens have and how their decision to avoid drugs and alcohol will help them reach their goal.

MARY: I'm so excited that we're all going to the state math tournament. This trip is going to be so much fun!

RYAN: Did you hear what happened last year on the trip?

SCOTT: No, what?

RYAN: A boy got caught using drugs. He was kicked out of the tournament, and he got suspended from school for a month. He was cut from the baseball team, too.

SCOTT: That was a really stupid thing to do. Everybody knows how drugs can mess up your life.

MARY: I don't want anything to do with that stuff—or with anyone who uses it. I have too many important things to do in my life to let drugs ruin it.

RYAN: Right—like going to this tournament.

SCOTT: If we study hard, our team might win a prize!

Practice

Read the scenario below. Then, on your own paper, list the steps Patrick could take to reach his goal. For each of the five goal-setting steps, include information about how avoiding drugs and alcohol will help Patrick reach his goal.

Patrick knows that his school has a zero-tolerance policy for drugs, tobacco, and alcohol use. Anyone who wants to participate in any team or school organization must remain substance free. This spring, Patrick wants to play in the school band. If he even associates with teens who use illegal substances, he won't be able to participate in the band.

Apply/Assess

Think of at least three negative consequences of using alcohol or drugs. Write each of these consequences on a separate note card. For example, you might write "losing my parents' trust" or "being infected with HIV." Put your cards face down on your desk and mix them up.

Now think of one of your personal goals. On a sheet of paper, write out the goal-setting steps that you plan to use to reach this goal. Then, turn over one of your cards and read what it says. Explain how the consequence listed on the card would affect your ability to achieve your goal.

COACH'S BOX

Goal Setting

1. Set a specific goal.
2. List the steps to reach your goal.
3. Get help from others.
4. Evaluate your progress.
5. Reward yourself.

Self-✓Check

- Have I identified at least three negative consequences of using alcohol or drugs?
- Does my plan use the steps for goal setting?
- Did I explain how my goal would be affected by the use of alcohol or drugs?

getting kicked off the team

getting arrested

flunking out of school

SUMMARY

LESSON·1 Alcohol is a drug that slows down the body's functions and reactions. Alcohol affects many parts of the body, including the brain, blood vessels, heart, liver, and stomach. People can become addicted to alcohol.

LESSON·2 Medicines are drugs that cure or prevent disease. Two types of medicines are prescription and over-the-counter. Medicines can have unwanted side effects. Medicines and other drugs are sometimes misused and abused.

LESSON·3 Stimulants, depressants, narcotics, hallucinogens, marijuana, and steroids are frequently abused and can lead to addiction.

LESSON·4 Staying away from alcohol and drugs will keep you healthy and ready for life. There are many good reasons to avoid alcohol and drugs.

Reviewing Vocabulary and Concepts

On a sheet of paper, write the numbers 1–8. After each number, write the term from the list that best completes each sentence.

- alcoholism
- antibiotics
- cirrhosis
- drug
- fetal alcohol syndrome (FAS)
- over-the-counter
- prescription
- tolerance

Lesson 1

1. Alcohol is a(n) _____ that slows down the body's functions and reactions.
2. Heavy drinking can cause _____, or destruction and scarring of liver tissue.
3. _____ is a disease in which the drinker develops a physical and mental need for alcohol.
4. Drinking alcohol during pregnancy may cause a baby to be born with _____.

Lesson 2

5. A(n) _____ medicine can only be used with written permission from a doctor.
6. _____ medicines can be purchased without a written order from a doctor.
7. Doctors often prescribe _____ for illnesses that are caused by bacteria.
8. A person develops a(n) _____ when his or her body becomes used to the effects of a medicine.

Lesson 3

On a sheet of paper, write the numbers 9–13. Write *True* or *False* for each statement. If the statement is false, change the underlined word or phrase to make it true.

9. The sickness that occurs when a person stops using an addictive substance is called <u>withdrawal</u>.

10. Amphetamines are a type of <u>hallucinogen</u>.

11. Drugs that slow down the body's functions and reactions are called <u>narcotics</u>.

12. <u>Anabolic steroids</u> are a group of drugs that relieve pain.

13. Many <u>inhalants</u> are common household products.

Lesson 4

On a sheet of paper, write the numbers 14–16. After each number, write the letter of the answer that best completes each statement.

14. An example of substance abuse would be
    a. using illegal drugs.
    b. using any drugs that are not medically necessary.
    c. using alcohol if you are under the legal drinking age.
    d. any of the above.

15. Starting your own business is an example of
    a. substance abuse.
    b. addiction.
    c. an alternative to drug use.
    d. refusal skills.

16. The group that offers help to teens with alcoholic parents is called
    a. Alateen.
    b. Al-Anon.
    c. Nar-Anon.
    d. a hospital.

Thinking Critically

Using complete sentences, answer the following questions on a sheet of paper.

17. **Explain** Why is it important to read the labels on all medicines?

18. **Speculate** The penalties for selling illegal drugs are usually higher than the penalties for possessing them. Why do you think this is the case?

19. **Compare** What are the similarities between alcohol addiction and drug addiction?

20. **Hypothesize** Why might joining a group like Al-Anon or Nar-Anon make it easier to deal with another person's substance abuse?

Career Corner

Pharmacist

Your pharmacist helps you use medicines wisely. Pharmacists work in drugstores, clinics, and hospitals. Their job is to fill prescriptions written by doctors and dentists. They create the labels that explain how to use medicines properly. They also answer customers' questions. A person must spend at least four years in a pharmacy program to enter this career. To learn more about how pharmacists help people maintain their health, visit Career Corner at health.glencoe.com.

Chapter 10

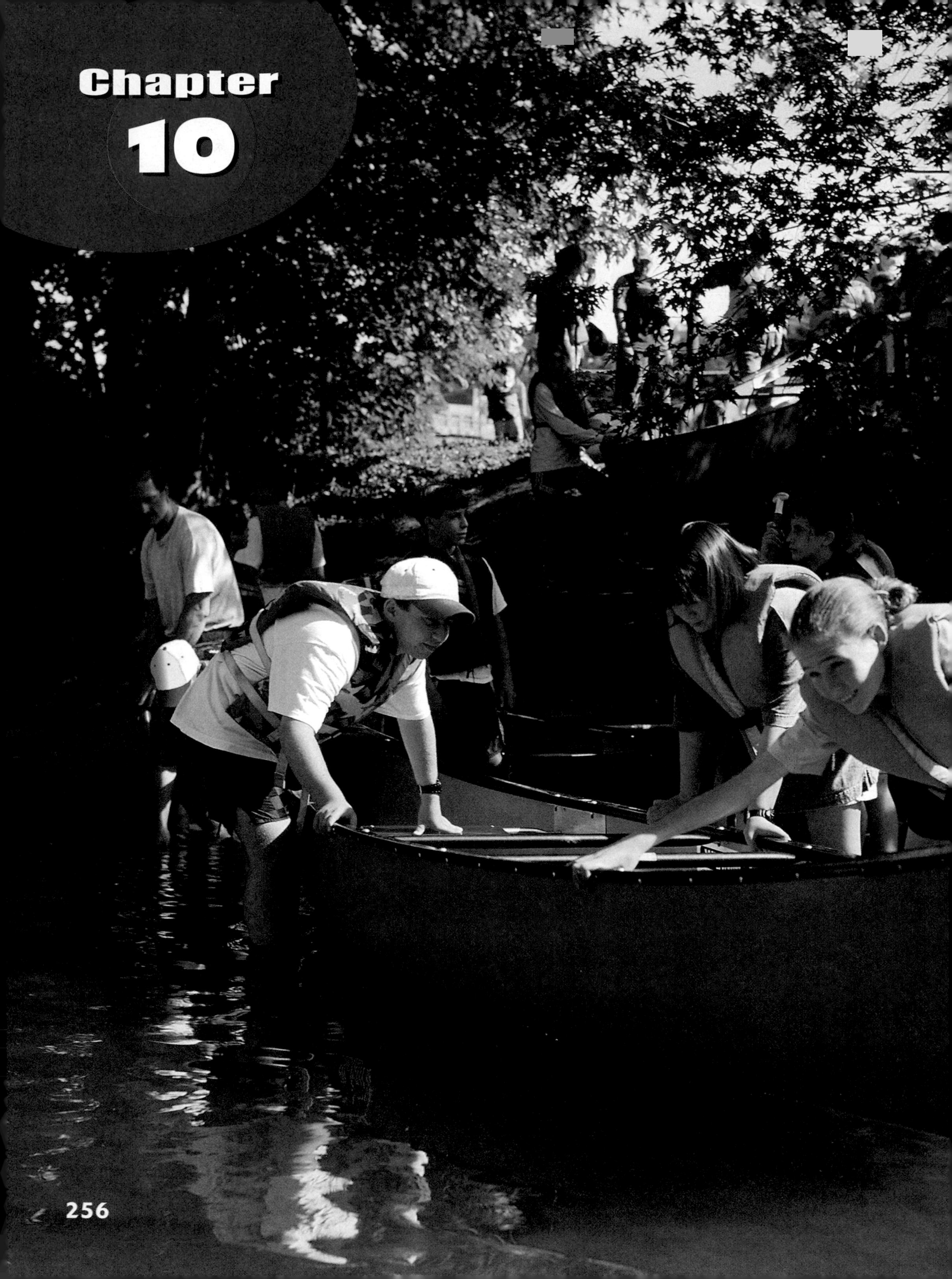

Safety and the Environment

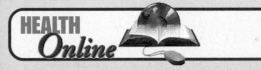

Personal Safety

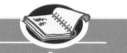

Quick Write

Describe how an injury you've had could have been prevented. Explain whether you think you could have avoided the injury and, if so, how.

LEARN ABOUT...

○ why it is important to make safety a habit.
○ what causes injuries.
○ how you can prevent unintentional injuries.

VOCABULARY

○ injury
○ unintentional injury
○ accident chain

Building Safe Habits

Your health and safety depend on practicing good safety habits. This means protecting yourself from **injury**, or *physical damage or harm to the body.* Some injuries are intentional— that is, they are the result of violence, in which one person deliberately harms another. Others are **unintentional injuries**, or *injuries caused by unexpected events.*

Many common activities, such as riding a bicycle or cutting fruit with a sharp knife, carry a risk of injury. However, good safety habits can help reduce the risk of an injury. That includes being careful, thinking ahead, and taking precautions. Staying safe means

● **staying away from risky behaviors.** Make the decision to avoid activities that lead to injuries.
● **ignoring peer pressure.** Do not give in to friends who want to take careless chances.

FIGURE 10.1

THE ACCIDENT CHAIN

Unsafe habits can lead to unintentional injury. *How could Tina have avoided this accident?*

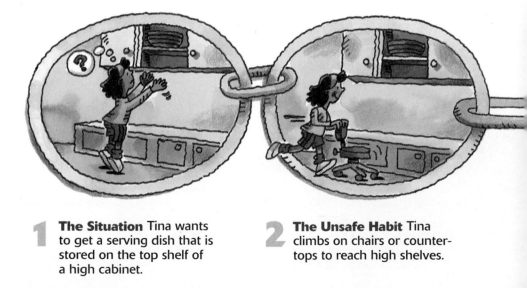

1 **The Situation** Tina wants to get a serving dish that is stored on the top shelf of a high cabinet.

2 **The Unsafe Habit** Tina climbs on chairs or countertops to reach high shelves.

- **thinking before you act and taking your time.** Being upset or excited can distract you and cause you to be careless.
- **knowing your limits.** Do not attempt to do more than you can do safely. For example, do not go into deep water if you do not know how to swim.

The Accident Chain

The unexpected events that cause unintentional injuries are known as accidents. Many accidents can be prevented. They often occur because of an **accident chain**, *a sequence of events that often leads to an unintentional injury.* **Figure 10.1** shows the accident chain in action.

Preventing Unintentional Injuries

Like most unintentional injuries, Tina's sprained wrist could have been prevented. She could have broken the accident chain by eliminating one of the first three links:

- **Change the situation.** If the dish had been on a lower shelf, Tina would not have had to climb up to reach it.
- **Change the unsafe habit.** Tina needs to break the unsafe habit of climbing on chairs and countertops.
- **Change the unsafe action.** Tina should always use a sturdy step stool to reach items on high shelves.

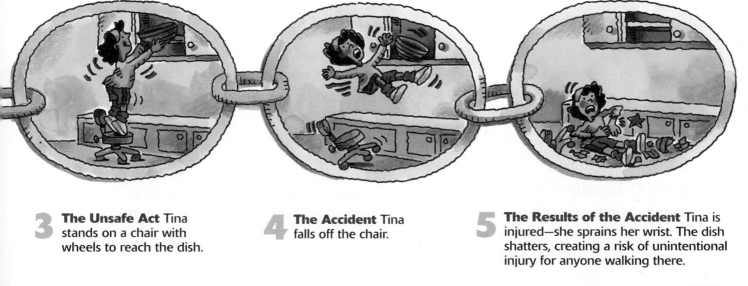

3 The Unsafe Act Tina stands on a chair with wheels to reach the dish.

4 The Accident Tina falls off the chair.

5 The Results of the Accident Tina is injured—she sprains her wrist. The dish shatters, creating a risk of unintentional injury for anyone walking there.

GOAL SETTING

Having Fun and Staying Safe

Soccer is Karen's favorite sport. Last season, she was injured twice. The first injury happened when she was late to practice. She didn't have time to warm up, so she strained a muscle in her leg. The second injury occurred because Karen forgot her soccer shoes. She wore her tennis sneakers instead, which caused her to slide into another player.

Karen's mom told her that if she keeps getting hurt, she won't be allowed to stay on the team. Karen knows she has to find a way to make it through this season without injuries.

What Would You Do?

Create a drawing representing the accident chain that led to one of Karen's injuries. Then show how she could use the steps for goal setting to avoid future injuries.

Finally, draw a new sequence that shows Karen breaking one or more of the links in the accident chain.

1. **SET A SPECIFIC GOAL.**
2. **LIST THE STEPS TO REACH YOUR GOAL.**
3. **GET HELP FROM OTHERS.**
4. **EVALUATE YOUR PROGRESS.**
5. **REWARD YOURSELF.**

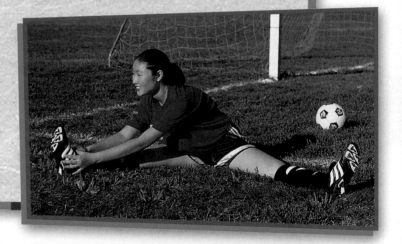

Lesson 1 Review

Using complete sentences, answer the following questions on a sheet of paper.

Reviewing Terms and Facts

1. **Vocabulary** What is an *unintentional injury?*
2. **Recall** List three basic guidelines that can help you avoid unintentional injuries.
3. **Describe** Define the *accident chain* and explain how it can be broken.

Thinking Critically

4. **Explain** Name an activity that carries a risk of unintentional injury. Explain why you think it is wise to know your limitations in that particular activity.
5. **Apply** Give an example of a situation in which peer pressure could lead someone to act unsafely. Explain how you would resist peer pressure in that situation.

Applying Health Skills

6. **Practicing Healthful Behaviors** Draw your own example of an accident chain and label each part. Exchange drawings with a classmate. Analyze your classmate's chain and name three ways to break it.

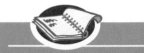
Safety at Home and Away

Safety in the Home

You probably think of your home as a comfortable, safe, and friendly place. However, most homes also have some **hazards**, or *possible sources of harm.* Following safety rules can help prevent injuries from home hazards. **Figure 10.2** on the next page shows some of the ways to make your home safer.

- **Preventing falls.** One goal of home safety is to prevent falls. Keep objects off the floor, where someone might trip over them. Always be sure rugs are fastened firmly to the floor and avoid running on wet or waxed floors. Keep a sturdy step stool around for reaching items on high shelves.

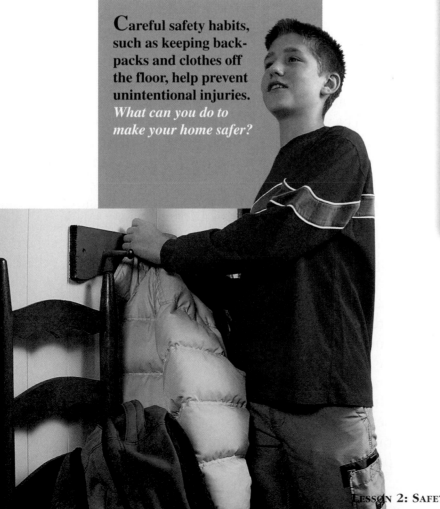

Careful safety habits, such as keeping backpacks and clothes off the floor, help prevent unintentional injuries. *What can you do to make your home safer?*

Quick Write

List two or three safety rules you follow on your way to and from school.

LEARN ABOUT...

- how to prevent unintentional injuries in your home.
- safety tips for traveling to and from your home.
- how to be safe in your school and community.

VOCABULARY

- hazard
- smoke alarm
- pedestrian
- Neighborhood Watch program

FIGURE 10.2
MAKING YOUR HOME SAFE

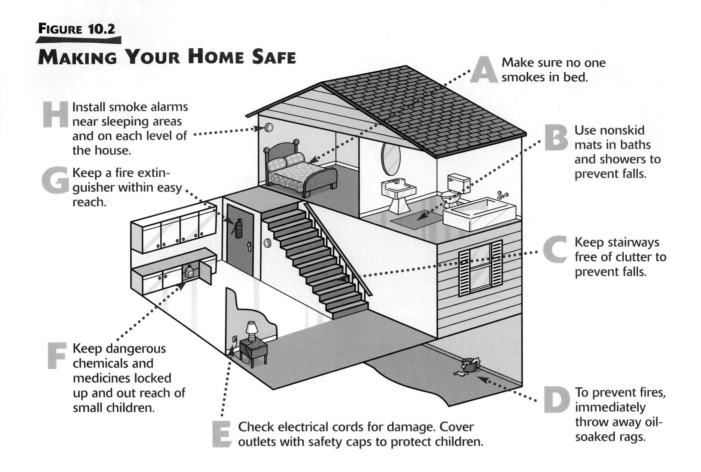

A Make sure no one smokes in bed.

H Install smoke alarms near sleeping areas and on each level of the house.

G Keep a fire extinguisher within easy reach.

B Use nonskid mats in baths and showers to prevent falls.

C Keep stairways free of clutter to prevent falls.

F Keep dangerous chemicals and medicines locked up and out reach of small children.

D To prevent fires, immediately throw away oil-soaked rags.

E Check electrical cords for damage. Cover outlets with safety caps to protect children.

Reading Check

Analyze word parts. Divide the words *bicycle* and *pedestrian* into parts. What do the parts tell you about the meanings of the words?

- **Electrical safety.** To avoid electrical hazards, always pull plugs out by the plug itself, not by the cord. Don't use appliances with damaged cords. In homes with small children, cover unused outlets. Keep electrical products away from water, and never use them if your skin is wet or if you are in a bathtub.

- **Fire safety.** Don't leave food cooking on the stove unattended. Turn pot handles inward, away from the edge. Keep small children away from the stove, and always put matches and cigarette lighters out of reach. In case a fire does occur, each level of the house should have a **smoke alarm**, *a device that makes a warning noise when it senses smoke.* Smother grease fires with a lid or baking soda, never with water. If your clothes catch fire, *stop, drop, and roll.* First, *stop* moving; if you run, the rush of air will fan the flames. Then *drop* to the floor and *roll* to smother the flames.

- **Gun safety.** If guns are kept in the home, they must always be stored in locked cabinets. Bullets should be stored separately. Never handle a gun without adult supervision. Never point a gun at a person.

Safety on the Road

You may encounter hazards on your way to and from home. Somctimes you will be a **pedestrian**, or *a person who travels on foot*. You may also be riding in a car, riding a bicycle, or skating. **Figure 10.3** shows how pedestrians and other travelers can share the road with drivers. Here are some other safety tips:

- **Use proper safety equipment.** Always wear a helmet. When using a skateboard, in-line skates, or a scooter, wear proper pads and gloves. Don't skate or ride a scooter after dark.
- **Dress appropriately**. Wear flat-soled shoes for riding a scooter. When cycling, wear clothes that won't catch in the bicycle chain.
- **Know where to ride.** Don't skate in traffic or in crowded pedestrian areas. Avoid wet, dirty, or uneven surfaces. On a bike, ride with traffic, single file, and obey traffic signals.
- **Be aware of others.** When cycling, check for cars before entering the traffic flow. Always watch for pedestrians.
- **Be visible to others.** Wear bright, reflective clothes. If you ride your bicycle at night, it should have lights and reflectors.
- **Ride carefully.** Keep your speed under control. Know how to stop. When skating, know how to fall properly.

FIGURE 10.3

Sharing the Road

Pedestrians, bicyclists, and drivers must share the road safely. Follow these basic safety rules.

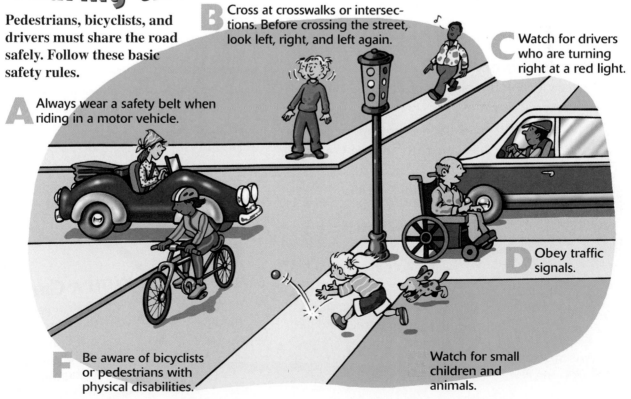

B Cross at crosswalks or intersections. Before crossing the street, look left, right, and left again.

C Watch for drivers who are turning right at a red light.

A Always wear a safety belt when riding in a motor vehicle.

D Obey traffic signals.

F Be aware of bicyclists or pedestrians with physical disabilities.

Watch for small children and animals.

Safety in Schools

Violence is a concern in some schools. Many schools are trying to reduce violence through measures such as:

- Peer mediation and crisis prevention programs.
- Violence prevention programs, which teach students to respect the feelings, opinions, and values of others.
- Counselors to talk to troubled students.
- Student assistance programs.
- Health education classes that teach conflict resolution.
- Police and security officers on campus.

Preventing Violence in Schools

Schools are also taking steps to eliminate guns and drugs, which can both contribute to violence. Some schools have removed lockers or added metal detectors to search for weapons. They may also use security guards, gun- and drug-sniffing dogs, or video cameras on school buses and school grounds. You can help, too. Tell your teacher or principal immediately if you know, or suspect, someone has a weapon or plans to cause trouble. It could save someone's life.

HEALTH SKILLS ACTIVITY

PRACTICING HEALTHFUL BEHAVIORS

Stranger Safety

To reduce your chances of being a victim, follow these safety rules:

- At home, do not open the door to anyone you don't know. Keep doors and windows locked. Never tell visitors or callers you are alone. Instead, say your parents are busy or can't come to the phone.
- If you are going out, tell your family your destination, route, and expected time of return.
- Never get into or go near a stranger's car. Never hitchhike.
- Do not enter a building with a stranger.
- Do not run errands or do other work for strangers.
- If someone tries to grab you, scream and run away. Go to the nearest place with people and ask them to call the police or your parents.

WITH A GROUP
Think of several situations that might be dangerous. Brainstorm safe responses to each situation.

Safety in Communities

To keep the streets safe, some communities have passed stricter laws against guns. They have also increased the punishments for violent crimes. In many areas, people have formed **Neighborhood Watch programs**. In these programs, *police train residents to look for and report suspicious activity in their neighborhood.* Communities may also try to protect teens by creating curfews, drug-free zones, and after-school and summer programs.

You can also help protect yourself. First, don't look like a target. Walk with purpose and confidence. Second, whenever possible, don't travel alone. Third, avoid unfamiliar areas and places that are known to be dangerous.

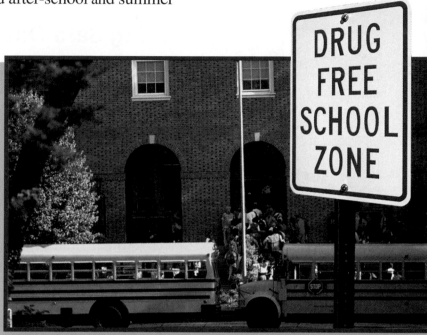

Many communities post signs such as this to keep the violence caused by drugs and drug dealers out of their area.

Lesson 2 Review

Using complete sentences, answer the following questions on a sheet of paper.

Reviewing Terms and Facts

1. **Vocabulary** What is meant by the term *hazard*?
2. **Recall** Describe four ways to protect your home from electrical hazards.
3. **Describe** How does a smoke alarm protect you in case of a fire?
4. **Give examples** State four ways communities can prevent violence.

Thinking Critically

5. **Hypothesize** Why is it important not to handle a gun without adult supervision?

6. **Explain** Why is obeying the rules of the road as important for bicyclists as it is for automobile drivers?
7. **Analyze** Why do you think teaching students to respect the feelings, opinions, and values of others can help prevent violence?

Applying Health Skills

8. **Advocacy** Be part of the solution to violence. Think of one way teens can help reduce the amount of violence in their school or community. Create a sign presenting your idea. Display the sign in the classroom or in the school hallway.

Safety Outdoors

Quick Write

List two or three things your family should do to prepare for storms or other weather emergencies common in your area.

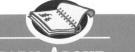

LEARN ABOUT...

- why you should use the buddy system.
- what you should know about water safety to prevent drowning.
- what tips you need to know for outdoor safety.
- how to be prepared for weather emergencies.

VOCABULARY

- hypothermia
- earthquake
- hurricane
- tornado

Being Safe Outdoors

It's always fun to enjoy the freedom of "the great outdoors." Outdoor fun can also be very healthful, as long as you follow some general safety rules.

- **Plan ahead.** Always make sure you have the right equipment and enough food and water.
- **Use the buddy system.** This is an agreement you have with one or more people to stay together.
- **Know your limits.** Be aware of your skills and abilities before you start an activity.
- **Use the proper equipment** for an activity.
- **Check the weather forecast.** Avoid extreme temperatures and electrical storms. Carry plenty of water and remember to wear sunscreen and other protection from the sun.
- **Warm up and cool down.** Warm up before exercising, and cool down afterward.

Knowing the rules and using the proper gear will make your outdoor activities safe and enjoyable. *What safety equipment are these teens using?*

Water and Boating Safety

Are you a fan of water activities? To avoid injury, you need to learn and follow water safety rules.

- Learn to swim well. Good swimmers are less likely to panic in an emergency.
- Never go in the water alone. Go to beaches or pools that have lifeguards, and always use the buddy system.
- If you ever feel you are in danger of drowning, stay calm. Call for help and use the technique in **Figure 10.4**.
- Use a pole, branch, rope, or life preserver to help someone in trouble. Don't go in the water yourself.
- Check water depth before diving. Never dive into shallow water or an aboveground pool. Take diving lessons.
- Wear a life jacket when boating. Be sure the boat is in good condition, and know how to operate it.
- Keep any boat steady to avoid falling in the water, which puts you at risk for **hypothermia** (hy·poh·THER·mee·uh), *a sudden and dangerous drop in body temperature.*

FIGURE 10.4

DROWNING PREVENTION

The technique shown here can help you stay afloat in warm water. In cold water, it is better to tread water slowly or float on your back to save energy.

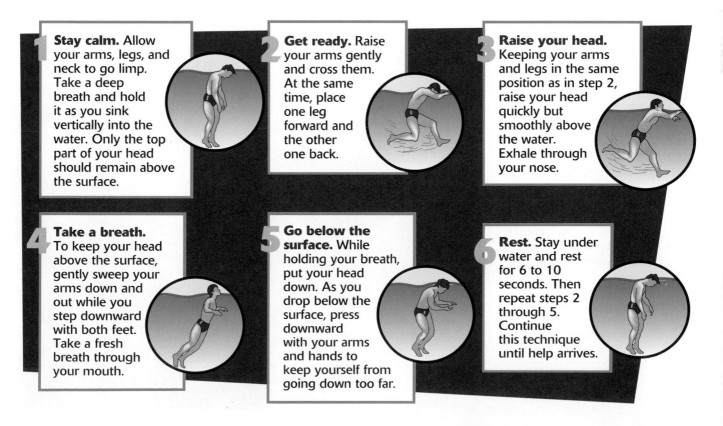

1 Stay calm. Allow your arms, legs, and neck to go limp. Take a deep breath and hold it as you sink vertically into the water. Only the top part of your head should remain above the surface.

2 Get ready. Raise your arms gently and cross them. At the same time, place one leg forward and the other one back.

3 Raise your head. Keeping your arms and legs in the same position as in step 2, raise your head quickly but smoothly above the water. Exhale through your nose.

4 Take a breath. To keep your head above the surface, gently sweep your arms down and out while you step downward with both feet. Take a fresh breath through your mouth.

5 Go below the surface. While holding your breath, put your head down. As you drop below the surface, press downward with your arms and hands to keep yourself from going down too far.

6 Rest. Stay under water and rest for 6 to 10 seconds. Then repeat steps 2 through 5. Continue this technique until help arrives.

Reading Check

Create your own chart about outdoor safety. Include information about Who, What, When, Where, Why, and How.

Hiking and Camping

You can make a hiking or camping trip safer and more fun if you bring the right clothing and equipment. For hiking, you need sturdy, well-cushioned shoes. You should break new shoes in for a few days before wearing them on the trail. If possible, layering two pairs of socks in your shoes can help prevent blisters. You should also wear clothing appropriate for the weather and the season.

When you go camping, make sure someone knows where you are going and when you plan to return. Carrying a cellular phone or walkie-talkie can help someone find you in an emergency. A compass and a flashlight (with extra batteries) will help prevent you from losing your way. You should also bring along plenty of fresh water and a first-aid kit in case of injuries. **Figure 10.5** shows some more steps you can take to stay safe while camping and hiking.

FIGURE 10.5

HIKING AND CAMPING SAFETY

These steps will help keep you safe while hiking or camping. *Why do you think you should not cook inside a tent?*

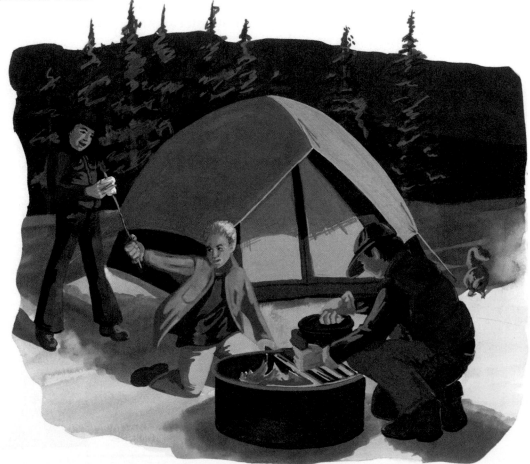

- Wear appropriate clothing to protect yourself from exposure to the sun and insects.
- Use proper equipment.
- Never camp alone.
- Stay in legal campsites and on marked trails.
- Learn which plants in the area are poisonous.
- Be aware of insects and animals you may encounter.
- Boil or filter stream or pond water before drinking.
- Never cook inside a tent.
- Keep all campfires in a pit and put them out thoroughly.

Winter Sports

Winter sports, such as ice-skating, skiing, and snowboarding, require the same attention to safety as other outdoor activities. In addition, they require protection against snow and cold. To stay warm, dress in several layers of clothing with a windproof jacket as the outermost layer. Layered clothing will trap warm air next to your body. Always wear a hat and gloves. Complete your outfit with a ski mask or scarf to protect your face.

Winter sports require appropriate clothing to protect against snow and cold temperatures.

Before starting a winter sport, check out your location. Be sure that ice is solid before you skate on it. There may be a "thin ice" sign or a red flag posted if the ice is too thin. You should have a clear path before you go downhill skiing or sledding. Ski only in approved, supervised areas.

If the weather is extremely cold, take extra measures to prevent frostbite (the freezing of the skin) and hypothermia. Gloves, boots, and extra socks help protect your hands and feet. If hypothermia or frostbite occurs, treat it at once by taking the person indoors. For hypothermia, cover the person with a blanket. Thaw frostbitten skin by soaking in warm, not hot, water for at least 30 minutes. Get medical help at a ski lodge or from a doctor as soon as possible.

Weather Emergencies

To be safe outdoors, you need to know what to do during unexpected events, such as storms. Being prepared will reduce risks and help you stay safe.

Floods

Floods, the most common of all natural disasters, can occur in all areas. During heavy rains, tune in to local radio or television stations for reports of rising water levels. Never walk or ride in a car through floodwater. You risk being swept away. Downed power lines pose a danger, too. Floodwaters often pollute tap water, so you should drink bottled water. After the flood, clean and disinfect everything that came in contact with the floodwater. Discard all contaminated food. Wear rubber or latex gloves during the cleanup. Make sure the water supply is safe before drinking any.

HEALTH SKILLS ACTIVITY

ACCESSING INFORMATION

Stay Tuned in an Emergency

Different kinds of weather emergencies occur in different areas of our country. Blizzards occur in cold climates. Hurricanes tend to strike on the southern and eastern coasts of the United States. Tornadoes tend to strike flat land areas. The National Weather Service (NWS) keeps an eye on the weather across the entire nation. It warns people when dangerous weather may be headed their way. Here are some facts about the NWS warning system:

- An *advisory* is for weather conditions that may pose a problem. People in the area are not in immediate danger. However, they should be careful.
- A *watch* is stronger than an advisory. It means that dangerous weather is possible. However, the emergency may not occur.
- The NWS issues a *warning* when dangerous weather is expected. People should find safe shelter right away.

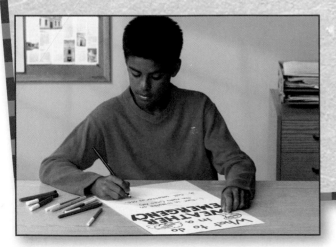

ON YOUR OWN

Find out how to get information during a weather emergency. Start by learning which local TV and radio stations broadcast updates in an emergency. You can also use the NWS Web site. Make a chart that shows how to find up-to-date information in an emergency. Post your chart in your home.

Earthquakes

An **earthquake** is *the shaking of the ground as rock below the surface moves.* If you are inside when this natural disaster strikes, stay there. Brace yourself in a doorway or crawl under a piece of sturdy furniture. Move away from objects that could fall or shatter. If you are outside during an earthquake, stand in the open. Stay away from buildings, trees, and power lines. Afterward, report any odor of gas that might indicate a leak.

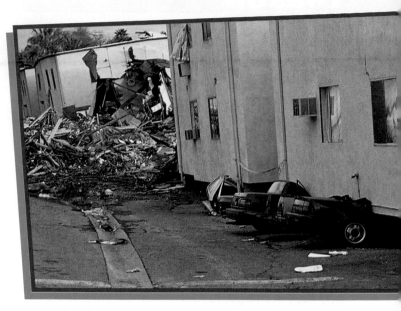

Hurricanes and Tornadoes

A **hurricane** (HER·uh·kayn) is *a strong tropical windstorm with driving rain.* If a hurricane is likely in your area, board up windows and bring in outdoor objects. Stay tuned to weather reports and be prepared to leave the area if necessary.

A **tornado** (tor·NAY·doh) is *a whirling, funnel-shaped windstorm that drops from the sky to the ground.* If a tornado warning is issued in your area, you should go to a storm cellar or basement. If you can't do that, go to a hallway, bathroom, or other inside area without windows. Don't stay in cars or mobile homes. If you are outdoors, try to find a ditch to lie in and cover yourself with a blanket or clothing.

Although natural disasters can strike with little warning, you can reduce your chances of injury by being prepared. *What safety precautions can you take during an earthquake?*

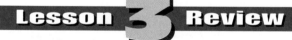

Lesson 3 Review

Using complete sentences, answer the following questions on a sheet of paper.

Reviewing Terms and Facts

1. **Recall** What is the first rule of water safety?
2. **Vocabulary** What is *hypothermia?*
3. **Give Examples** List four safety rules for hiking and camping.
4. **Distinguish** In the NWS warning system, what is the difference between a *watch* and a *warning?*

Thinking Critically

5. **Explain** What would you do if your "buddy" wanted to swim out farther than you thought you were able to swim safely?
6. **Apply** How would you protect yourself from frostbite if you wanted to go sledding with your friends?

Applying Health Skills

7. **Practicing Healthful Behaviors** Draw a layout of your home. On the sketch, indicate the best places to go for safety in the event of a tornado or an earthquake.

First Aid for Emergencies

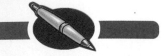
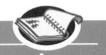
What Is First Aid?

Knowing what to do in emergencies is as important as preventing them. Taking the right steps to help an injured person can prevent further injury or even death. **First aid** is *the care first given to an injured or ill person until regular medical care can be supplied.* A person needs proper training to give first aid. **Figure 10.6** shows the first steps to take in an emergency.

FIGURE 10.6

WHAT TO DO IN AN EMERGENCY

In an emergency situation, you should follow the Red Cross guidelines, which can be remembered with the words "CHECK-CALL-CARE."

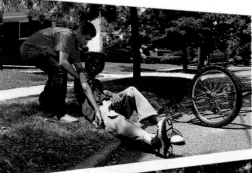

1 **CHECK the scene and the victim.** To avoid further injury, move the victim only if he or she is in danger. However, do not put your own life at risk to help the victim.

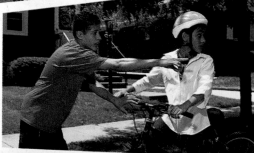

2 **CALL for help.** In most areas, you can dial 911 for Emergency Medical Services (EMS). If possible, stay with the victim and ask a passerby for help.

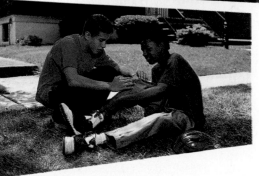

3 **CARE for the person until help arrives.** Use the first aid steps discussed in this lesson to treat the victim's injuries.

Basic Techniques

Some emergencies are life-threatening. For example, a victim's life is in danger if the person has stopped breathing, is bleeding severely, is choking, has swallowed poison, or has been severely burned. These victims often cannot wait for professional help to arrive. By learning a few basic techniques, you may be able to save a life.

If the victim's heart has stopped, medical professionals may perform **cardiopulmonary resuscitation (CPR)**. CPR is *a rescue measure that attempts to restore heartbeat and breathing.* Only people with special training should perform CPR.

Rescue Breathing

You can check for breathing by putting your ear and cheek close to the victim's nose and mouth. Listen and feel for air exhaled. Look to see if the chest is rising and falling. If the victim is not breathing, call for help immediately. Then perform **rescue breathing**, *a substitute for normal breathing in which someone forces air into the victim's lungs.* **Figure 10.7** shows how to perform rescue breathing on an adult. The process is different for infants and younger children.

FIGURE 10.7

RESCUE BREATHING FOR ADULTS AND OLDER CHILDREN

When a victim is not breathing, immediately call 911. Then begin rescue breathing if the person has a pulse.

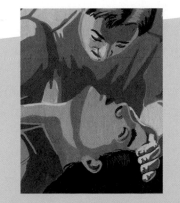

1. Point the victim's chin upward by gently lifting it up with your fingers and tilting the head back. The airway will now be open.

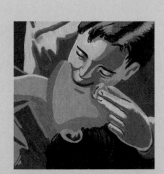

2. Pinch the victim's nostrils shut. Cover the victim's mouth with your own, forming a tight seal. Give two slow breaths each about 2 seconds long. Make sure the victim's chest rises during each breath.

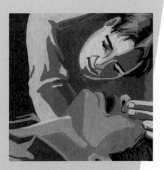

3. Watch for the victim's chest to fall and listen for air flowing from the lungs. If the victim begins breathing normally, stop. Otherwise, give one rescue breath every 5 seconds until help arrives.

FIGURE 10.8

LOCATION OF PRESSURE POINTS

The dots in this illustration are pressure points. Applying pressure to the nearest pressure point can help stop the flow of blood to a wounded area.

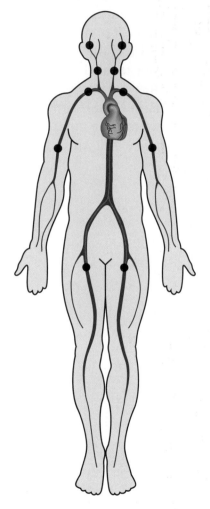

Bleeding

Nosebleeds, or sudden bleeding from one or both nostrils, are fairly common. Sitting upright and pinching your nostrils with your thumb and forefinger for 10 minutes will stop a common nosebleed.

A much more serious problem is severe bleeding due to injury. Treating bleeding is difficult because it can be dangerous to touch another person's blood. If possible, wear gloves. You can use the following first aid techniques for bleeding:

- Lay the victim down and try to elevate his or her legs to reduce the risk of fainting. If possible, carefully raise the wounded body part above the victim's heart. This technique slows the blood coming from the heart to the wound. Use it only if the body part has no broken bones.
- Apply direct, steady pressure to the wound. Press down firmly on the wound with a clean cloth. If necessary, add more cloth without removing the first cloth.
- At the same time, apply pressure to the main artery supplying blood to the wound. **Figure 10.8** shows several pressure points that can be used to stop bleeding. Push on the pressure point until you feel the bone, and hold the pressure.
- After the bleeding has stopped, cover the wound with a clean cloth to prevent infection. If the victim needs professional medical treatment, leave the bandages in place and get him or her to the emergency room as quickly as possible.

Choking

Choking is *a condition that occurs when a person's airway becomes blocked.* A choking victim can die in minutes because air cannot get to the lungs. The universal sign for choking—grabbing the throat between the thumb and forefinger—helps you recognize a choking victim. Victims may also gasp for breath or be unable to speak. Their faces may turn red, then bluish.

If an infant is choking, position the victim on his or her abdomen along your forearm, bracing your arm against your thigh. Support the infant's head with your hand, and point the head down. Then give up to five blows with the heel of your hand between the victim's shoulder blades. Sweep your finger through the victim's mouth and remove the dislodged object. If the object is still stuck, turn the victim on his or her back. Support the victim's shoulders and neck with one hand. With the other, place two fingers in the middle of the child's breast-bone and press quickly up to five times. Alternate five back blows and five chest thrusts until the object is dislodged.

To help an adult or older child, ask, "Are you choking?" If the victim nods or does not respond, you can help by using **abdominal thrusts**. Apply *quick upward pulls into the diaphragm to force out the object blocking the airway.* **Figure 10.9** illustrates this technique.

If you are choking and no one is there to help you, make a fist and thrust it quickly into your upper abdomen. This will force out the object blocking your airway. You can also try shoving your abdomen against the back or arm of a chair.

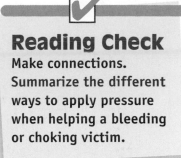

Reading Check
Make connections. Summarize the different ways to apply pressure when helping a bleeding or choking victim.

FIGURE 10.9

ABDOMINAL THRUSTS

Use these steps to help a victim who is choking. If the person can talk or cough, or you can hear breathing, don't do anything. *Why might it be dangerous to perform abdominal thrusts on a person who is not choking?*

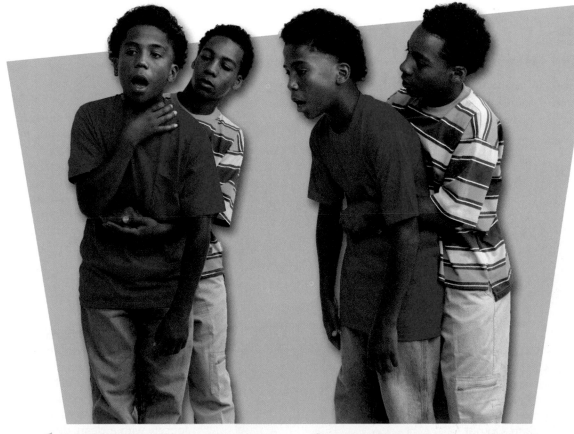

1 Stand behind the victim. Wrap your arms around his or her waist and bend victim slightly forward. Place your fist slightly above the person's navel.

2 Hold your fist with your other hand and press it hard into the abdomen with an upward thrust. Repeat until the object is coughed up.

Poisoning

If you think someone has swallowed poison, seek professional help. Call either 911, your doctor, or a **poison control center,** *a place that helps people deal with poisons.* The inside cover of your telephone book usually gives the number of the center. Follow the directions you receive.

Keep the person warm and breathing while you wait for an ambulance. Remove extra traces of poison from around the victim's mouth with a damp, clean cloth wrapped around your finger. Be sure to save the container of poison. Show it to the ambulance team. Tell them all you know about what happened.

Burns

Burns are identified by how much they damage the skin. Use **Figure 10.10** to help you identify the three types of burns. Note the differences in first aid treatment.

FIGURE 10.10

TYPES OF BURNS

Different kinds of burns require different treatments. *How would you treat a first-degree burn?*

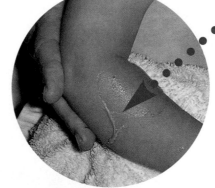

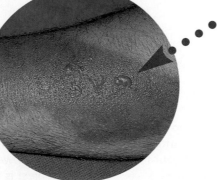

A **first-degree burn** is *a burn in which only the outer part of the skin is burned and turns red.* Cool the burned area with cold water for at least 15 minutes and wrap it loosely in a clean, dry dressing.

A **second-degree burn** is *a more serious type of burn in which the burned area blisters or peels.* Cool the burn in cold water (not ice) and elevate the burned area. Wrap loosely with a clean, dry dressing. Do not pop blisters or peel loose skin.

A **third-degree burn** is *a very serious burn in which deeper layers of skin and nerve endings are damaged.* Perform rescue breathing if necessary. Cover the burn with a cool, moist cloth. Do not apply water, ice, or ointments.

ACCESSING INFORMATION

Minor Injury Lookout

Minor unintentional injuries can occur in your own home or on outings. Some can be treated at home. Here are some tips for treating minor injuries.

- **Sprains.** A sprained joint, such as a wrist or ankle, is one that has been stretched or twisted or has torn ligaments. Treatment includes the R.I.C.E. procedure: Rest, Ice, Compression, and Elevation.

- **Bites and Stings.** These injuries can cause bumps and itching on the skin. The bites of some snakes, spiders, scorpions, and flying insects, however, can affect the entire body. For these, get immediate professional help.

- **Poisonous Plants.** Plants such as poison ivy, poison oak, and poison sumac can cause redness, itching, and swelling if your skin comes in contact with them. You can treat these symptoms with soap and water, rubbing alcohol, special creams, and calamine lotion. Severe cases require a doctor's care.

> **WITH A GROUP**
> Use the Internet and library resources to research one of these types of injuries further. Suggestions include recognizing poisonous plants or dangerous snakes found in your area. Make an illustrated poster and present it to the class.

Lesson 4 Review

Using complete sentences, answer the following questions on a sheet of paper.

Reviewing Terms and Facts

1. **Vocabulary** Define the term *first aid*. Use it in an original sentence.
2. **List** Name the three basic first-aid steps to follow in an emergency.
3. **Recall** How can you check to make sure a victim is breathing?
4. **Identify** Give the three methods used to control severe bleeding.
5. **Distinguish** What is the difference between a first-degree burn, a second-degree burn, and a third-degree burn?

Thinking Critically

6. **Compare and Contrast** How is the method used to help someone else who is choking similar to and different from the method used to help yourself if you are choking?
7. **Analyze** Why do you think it is important to save the container if someone has swallowed poison?

Applying Health Skills

8. **Advocacy** Work with a partner to create a first-aid handbook for baby-sitters. Include first aid for emergencies that may occur with young children, such as choking, bleeding, and swallowing poisons. Also include local emergency phone numbers. Share your handbook with the class.

Protecting Your Environment

Quick Write

Write a short essay describing one or more environmental threats you have observed.

LEARN ABOUT...

- the causes of air, water, and land pollution.
- what happens to garbage after it is thrown away.
- what you can do to protect the environment.

VOCABULARY

- environment
- pollution
- fossil fuel
- ozone
- smog
- acid rain
- recycling
- conservation
- biodegradable

Our Environment

Look around you. Everything you see, plus many other things you cannot see (such as the air), are part of your **environment** (en·VY·ruhn·ment). In fact, *you and all living and nonliving things around you* make up the environment. What types of things do you see in the environment? You see living things like people, plants, and animals. You see rivers, hills, and valleys. You also see schools, homes, and other things made by people.

Pollution

In order for you to remain healthy, you need to live in a healthy environment. Unfortunately, the way people live can damage the environment. **Pollution** (puh·LOO·shuhn) is *the changing of the air, water, and land from clean and safe to dirty and unsafe.* Pollution affects the air you breathe, the water you drink, and the land you live on.

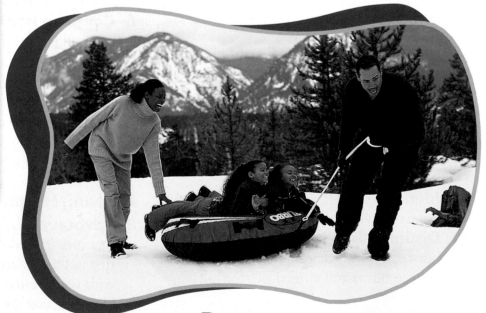

People who care about nature want to protect it from pollution. *Describe a natural area you like to visit.*

Air Pollution

Some natural events, such as erupting volcanoes, release gases that pollute the air. Other air pollution is caused by humans. Humans damage the air mostly by burning **fossil** (FAH·suhl) **fuels**. These are *the coal, oil, and natural gas used to power the engines of motor vehicles and factories.*

Air pollution can cause your eyes to water, give you headaches, and make you dizzy or tired. It can also damage your lungs, causing diseases that make it difficult to breathe. Air pollution is responsible for a variety of environmental problems.

- **Ozone** (OH·zohn) is *a special form of oxygen.* A layer of ozone in the upper atmosphere helps to protect the earth from the sun's harmful rays. Certain chemicals in air pollution have begun to damage this protective layer.
- Although the ozone high above the earth protects people, ozone at ground level can be very harmful. It is a major part of **smog**, *a yellow-brown haze that forms when sunlight reacts with impurities in car exhaust.* Over long periods, breathing smog can cause serious damage to your lungs.
- **Acid rain** is *rainfall that contains air pollution from the burning of fossil fuels.* Over time, it can destroy large forests, wildlife, and plant life.

Water Pollution

All humans, animals, and plants need water to survive. Water can become polluted in many ways. For example, chemicals dumped in rivers and streams can damage the water supply. Large oil spills foul beaches and harm wildlife. Fertilizers used in farm fields can seep into the water supply. Food, human waste, detergents, and other products washed down drains end up in rivers and oceans.

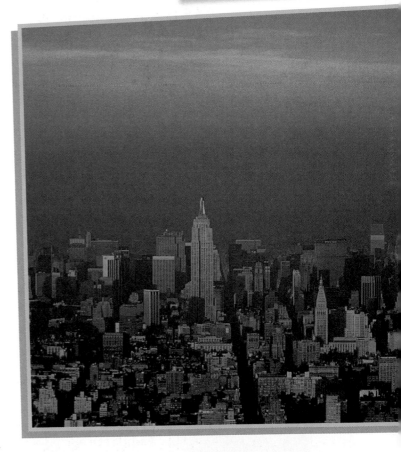

Reading Check

Think about what these words have to do with safety and the environment: pollution, fossil fuel, smog, acid rain, recycling, conservation. Find other words that fit with these. Then group the words into different categories.

Local news programs will often alert residents on days when smog reaches harmful levels. *Why should you limit physical activity on smoggy days?*

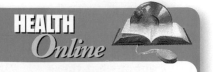

Water polluted in these ways threatens the life and health of plants and animals alike. People can become sick when they drink polluted water or eat fish that have absorbed these wastes and chemicals. In some parts of the world, unclean water spreads deadly diseases, such as cholera (KAH·luh·ruh) and typhoid. These illnesses threaten whole communities.

Land Pollution

As a good citizen, you do your part to pick up after yourself and properly dispose of wastes. Even properly discarded wastes, however, have to go somewhere (see **Figure 10.11**). Solid wastes often go to landfills. Harmful substances from landfills can leak into the soil and the water supply. Some communities burn their trash. Burning trash can pollute the air, however, so many communities do not allow it.

Some types of waste present special problems. Hazardous wastes can cause serious illnesses or environmental damage. They include plastics, paints, acids, and chemicals used to kill insects. Nuclear wastes, the chemicals left over from nuclear power plants and factories, can be very dangerous. They sometimes take thousands or even millions of years to break down naturally.

FIGURE 10.11

HOW WE DISPOSE OF WASTE

Solid wastes are usually buried in landfills, burned in incinerators, or stored in special locations designated for hazardous materials.

Landfill. Communities build landfills to bury their wastes. Special linings are designed to prevent pollution from leaking into water under the site.

Incineration. This involves burning waste at high temperatures in a special kind of furnace. Burning waste reduces the volume of trash. It can also produce energy, reducing the need for fossil fuels. However, it can cause air pollution, and the ashes are dangerous.

Hazardous Waste Storage. Hazardous wastes are often stored in containers, tanks, or buildings. Later, they are treated and placed in special landfills.

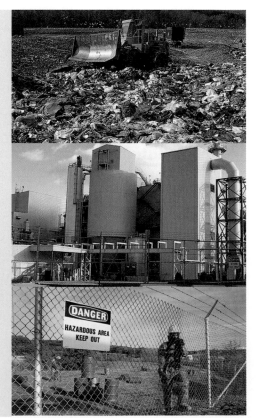

What You Can Do

You can do your part to dispose of trash by reducing the amount you create. The best way to do that is by reusing as many items as possible. Also, recycle whatever you can. **Recycling** means *recovering and changing items so they can be used for other purposes.*

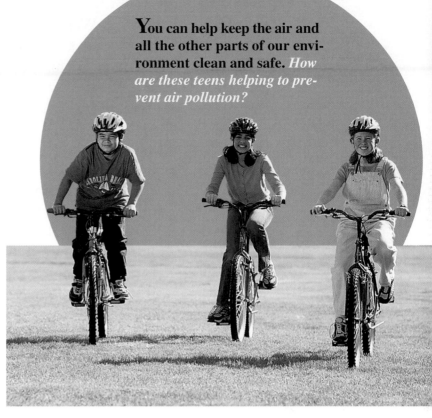

You can help keep the air and all the other parts of our environment clean and safe. *How are these teens helping to prevent air pollution?*

Protecting the Air

Exhaust from motor vehicles is a major source of air pollution. Driving less, therefore, is one way to help clean up the air. You and your family might use buses, trains, or subways instead of driving. You can also walk, take your bicycle, or carpool to cut the number of cars on the road.

Another way to help is by conserving energy. **Conservation** is *the saving of resources.* If we burn less fossil fuel for energy, we create less air pollution. Your family can conserve energy by turning off electric lights and appliances when they are not in use. You can also seal off leaks around windows and doors that can let heat escape. Keep windows closed while the heat or air conditioning is on. Towel dry or air dry dishes instead of heat drying them in a dishwasher.

Protecting the Water

Do you turn the water off while you brush your teeth? If you do, you are helping to protect our water supply by using less of it. You can also save water by taking shorter showers and repairing leaky faucets.

To keep our water clean, you and your friends can remove litter from rivers and lakes. Also try to use cleaning supplies that are **biodegradable** (by·oh·di·GRAY·duh·buhl) or *able to break down naturally without causing pollution.* Any detergents and cleaning supplies you dump down the drain end up in our rivers, lakes, and oceans.

Reducing Waste

If you want to cut down on the amount of trash you create, there are three basic steps you can take: reduce, reuse, and recycle.

- **Reduce.** Buy products that have less packaging to throw away. Also, consider whether you need an item at all. Maybe something you already have would do just as well.
- **Reuse.** Use items more than once. For example, a glass can replace several paper cups. You can also reuse items in new ways, such as turning a glass bottle into a vase.
- **Recycle.** Everyday materials such as glass, paper, and aluminum can be used to manufacture new items.

To help make recycling successful, people must buy recycled products. These products are often labeled with the recycling symbol shown in **Figure 10.12**. By buying these goods, you "complete the cycle."

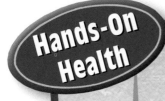

Hands-On Health

ARE YOU EARTH-FRIENDLY?

How do you rate as a friend of the environment? Take this conservation inventory to find out.

WHAT YOU WILL NEED
- pencil or pen
- paper

WHAT YOU WILL DO
1. Write the letters a.–j. on your paper.
2. Write *yes* or *no* for each of the following statements:
   a. I take quick showers.
   b. I turn off lights and appliances that are not in use.
   c. I close windows at night to keep cold air out.
   d. I don't let water run when I'm brushing my teeth.
   e. I recycle products whenever possible.
   f. I bring my own bags to the store.
   g. I find new ways to use old items.
   h. I put litter in trash containers.
   i. I encourage my family to carpool.
   j. I walk or ride my bicycle whenever possible instead of asking for a ride.

IN CONCLUSION
Give yourself 1 point for each yes answer. Add up your score and see how you rate.
3 or less: Energy Eater
4 to 7: Average Earth Friend
8 or more: Conservation Star
List ways you can improve your rating.

FIGURE 10.12

REDUCE, REUSE, RECYCLE

The recycling symbol is made up of three arrows. It reminds you that one item can be used many times. Look for the recycling symbol on products you buy.

Reduce
Buy items that can be reused, refilled, or recycled. Avoid products with excess packaging. Use fewer disposable items. Choose biodegradable products whenever possible. Buy in large quantities to save on packaging.

Recycle
Learn where you can recycle different materials such as aluminum, glass, plastic, paper, batteries, motor oil, and yard waste. Help start a curbside recycling program if your area does not have one. Take items to recycling centers. Complete the cycle by buying products made of recycled materials.

Reuse
Reuse grocery bags when you go shopping. Use empty cans for storage. Save old rags to use for cleaning. Repair broken items instead of buying new ones. Use your imagination to find new uses for items.

Lesson 5 Review

Using complete sentences, answer the following questions on a sheet of paper.

Reviewing Terms and Facts

1. **Describe** Which of the following are harmful to the environment: pollution, ozone layer, smog, acid rain, conservation?
2. **Recall** In what three ways do communities dispose of solid waste materials?
3. **Vocabulary** What are *biodegradable* products? Use this term in a statement about the environment.

Thinking Critically

4. **Compare and Contrast** Describe the similarities and differences between reducing, reusing, and recycling.
5. **Invent** Think about the kind of container your milk comes in. How could you reuse the container?

Applying Health Skills

6. **Goal Setting** Create a chart showing the different ways you plan to protect the environment. Use these four headings on your chart: At Home, At School, On the Road, When Shopping. Explain your goal for the environment.

APPLYING FIRST AID SKILLS

Model

Many injuries are minor and can be treated in the home. Others are major, requiring the attention of a medical professional. Knowing the difference between problems you can treat and problems that need professional help is an important health skill. Read about how Martin responds to an unintentional injury.

While riding his bike, Martin falls and hurts his knee. The first thing he does is to examine the wound. He sees that his knee is skinned but not bleeding much. Martin decides that this is a minor injury. He goes into the house and washes his knee with soap and water. Then he applies antibiotic ointment and covers the wound with a bandage. In ten minutes, he is feeling fine and ready to get back on his bike.

Practice

Read the following scenario about a teen dealing with an injury. Determine whether the injury is a major injury or a minor injury. Then decide what actions Jen should take.

Jen is babysitting her little sister Kayla. Kayla accidentally touches the stove burner while Jen is preparing their lunch. Kayla starts crying, but Jen can see that the burn is just slightly pink. There are no blisters or discolored skin.

Apply/Assess

Choose one of the scenarios below. Tell whether the injury is a major or minor injury and explain why. Then write a description of how you would care for the injury. Assume that basic first aid materials, such as soap and water, bandages, and antibiotic ointment, are available.

Michael is mowing the lawn. The mower hits a sharp stone and sends it flying back into his leg. Michael's leg hurts a lot and there is blood flowing from the wound.

Lisa is playing ball with her friends. As she runs to make a catch, she trips and falls. When she gets up, she finds that her nose is bleeding.

Mario is helping his parents cook dinner. He accidentally spills a bowl of hot soup on himself. Mario's hand is red and blistered.

Practicing Healthful Behaviors

Basic first aid skills include:
- Caring for major and minor wounds.
- Caring for major and minor burns.

Self-Check

- Did I recognize the differences between major and minor injuries?
- Did I describe the correct first aid procedures?

REUSE TO REDUCE WASTE

Model

When Amy looked in her family's trashcan, she saw items that she thought could still be useful. She started encouraging her family members to look carefully at every item before throwing it away. As a result, the members of Amy's family changed their habits. They gave useable items to charity instead of throwing them away. They recycled cans, bottles, and newspapers. They also found creative ways to reuse objects. Chipped mugs became pencil cups. Grocery bags were used to line wastebaskets.

When Amy saw how much they had reduced their trash, she was so excited that she started sharing her family's ideas with others. Now all her friends are eager to start reusing, too!

Practice

In groups of four, discuss some of the things your families regularly throw into the trash. On a sheet of paper, write down as many of these items as you can. Then select two or three items from your list and brainstorm ways to reuse each item. Write the name of each item at the top of your paper and underline it. Below, list all the ways you find to reuse it. Remember that giving away intact items is a good way to reuse them.

1. What ways did you think of to reuse different items?
2. Which of your ideas do you think would be most practical?
3. How could you persuade others to reuse items in the ways you suggested?

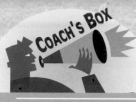

COACH'S BOX

Advocacy

The skill of advocacy asks you to
- take a clear stand on an issue.
- persuade others to make healthy choices.
- be convincing.

Apply/Assess

Work with your group to create a collage that encourages others to reuse. Each member of the group should choose one of the ideas you thought of in the Practice section. Think of a way to convince others that your idea is a good way to reuse. One way would be to draw a picture of the reused item. You could also write out a list of directions for creating it. Photos clipped from newspapers or magazines can help you illustrate your idea. Attach all your drawings and other materials to a large piece of poster board to form a group collage. Finish your collage by attaching a list of all the benefits of reusing.

Self-√Check

- Does our collage clearly show how objects can be reused?
- Does our collage explain why reusing materials is important?
- Would our collage persuade others in our age group to reuse items?

SUMMARY

LESSON•1 Many unintentional injuries result from the accident chain. Knowing how to break the accident chain will decrease your risk of unintentional injury.

LESSON•2 Removing hazards can help prevent accidents and injuries in the home. To stay safe on the road, follow safety rules and traffic laws. Schools and communities are working to reduce violence and other dangers.

LESSON•3 To stay safe during outdoor activities, plan ahead, use the buddy system, and communities can work to prevent violence. Take safety precautions. Learning about weather emergencies can help you prepare and stay safe.

LESSON•4 First aid is the care a person receives in an emergency before professional medical help arrives. Basic first-aid techniques can save lives.

LESSON•5 Your health depends on the health of the environment. Pollution threatens our air, water, and land. Using resources wisely can reduce these dangers.

- accident chain
- injury
- drowning
- unintentional injuries
- pedestrian
- tornado
- Neighborhood Watch program
- hurricane
- falls
- earthquake

Reviewing Vocabulary and Concepts

On a sheet of paper, write the numbers 1–10. After each number, write the term from the list that best completes each sentence.

Lesson 1

1. Injuries caused by unexpected events are known as _____.

2. Good safety habits protect you from _____, or physical harm.

3. Changing an unsafe habit is one way to break the _____.

Lesson 2

4. A(n) _____ is a person who travels on foot.

5. In a(n) _____, police train residents to look for and report suspicious activity in their community.

6. Keeping objects off the floor is a good way to prevent _____.

Lesson 3

7. The six steps of _____ prevention are: stay calm, get ready, raise your head, take a breath, go below the surface, and rest.

8. A(n) _____ is the shaking of the ground as rock below the surface moves.

9. A strong windstorm with driving rain is called a(n) _____.

10. If you are warned of a(n) _____ in your area, go down to a storm cellar or basement.

On a sheet of paper, write the numbers 11–20. Write *True* or *False* for each statement below. If the statement is false, change the underlined word or phrase to make it true.

Lesson 4

11. <u>Cardiopulmonary resuscitation (CPR)</u> is a substitute for normal breathing in which someone forces air into the victim's lungs.

12. Applying pressure to a main <u>artery</u> can help stop severe bleeding.

13. You can help an adult who is choking by giving <u>abdominal thrusts.</u>

14. A <u>poison control center</u> is one place that helps people deal with poisons.

15. In a <u>third-degree burn,</u> only the outer part of the skin turns red.

Lesson 5

16. You and the living and nonliving things around you make up the <u>environment</u>.

17. When the air, water, and land change from clean and safe to dirty and unsafe, it is known as <u>conservation</u>.

18. <u>Smog</u> forms when sunlight reacts with impurities in car exhaust.

19. Turning off electric lights and appliances when they are not in use is an example of <u>recycling</u>.

20. Everyday materials such as aluminum, glass, and paper <u>cannot</u> be recycled.

Thinking Critically

Using complete sentences, answer the following questions on a sheet of paper.

21. Suggest Identify three possible causes of accidents in the kitchen?

22. Explain Why is it important to be aware of your limits before engaging in an activity such as boating?

23. Analyze What is your opinion on allowing student lockers to be searched for drugs and weapons?

24. Classify A friend has burned his arm with hot chocolate. His skin has blisters. What degree of burn is this, and what kind of first aid is needed?

25. Hypothesize Which is better for the environment: to buy individual serving packages of snacks and meals or to buy larger packages? Why?

Career Corner

Occupational Safety and Health Specialist

Would you like to help keep people safe while they work? Are you good at solving problems? Then you might want to think about a career in occupational safety and health. In this career, you will look at hazards in the workplace and find ways to prevent or eliminate them. You'll need a four-year degree in occupational safety and health. Visit Career Corner at health.glencoe.com to learn more about this and other health careers.

Glossary

The Glossary contains all the important terms used throughout the text. It includes the **boldfaced** terms listed in the "Vocabulary" lists at the beginning of each lesson, which also appear in text and art.

The Glossary lists the term, the pronunciation (in the case of difficult terms), the definition, and the page on which the term is defined. The pronunciations here and in the text follow the system outlined below. The column headed "Symbol" shows the spelling used in this book to represent the appropriate method.

PRONUNCIATION KEY

Sound	As In	Symbol	Example
ă	hat, map	a	abscess (AB·ses)
ā	age, face	ay	atrium (AY·tree·uhm)
a	care, their	eh	capillaries (KAP·uh·lehr·eez)
ä, ŏ	father, hot	ah	biopsy (BY·ahp·see)
ar	far	ar	cardiac (KAR·dee·ak)
ch	child, much	ch	barbiturate (bar·BI·chuh·ruht)
ĕ	let, best	e	vessel (VE·suhl)
ē	beat, see, city	ee	acne (AK·nee)
er	term, stir, purr	er	nuclear (NOO·klee·er)
g	grow	g	malignant (muh·LIG·nuhnt)
ĭ	it, hymn	i	bacteria (bak·TIR·ee·uh)
ī	ice, five	y	benign (bi·NYN)
		eye	iris (EYE·ris)
j	page, fungi	j	cartilage (KAR·tuhl·ij)
k	coat, look, chorus	k	defect (DEE·fekt)
ō	open, coat, grow	oh	aerobic (ehr·OH·bik)
ô	order	or	organ (OR·guhn)
ȯ	flaw, all	aw	palsy (PAWL·zee)
oi	voice	oy	goiter (GOY·ter)
ou	out	ow	fountain (FOWN·tuhn)
s	say, rice	s	dermis (DER·mis)
sh	she, attention	sh	conservation (kahn·ser·VAY·shuhn)
ŭ	cup, flood	uh	bunion (BUHN·yuhn)
u	put, wood, could	u	pulmonary (PUL·muh·nehr·ee)
ü	rule, move, you	oo	attitudes (AT·i·toodz)
w	win	w	warranty (WAWR·uhn·tee)
y	your	yu	urethra (yu·REE·thruh)
z	says	z	hormones (HOR·mohnz)
zh	pleasure	zh	transfusion (trans·FYOO·zhuhn)
ə	about, collide	uh	addiction (uh·DIK·shuhn)

A

Abdominal thrusts Quick upward pulls into the diaphragm to force out an object blocking the airway. (page 275)

Abstinence (AB·sti·nuhns) Refusing to participate in health-risk behaviors. (page 39)

Abuse (uh·BYOOS) A pattern of mistreatment of another person. (page 58)

Accident chain A sequence of events that often leads to an unintentional injury. (page 259)

Acid rain Rainfall that contains air pollution from the burning of fossil fuels. (page 279)

Acne (AK·nee) A skin condition caused by overly active oil glands. (page 90)

Addiction The body's physical or mental need for a drug or other substance. (page 213)

Adolescence (a·duhl·EH·suhns) The period between childhood and adulthood. (page 165)

Adrenaline (uh·DRE·nuhl·in) A hormone that prepares the body to respond to a stressor. (page 42)

Advertisement A message used to persuade consumers to buy goods or services. (page 101)

Aerobic exercise Rhythmic, nonstop, moderate to vigorous activities that work the heart. (page 134)

AIDS An HIV infection combined with severe immune system problems. (page 192)

Alcohol (AL·kuh·hawl) A substance that is produced by a chemical reaction in some foods. (page 230)

Alcoholism The physical and mental need for alcohol. (page 233)

Allergen (AL·er·juhn) A substance that causes an allergic reaction. (page 199)

Allergy The body's sensitivity to certain substances. (page 199)

Alternative Another way of thinking or acting. (page 248)

Anabolic steroids (a·nuh·BAH·lik STIR·oydz) Synthetic drugs based on a male hormone. (page 245)

Anaerobic exercise Intense physical activity that requires short bursts of energy. (page 134)

Anorexia nervosa (an·uh·REK·see·uh ner·VOH·suh) An eating disorder in which a person has an intense fear of weight gain and starves himself or herself. (page 131)

Antibiotic (an·ti·by·AH·tik) A medicine that kills or stops the growth of certain germs. (page 235)

Antibodies Chemicals produced specifically to fight a particular invading substance. (page 185)

Asthma (AZ·muh) A chronic breathing disease caused by allergies, physical exertion, air pollution, or other factors. (page 200)

Astigmatism A condition in which the shape of the cornea or of the lens causes objects to look wavy or blurred. (page 96)

B

Behavior How you act in situations that occur in your life. (page 169)

Biodegradable (by·oh·di·GRAY·duh·buhl) Able to break down naturally without causing pollution. (page 281)

Blood pressure The force of the blood pushing against the walls of the blood vessels. (page 158)

Body language Facial expressions, gestures, and posture. (page 67)

Body system A group of organs that perform a body function. (page 151)

Glossary

Brain The organ that controls your senses, thoughts, and actions. (page 161)

Bulimia nervosa (boo·LEE·mee·uh ner·VOH·suh) An eating disorder in which a person repeatedly eats large amounts of food and then purges by vomiting or using laxatives. (page 132)

C

Calcium A mineral that helps your body build healthy teeth and bones. (page 127)

Calorie A unit of heat that measures the energy available in foods. (page 130)

Cancer A disease caused by abnormal cells that grow out of control. (page 198)

Carbohydrate (kar·bo·HY·drayt) The main source of energy for your body. (page 117)

Carbon monoxide (KAR·buhn muh·NAHK·syd) A poisonous, odorless gas produced when tobacco burns. (page 212)

Cardiopulmonary resuscitation (CPR) A rescue measure that attempts to restore heartbeat and breathing. (page 273)

Cell The basic building block of life. (page 150)

Character The way you think, feel, and act. (page 17)

Choking A condition that occurs when a person's airway becomes blocked. (page 274)

Cholesterol (kuh·LES·tuh·rawl) A waxlike substance our bodies produce and need in small amounts. (page 129)

Chromosomes (KROH·muh·sohmz) Pairs of tiny, threadlike pieces of matter that carry the codes for inherited traits. (page 170)

Chronic (KRAH·nik) Long-lasting. (page 196)

Circulatory system A body system that allows the body to transport, or move, materials from one place to another. (page 157)

Cirrhosis (suh·ROH·sis) Destruction and scarring of liver tissue. (page 231)

Communicable (kuh·MYOO·ni·kuh·buhl) **disease** A disease that can be spread. (page 182)

Communication The sharing of thoughts and feelings between two or more people. (page 66)

Compromise Each person giving up something in order to reach a solution that satisfies everyone. (page 72)

Conflict A problem in a relationship. (page 70)

Consequence A result. (page 14)

Conservation The saving of resources. (page 281)

Consumer Someone who buys products or services. (page 100)

Contagious (cuhn·TA·jus) Able to spread to others by direct or indirect contact. (page 187)

Cool-down Some gentle activity to slow down after exercise. (page 141)

Coupon (KOO·pahn) A slip of paper that saves you money on certain brands. (page 102)

Cumulative (KYOO·myuh·luh·tiv) **risk** The addition of one risk factor to another, increasing the chance of harm or loss. (page 17)

Cuticle (KYOO·ti·kuhl) A nonliving band of epidermis surrounding fingernails and toenails. (page 92)

D

Dandruff Flaking of the outer layer of dead skin cells on the scalp. (page 92)

Decibel A measurement of the loudness of sound. (page 98)

Decision A choice that you make. (page 14)

Depressant A drug that slows down the body's functions and reactions. (page 242)

Dermatologist (DER·muh·TAH·luh·jist) A doctor who treats skin disorders. (page 91)

Dermis The thicker inner layer of the skin. (page 89)

Diabetes (dy·uh·BEE·teez) A disease that prevents the body from using the sugars and starches in food for energy. (page 201)

Diaphragm (DY·uh·fram) A large muscle at the bottom of the chest. (page 160)

Digestive (dy·JEHS·tiv) **system** A body system that breaks down the food you eat into a form that your body cells can use as fuel. (page 163)

Discount store A store that offers lower prices, but has fewer salespeople and services. (page 102)

Disease (dih·ZEEZ) An unhealthy condition of the body or mind. (page 182)

Distress Negative stress. (page 42)

Drug Any substance that changes the structure or function of the body or mind. (page 230)

Drug abuse (uh·BYOOS) Using drugs in ways that are unhealthy or illegal. (page 239)

Drug misuse Taking medicine in a way that is not intended. (page 239)

Earthquake The shaking of the ground as rock below the surface moves. (page 271)

Egg cell The reproductive cell in the female body. (page 171)

Emotion A feeling. (page 36)

Empathy The ability to identify and share another person's feelings. (page 62)

Emphysema (em·fuh·SEE·muh) A disease that occurs when the tiny air sacs in the lungs lose their elasticity, or ability to stretch. (page 214)

Endocrine (EHN·duh·krin) **system** A body system made up of glands throughout the body that produce hormones. (page 165)

Endurance (en·DER·uhns) How long you can engage in physical activity without becoming overly tired. (page 134)

Environment (en·VY·ruhn·ment) You and all living and nonliving things around you. (page 278)

Epidermis The thinner outer layer of the skin. (page 89)

Eustress (YOO·stres) Positive stress. (page 42)

Excretory (EK·skruh·tohr·ee) **system** A body system that gets rid of some of the wastes your body produces and maintains fluid balance. (page 164)

Exercise Planned, structured, repetitive physical activity that improves or maintains physical fitness. (page 136)

Family The basic unit of society. (page 54)

Farsightedness The ability to see objects at a distance, while close objects look blurry. (page 96)

Fat A source of energy found in food. (page 118)

Fatigue (fuh·TEEG) Extreme tiredness. (page 43)

Fertilization The joining together of an egg cell and a sperm cell. (page 171)

Glossary

Fetal (FEE·tuhl) **alcohol syndrome (FAS)** A group of permanent physical and mental problems caused by a mother's use of alcohol while pregnant. (page 233)

Fiber The tough, stringy part of raw fruits, raw vegetables, whole wheat, and other grains, which you cannot digest. (page 117)

First aid The care first given to an injured or ill person until regular medical care can be supplied. (page 272)

First-degree burn A burn in which only the outer part of the skin is burned and turns red. (page 276)

Flexibility The ability to move body joints through a full range of motion. (page 135)

Fluoride (FLAWR·eyed) A substance that fights tooth decay. (page 87)

Food Guide Pyramid A daily guideline to help you choose what and how much to eat to get the nutrients you need. (page 121)

Fossil fuels The coal, oil, and natural gas used to power the engines of motor vehicles and factories. (page 279)

Fraud Deliberate deceit or trickery. (page 103)

Friendship A special type of relationship between people who enjoy being together. (page 61)

G

Generic (juh·NEHR·ic) Sold in plain packages. (page 102)

Genes (JEENZ) The basic units of heredity. (page 170)

Gestures Movements of the hands, arms, and legs. (page 67)

Goal Something that you hope to accomplish. (page 20)

H

Habit A pattern of behavior that you follow almost without thinking. (page 7)

Hallucinogen (huh·LOO·suhn·uh·jen) An illegal drug that causes the user's brain to distort images and to see and hear things that aren't real. (page 243)

Hazard A possible source of harm. (page 261)

Health A combination of physical, mental, emotional, and social well-being. (page 4)

Health insurance A monthly or yearly fee to an insurance company that agrees to pay for some or most costs of medical care. (page 106)

Heart The muscle that acts as the pump for the circulatory system. (page 158)

Heredity (huh·REHD·ih·tee) The process by which parents pass traits to their children. (page 170)

HIV The virus that causes AIDS. (page 192)

Hormones (HOR·mohnz) Powerful chemicals, produced by glands, that regulate many body functions. (page 37)

Hurricane (HER·uh·kayn) A strong tropical windstorm with driving rain. (page 271)

Hypothermia (hy·poh·THER·mee·uh) A sudden and dangerous drop in body temperature. (page 267)

I

Immune (i·MYOON) **system** A group of cells, tissues, and organs that fights disease. (page 185)

Immunity A resistance to infection. (page 185)

Infection The result of pathogens invading the body, multiplying, and harming some of your body's cells. (page 183)

Inhalant (in·HAY·luhnt) A substance whose fumes are inhaled to produce hallucinations. (page 244)

Injury Physical damage or harm to the body. (page 258)

Insulin A hormone produced by the pancreas. (page 201)

Joint A place where one bone meets another. (page 155)

L

Long-term goal A goal that you hope to achieve within a period of months or years. (page 20)

Lungs The main organs of the respiratory system. (page 159)

Lymphocyte (LIM·fuh·syt) A white blood cell that attacks pathogens. (page 185)

M

Managed care A health insurance plan that saves money by limiting people's choice of doctors. (page 107)

Marijuana (mar·uh·WAHN·uh) An illegal drug that comes from the hemp plant. (page 244)

Media The various methods of communicating information, including newspapers, magazines, radio, television, and the Internet. (page 219)

Medicine A drug that is used to cure or prevent diseases or other conditions. (page 234)

Mineral (MIN·uh·ruhl) An element in food that helps your body work properly. (page 120)

Muscular system All the muscles in your body. (page 156)

Narcotics (nar·KAH·tics) Certain drugs that relieve pain. (page 243)

Nearsightedness The ability to see objects close to you, while distant objects look blurry. (page 96)

Neglect The failure of parents to provide basic physical and emotional care for their children. (page 58)

Neighborhood Watch program A program in which police train residents to look for and report suspicious activity in their neighborhood. (page 265)

Nervous system The control and communication system of the body. (page 161)

Neuron (NOO·rahn) A cell that carries electrical messages. (page 161)

Nicotine (NI·kuh·teen) A drug that speeds up the heartbeat and affects the central nervous system. (page 212)

Noncommunicable disease A disease that does not spread. (page 182)

Nurture To provide for someone's physical, emotional, mental, and social needs. (page 55)

Nutrient (NOO·tree·ent) A substance in food that your body needs. (page 117)

Nutrition (noo·TRI·shun) The science that studies the substances in food and how the body uses them. (page 116)

Glossary

O

Organ A structure that is made up of different types of tissues that do a particular job. (page 151)

Orthodontist A dentist who specializes in dealing with irregularities of the teeth and jaw. (page 88)

Over-the-counter (OTC) medicine A medicine available without a written order from a doctor. (page 234)

Ozone (OH·zohn) A special form of oxygen. (page 279)

P

Pathogens Disease-causing germs. (page 183)

Pedestrian A person who travels on foot. (page 263)

Peer mediation (mee·dee·AY·shuhn) A process in which a specially trained student listens to both sides of an argument and then helps the opposing sides reach a solution. (page 73)

Peer pressure The influence you feel to go along with the behavior and beliefs of your peer group. (page 63)

Peers Your friends and other people in your age group. (page 63)

Personality The sum total of your feelings, actions, habits, and thoughts. (page 169)

Physical activity Any kind of movement that causes your body to use energy. (page 133)

Physical fitness The ability to handle everyday physical work and play without becoming tired. (page 136)

Plaque (PLAK) A soft, colorless, sticky film containing bacteria that grows on your teeth. (page 86)

Poison control center A place that helps people deal with poisons. (page 276)

Pollution (puh·LOO·shuhn) The changing of the air, water, and land from clean and safe to dirty and unsafe. (page 278)

Prescription (pri·SKRIP·shuhn) **medicine** A medicine sold only with a written order from a doctor. (page 234)

Prevention Keeping something from happening. (page 8)

Protein A nutrient essential for the growth and repair of all the cells in your body. (page 118)

Puberty (PYOO·ber·tee) The time when you begin to develop certain physical traits of the adults of your gender and become physically able to reproduce. (page 166)

R

Recycling Recovering and changing items so they can be used for other purposes. (page 281)

Refusal skills Methods for saying no. (page 64)

Reinforce To support. (page 33)

Relationship (ri·LAY·shuhn·ship) A connection you have with another person. (page 60)

Reliable Dependable. (page 62)

Rescue breathing A substitute for normal breathing in which someone forces air into the victim's lungs. (page 273)

Respiratory system A body system that enables you to breathe. (page 159)

Risk The chance of harm or loss. (page 14)

S

Saturated (SAT·chur·ay·tuhd) **fat** A type of fat found mostly in animal products such as butter, meat, milk, and egg yolks. (page 129)

Second-degree burn A serious type of burn in which the burned area blisters or peels. (page 276)

Secondhand smoke Tobacco smoke that stays in the air. (page 217)

Self-concept The view you have of yourself. (page 32)

Self-esteem The ability to like and respect yourself. (page 35)

Sexual abuse An adult displaying sexual material to a child, touching a child's private body parts, or engaging in any kind of sexual activity with a child or teen. (page 58)

Sexually transmitted infections (STIs) Communicable diseases that are passed from one person to another through sexual contact. (page 191)

Short-term goal A goal that you plan to accomplish in a short time. (page 20)

Side effect Any reaction to a medicine other than the one intended. (page 235)

Skeletal system A framework of bones and the tissues that connect those bones. (page 154)

Smog A yellow-brown haze that forms when sunlight reacts with impurities in car exhaust. (page 279)

Smoke alarm A device that makes a warning noise when it senses smoke. (page 262)

Snuff Finely ground tobacco that is inhaled or held in the mouth between the lower lip and gum. (page 216)

Sodium A mineral that helps control the amount of fluid in your body. (page 129)

Sound waves Vibrations or movements in the air. (page 97)

Specialist (SPEH·shuh·list) A doctor trained to handle particular health problems. (page 104)

Sperm cell The reproductive cell in the male body. (page 171)

Spinal cord A tube of neurons that runs up the spine. (page 161)

Stimulant (STIM·yuh·luhnt) A drug that speeds up the body's functions. (page 241)

Strength The ability of your muscles to exert a force. (page 134)

Stress Your body's response to changes around you. (page 41)

Stressor An object, person, place, or event that triggers stress. (page 42)

Substance abuse Use of illegal or harmful drugs, including any use of alcohol while under the legal drinking age. (page 246)

T

Tar A thick, oily, dark liquid that forms when tobacco burns. (page 212)

Target pulse rate The level at which your heart and lungs receive the most benefit from a workout. (page 140)

Tartar A hard material that forms when plaque builds up on teeth. (page 87)

Third-degree burn A very serious burn in which deep layers of skin and nerve endings are damaged. (page 276)

Tissue A group of similar cells that do the same kind of work. (page 150)

Tolerance (TAHL·er·ence) The ability to accept other people as they are. (page 71)

Tolerance (TAHL·er·ence) A condition in which the body becomes used to the effects of a medicine and needs greater amounts to get the same effects. (page 235)

Glossary

Tornado (tor·NAY·doh) A whirling, funnel-shaped windstorm that drops from the sky to the ground. (page 271)

Tumor A mass of abnormal cells. (page 198)

U

Umbilical (uhm·BIL·i·kuhl) **cord** A tube that connects the lining of the uterus to the unborn baby. (page 172)

Unintentional injury An injury caused by unexpected events. (page 258)

Uterus (YOO·tuh·ruhs) A pear-shaped organ inside a woman's body that expands as a baby grows. (page 172)

V

Vaccine (vak·SEEN) A preparation of killed or weakened germs. (page 188)

Values Beliefs you feel strongly about that help guide the way you live. (page 17)

Violence The use of physical force to harm someone or something. (page 74)

Vitamin (VI·tuh·min) A substance that helps regulate body functions. (page 118)

Voluntary health group An organization that works to treat and eliminate certain diseases. (page 106)

W

Warm-up Some gentle activity that prepares your body for exercise. (page 140)

Warranty A promise to make repairs or refund money if a product does not work as claimed. (page 102)

Wellness A state of well-being, or balanced health. (page 7)

Withdrawal A series of mental and physical symptoms that occur when a person stops using an addictive substance. (page 240)

Glosario

A

Abdominal thrusts/presiones abdominales Presiones rápidas y hacia arriba sobre el diafragma, para desalojar un objeto que bloquea la vía respiratoria.

Abstinence/abstinencia Privarse de la participación en actividades que pongan en riesgo la salud.

Abuse/abuso El maltratamiento repetitivo de otra persona.

Accident chain/cadena de accidentes Una secuencia de sucesos que muchas veces termina en un daño no intencionado.

Acid rain/lluvia ácida Lluvia contaminada debido a la quema de combustibles fósiles.

Acne/acné Una enfermedad de la piel causada por actividad excesiva en las glándulas sebáceas.

Addiction/adicción La dependencia física o mental de drogas u otras sustancias.

Adolescence/adolescencia El período de vida entre la niñez y la adultez.

Adrenaline/adrenalina Una hormona que facilita la reacción del cuerpo a un estresante.

Advertisement/anuncio Un mensaje público para persuadir a los consumidores que compren bienes o servicios.

Aerobic exercise/ejercicio aeróbico Actividad rítmica de intensidad moderada o vigorosa que hace que el corazón trabaje.

AIDS/SIDA Una combinación de una infección del virus VIH y problemas severos del sistema de defensas.

Alcohol/alcohol Una sustancia producida por una reacción química en ciertos alimentos.

Alcoholism/alcoholismo La necesidad física y mental de consumir alcohol.

Allergen/alergeno Una sustancia que causa una reacción alérgica.

Allergy/alergia La sensibilidad del cuerpo a ciertas sustancias.

Alternative/alternativa Otra manera de pensar o actuar.

Anabolic steroids/esteroides anabólicos Drogas sintéticas basadas en una hormona masculina.

Anaerobic exercise/ejercicio anaeróbico Intensa actividad física que requiere explosiones breves de energía.

Anorexia nervosa/anorexia nerviosa Un trastorno de la alimentación en que una persona tiene miedo intenso de aumentar de peso y por consiguiente deja de comer.

Antibiotic/antibiótico Una medicina que produce la muerte de o impide el desarrollo de ciertos gérmenes.

Antibodies/anticuerpos Sustancias químicas producidas con el fin de combatir una sustancia invasora específica.

Asthma/asma Una enfermedad crónica respiratoria causada por alergias, esfuerzos físicos, la contaminación u otros factores.

Astigmatism/astigmatismo Una condición en la que la forma irregular de la córnea o las lentes del ojo causan que los objetos se ven distorsionados o borrosos.

B

Behavior/conducta Manera en que una persona actúa frente a las situaciones de la vida.

Glosario

Biodegradable/biodegradable Que se descompone naturalmente, sin causar contaminación.

Blood pressure/presión arterial La fuerza que ejerce la sangre contra las paredes de los vasos sanguíneos.

Body language/expresión corporal Expresiones faciales, gestos y postura.

Body system/aparato corporal Un grupo de órganos que ejecuta una función del cuerpo.

Brain/cerebro El órgano que controla los sentidos, los pensamientos, y las acciones.

Bulimia nervosa/bulimia nerviosa Un trastorno de la alimentación en el cual una persona come grandes cantidades y después se induce el vómito o toma un laxante.

C

Calcium/calcio Un mineral que ayuda al cuerpo formar dientes y huesos sanos.

Calorie/caloría Una unidad de calor que mide la energía disponible en los alimentos.

Cancer/cáncer Una enfermedad causada por el crecimiento incontrolado de células anormales.

Carbohydrate/carbohidrato La fuente principal de la energía del cuerpo.

Carbon monoxide/monóxido de carbono Un gas venenoso e inodoro que se produce al quemar tabaco.

Cardiopulmonary resuscitation (CPR)/resucitación cardiopulmonar Una medida de primeros auxilios que intenta restaurar el ritmo cardíaco y la respiración.

Cell/célula La unidad fundamental de los seres vivos.

Character/carácter La manera en que una persona piensa, se siente y actúa.

Choking/ahogo Una situación que ocurre cuando la vía respiratoria de una persona está bloqueada.

Cholesterol/colesterol Una sustancia parecida a la cera que se produce el cuerpo y que el cuerpo necesita en pequeñas cantidades.

Chromosomes/cromosomas Pares de materia filiforme minúscula que contienen los códigos genéticos de las características hereditarias.

Chronic/crónico Duradero.

Circulatory system/aparato circulatorio Un aparato corporal por medio del cual el cuerpo hace circular, o trasladar, materias de un lugar a otro.

Cirrhosis/cirrosis La destrucción y cicatrización del tejido del hígado.

Communicable disease/enfermedad contagiosa Una enfermedad que se puede transmitir.

Communication/comunicación El intercambio de pensamientos y sentimientos entre dos o más personas.

Compromise/acuerdo Un pacto en el que las personas involucradas sacrifican algo que desean para llegar a una solución que satisfaga a todos.

Conflict/conflicto Un problema en una relación.

Consequence/consecuencia Un resultado.

Conservation/conservación La protección de los recursos naturales.

Consumer/consumidor Una persona que compra productos o servicios.

Contagious/contagioso Que se puede transmitir por el contacto directo o indirecto.

Cool-down/enfriamiento Actividad no vigorosa para calmarse después de hacer ejercicio.

Coupon/cupón Un papel que se puede intercambiar por un descuento en ciertos productos.

Cumulative risk/riesgo acumulativo El añadido de un riesgo a otro que aumenta la posibilidad de daño o pérdida.

Cuticle/cutícula Una franja de epidermis no viva que rodea la parte inferior de las uñas.

Dandruff/caspa Escamas de piel muerta en la superficie del cuero cabelludo.

Decibel/decibel Una unidad de medida del volumen del sonido.

Decision/decisión La selección que hace una persona.

Depressant/depresor Una droga que disminuye las funciones y reacciones del cuerpo.

Dermatologist/dermatólogo Un médico que trata enfermedades de la piel.

Dermis/dermis La capa más gruesa y profunda de la piel.

Diabetes/diabetes Una enfermedad que le impide al cuerpo utilizar los azúcares y las harinas de los alimentos para crear energía.

Diaphragm/diafragma Un músculo grande situado en la parte inferior del pecho.

Digestive system/aparato digestivo Un aparato corporal que descompone los alimentos en sustancias que las células del cuerpo puedan usar como energía.

Discount store/tienda de rebajas Una tienda que vende mercancía a precios rebajados pero tiene menos empleados y servicios.

Disease/enfermedad Una condición no sana del cuerpo o de la mente.

Distress/angustia El estrés negativo.

Drug/droga Cualquier sustancia que altera la estructura o el funcionamiento del cuerpo o de la mente.

Drug abuse/abuso de drogas El uso de drogas de manera malsana o ilegal.

Drug misuse/mal uso de las drogas El tomar medicina de manera indebida.

Earthquake/terremoto El sacudimiento de la tierra mientras la capa de roca por debajo de la superficie terrestre se mueve.

Egg cell/óvulo La célula reproductora del cuerpo femenino.

Emotion/emoción Un sentimiento.

Empathy/empatía La habilidad de identificar y comprender los sentimientos de otra persona.

Emphysema/enfisema Una enfermedad que ocurre cuando los pequeños sacos de aire en los pulmones pierden la elasticidad o la capacidad de estirarse.

Endocrine system/aparato endocrino Un aparato corporal que comprende las glándulas que producen hormonas.

Endurance/resistencia La cantidad de tiempo que uno puede hacer actividad física sin cansarse demasiado.

Environment/medio ambiente Todas las cosas vivas y no vivas que te rodean.

Epidermis/epidermis La capa delgada más externa de la piel.

Eustress/tensión positiva Estrés positivo.

Excretory system/aparato excretor Un aparato corporal que expulsa algunos de los desechos producidos en el cuerpo y que mantiene en él el balance del líquido.

Exercise/ejercicio Actividad física, planeada, repetida y orquestada que mejora o mantiene la buena salud.

F

Family/familia La unidad básica de la sociedad.

Farsightedness/hipermetropía La capacidad de ver claramente los objetos a la distancia, mientras los objetos cercanos se ven borrosos.

Fat/grasa Una fuente de energía en los alimentos.

Fatigue/fatiga Cansancio extremo.

Fertilization/fertilización La unión de un óvulo y un espermatozoide.

Fetal alcohol syndrome/síndrome de alcoholismo fetal Un grupo de defectos permanentes físicos y mentales, causados por el uso del alcohol de la madre durante el embarazo.

Fiber/fibra La parte no digerible de las frutas y vegetales crudos, el trigo integral y otros granos.

First aid/primeros auxilios Los cuidados que se dan a una persona herida o enferma, durante una emergencia hasta se obtiene ayuda médica regular.

First-degree burn/quemadura de primer grado Una quemadura en que sólo la capa exterior de la piel se quema y enrojece.

Flexibility/flexibilidad La habilidad de mover las articulaciones libremente en todas las direcciones posibles.

Fluoride/fluoruro Una sustancia que previene las caries.

Food Guide Pyramid/Pirámide de alimentos Una guía que ayuda a elegir los alimentos y a decidir cuánto se debe comer diariamente para obtener los nutrientes necesarios.

Fossil fuels/combustibles fósiles El carbón, petróleo, y gas natural que se usan para hacer funcionar las fábricas y los motores de vehículos.

Fraud/fraude Engaño o decepción intencional.

Friendship/amistad La relación especial entre personas que disfrutan de pasar tiempo juntos.

G

Generic/genérico Vendido en empaques simples.

Genes/genes Las unidades básicas de la herencia.

Gestures/gestos Movimientos de las manos, los brazos y las piernas.

Goal/meta Un objetivo que una persona trata de alcanzar.

H

Habit/hábito Una manera de actuar que uno hace casi sin pensar.

Hallucinogen/alucinógeno Una droga ilegal que afecta el cerebro de manera que la persona que la usa ve imágenes deformadas, y oye y ve cosas irreales.

Hazard/peligro Una fuente posible de daño.

Health/salud Una combinación de bienestar físico, mental, emocional y social.

Health insurance/seguro de salud Un precio mensual o anual que se paga a una compañía de seguros que se encarga de pagar parte o la mayor parte de los gastos médicos.

Heart/corazón El músculo que sirve de bomba para el aparato circulatorio.

Heredity/herencia El proceso mediante el cual los padres transfieren sus características a sus hijos.

HIV/VIH El virus que causa el SIDA.

Hormones/hormonas Sustancias químicas potentes producidas en las glándulas que regulan muchas funciones del cuerpo.

Hurricane/huracán Una tormenta tropical fuerte con vientos y lluvia.

Hypothermia/hipotermia Un descenso rápido y peligroso de la temperatura del cuerpo.

Immune system/sistema de defensas Un grupo de células, tejidos y órganos que protegen contra enfermedades.

Immunity/inmunidad Una resistencia a un agente infeccioso.

Infection/infección El resultado de agentes patógenos cuando invaden el cuerpo, se multiplican y hacen daño a algunas de las células del mismo.

Inhalant/inhalante Una sustancia cuyos vapores se aspiran para producir efectos alucinógenos.

Injury/herida Daño físico o perjuicio al cuerpo.

Insulin/insulina Una hormona producida por el páncreas.

Joint/articulación Un lugar donde se unen dos huesos.

Long-term goal/meta a largo plazo Un objetivo que una persona trata de alcanzar durante un período de meses o años.

Lungs/pulmones Los órganos principales del aparato respiratorio.

Lymphocyte/linfocito Un glóbulo blanco que ataca los agentes patógenos.

Managed care/asistencia médica administrada Un plan de seguro médico que limita la selección de médicos y así ahorra más dinero.

Marijuana/marihuana Una droga ilegal que proviene de la planta de cáñamo.

Media/media Los varios métodos de comunicación, incluyendo periódicos, revistas, radio, televisión y la internet.

Medicine/medicina Una droga que se usa para curar o prevenir enfermedades u otros trastornos.

Mineral/mineral Una sustancia que se encuentra en los alimentos que ayuda al buen funcionamiento del cuerpo.

Muscular system/aparato muscular Todos los músculos del cuerpo.

N

Narcotics/narcóticos Ciertas drogas que alivian el dolor.

Nearsightedness/miopía La capacidad de ver claramente los objetos cercanos, mientras los objetos lejanos se ven borrosos.

Neglect/negligencia La ausencia de cuidados básicos, físicos y emocionales por la parte de los padres para con los hijos.

Glosario

Neighborhood Watch program/ programa de vigilancia en el barrio
Un programa en el cual la policía les enseña a los residentes a vigilar y reportar cualquier actividad sospechosa en el barrio.

Nervous system/sistema nervioso
El aparato de control y comunicación del cuerpo.

Neuron/neurona Una célula que lleva mensajes eléctricos.

Nicotine/nicotina Una droga que acelera el ritmo cardíaco y afecta el sistema nervioso central.

Noncommunicable disease/ enfermedad no contagiosa
Una enfermedad que no se transmita.

Nurture/criar Proveer las necesidades físicas, emocionales, mentales y sociales de una persona.

Nutrient/nutriente Una sustancia en los alimentos que necesita el cuerpo.

Nutrition/nutrición La ciencia que estudia las sustancias en los alimentos y cómo las utiliza el cuerpo.

Organ/órgano Una estructura formada por diferentes clases de tejidos que ejecutan una función específica.

Orthodontist/ortodoncista Un dentista quien se especializa en tratamientos de defectos de los dientes y la mandíbula.

Over-the-counter medicine/ medicamento sin receta
Una medicina disponible sin receta de un médico.

Ozone/ozono Una forma especial del oxígeno.

Pathogens/agentes patógenos Gérmenes que causan enfermedades.

Pedestrian/peatón Una persona que se traslada a pie.

Peer mediation/mediación de contemporáneos
Un proceso mediante el cual un estudiante especialmente entrenado escucha las dos partes de una discusión y luego ayuda a los oponentes a encontrar una solución.

Peer pressure/presión de contemporáneos
La influencia que uno siente, de tener que seguir las acciones y el pensamiento de los miembros del grupo de contemporáneos.

Peers/contemporáneos Amigos y otras personas de la misma edad.

Personality/personalidad La suma total de los sentimientos, conducta, hábitos y pensamientos de una persona.

Physical activity/actividad física
Cualquier movimiento que cause que el cuerpo use energía.

Physical fitness/buen estado físico
La capacidad de jugar y hacer trabajos físicos normales sin cansarse.

Plaque/placa Una película pegajosa, blanda e incolora que contiene bacterias que crece en los dientes.

Poison control center/centro para el control de venenos
Un lugar que ayuda a la gente en cuanto a los venenos.

Pollution/polución El cambio en el aire, el agua y la tierra de estar limpios y sanos a sucios y nocivos.

Prescription medicine/medicamento con receta Una droga que sólo puede ser vendida con la receta escrita de un médico.

Prevention/prevención Prevenir que ocurra algo.

Protein/proteína Un nutriente esencial para el desarrollo y la reparación de todas las células en el cuerpo.

Puberty/pubertad La etapa de la vida, en la cual una persona comienza a desarrollar ciertas características físicas propias de los adultos del mismo sexo y llega a ser capaz físicamente de reproducirse.

Recycling/reciclaje Recuperar y cambiar un objeto con el fin de usarse con otro propósito.

Refusal skills/destrezas de negación Métodos para decir no.

Reinforce/reforzar Fortalecer.

Relationship/relación Una conexión que una persona tiene con otra.

Reliable/seguro De confianza.

Rescue breathing/respiración de rescate Un método que reemplaza la respiración normal en el cual otra persona le llena los pulmones de aire a la víctima.

Respiratory system/aparato respiratorio Un aparato corporal que permite la respiración.

Risk/riesgo La posibilidad de daño o pérdida.

Saturated fat/grasa saturada Un tipo de grasa que se encuentra mayormente en los productos animales como la mantequilla, la carne, la leche y la yema del huevo.

Second-degree burn/quemadura de segundo grado Un tipo de quemadura seria en la que se forman ampollas o se despelleja la piel quemada.

Secondhand smoke/humo secundario El humo del tabaco que se queda en el aire.

Self-concept/autoimagen La imagen que uno tiene sobre sí mismo.

Self-esteem/autoestima La capacidad de una persona de estar contenta y respetarse a sí misma.

Sexual abuse/abuso sexual El mostrar materiales sexuales un adulto a un niño, el tocar un adulto las partes pudendas de un niño, o participar en cualquier actividad sexual con un niño o adolescente.

Sexually transmitted infections (STIs)/infecciones transmitidas sexualmente Infecciones transmisibles que se pasan de una persona a otra, a través de contacto sexual.

Short-term goal/meta a corto plazo Un objetivo que una persona trata de alcanzar, dentro de un corto período de tiempo.

Side effect/efecto secundario Cualquier reacción a una medicina que no se espera.

Skeletal system/sistema esquelético Una estructura de huesos y los tejidos que los conectan.

Smog/smog Una neblina amarillenta-café que se forma cuando la luz solar reacciona con las impurezas en el gas de escape que viene de los autos.

Glosario

Smoke alarm/alarma de humo Un aparato que hace un ruido de advertencia cuando detecta humo.

Snuff/rapé Tabaco finamente molido que se aspira por la nariz o se pone en la boca entre el labio inferior y la encía.

Sodium/sodio Un mineral que ayuda a controlar la cantidad de líquidos en el cuerpo.

Sound waves/ondas sonoras Vibraciones en el aire.

Specialist/especialista Médico que está entrenado para diagnosticar y tratar problemas específicos de la salud.

Sperm cell/espermatozoide La célula reproductora en el cuerpo masculino.

Spinal cord/médula espinal Un tubo de neuronas que se encuentra a lo largo de la columna vertebral.

Stimulant/estimulante Una droga que acelera las funciones del cuerpo.

Strength/fuerza La capacidad de los músculos de ejercer un poder.

Stress/estrés La reacción del cuerpo a los cambios a su alrededor.

Stressor/estresante Un objeto, persona, lugar o suceso que causa estrés.

Substance abuse/abuso de sustancias Uso de drogas ilegales o dañinas, incluso cualquier uso del alcohol por menores.

T

Tar/alquitrán Una sustancia oscura, aceitosa y pegajosa que se forma cuando se quema tabaco.

Target pulse rate/ritmo deseado del pulso El nivel en el cual el corazón y los pulmones obtienen el mayor beneficio, durante el ejercicio.

Tartar/sarro Una sustancia dura que se forma en los dientes cuando la placa se acumula.

Third-degree burn/quemadura de tercer grado Una quemadura muy seria que daña las capas más profundas de la piel y las terminaciones nerviosas.

Tissue/tejido Un grupo de células similares que tienen la misma función.

Tolerance/tolerancia La habilidad de aceptar a la gente como es.

Tolerance/tolerancia Un estado en el cual el cuerpo se acostumbra tanto a los efectos de una medicina, que necesita mayores cantidades para que la medicina produzca los mismos efectos.

Tornado/tornado Una tormenta en forma de torbellino, que gira en grandes círculos y que cae del cielo a la tierra.

Tumor/tumor Una masa de células anormales.

U

Umbilical cord/cordón umbilical Un tubo que une el revestimiento del útero al bebé antes de nacer.

Unintentional injury/daño no intencionado Un daño causado por sucesos inesperados.

Uterus/útero Un órgano femenino en forma de pera que se expande mientras crece el bebé.

V

Vaccine/vacuna Una preparación de gérmenes muertos o debilitados.

Values/valores Creencias fuertes que guían a una persona en su forma de vivir.

Violence/violencia El uso de fuerza física con la intención de causarle daño a alguien o a alguna cosa.

Vitamin/vitamina Una sustancia que ayuda a regular las funciones del cuerpo.

Voluntary health group/grupo de voluntarios para la salud Una organización que se dedica al tratamiento o a la eliminación de ciertas enfermedades.

 W

Warm-up/calentamiento Alguna actividad no muy vigorosa que prepara el cuerpo para hacer ejercicio.

Warranty/garantía Una promesa de que el producto será reparado o que se hará un reembolso en caso de que el producto no funcione de la manera prometida.

Wellness/bienestar Un estado de buena salud, o salud balanceada.

Withdrawal/síntomas de carencia de drogas Una serie de síntomas mentales y físicos que ocurren cuando una persona deja de tomar una sustancia adictiva.

Index

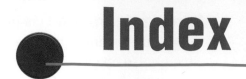

Note: Page numbers in *italics* refer to art and marginal features.

Index

Community health, 104–7
Comparison shopping, 102
Compromise, 72
Conflict resolution, *9,* 11, 70, 72–75, 78–79
Conflict(s), 70–71, 74–75
Connecting neurons, 161
Consequence, definition of, 14
Conservation, 281, 282
Consideration, *62*
Consumer, definition of, 100
Consumer skills, 100–103
Contact lenses, 96, 97
Contagious diseases, 187
Cool-down exercises, 141
Cornea, *95*
Counseling, 59
Couples (family units), 55
Coupons, 102
CPR (cardiopulmonary resuscitation), 273
Crack, 242, 247
Crisis centers, 59
Cumulative risk, 17
Cuticle, 92

D

Daily Value, 119
Dandruff, 92
Deafness, 99
Death of family member, 57
Decision making, *9,* 12, 14–19
    about family responsibilities, 57
    analyzing influences on, 24–25
    avoiding alcohol, 250–51
    buying decisions, *100*
    and character, 14, *17,* 19
    food choices, 142–43
    and good character, *17*
    H.E.L.P. criteria for, 16
    process of, 15–18
    steps in, 16–18, 26–27
    using steps in, 18

Decisions, definition of, 14
Dental checkups, 88
Dental hygienists, 88, 113
Dentists, 88
Depressants, 242
Depression, 232, 243, 245
Dermatologists, 91
Dermis, 89
Development. *See* Growth and development
Diabetes, 201
Diaphragm, 160
Dietary Guidelines for Americans (USDA), 128–29
Dietetic technicians, 147
Differences, acceptance of, 75
Digestive system, 152, *153,* 163
Discount stores, 102
Diseases, 182–201
    caused by tattoos/piercings, 91
    communicable, 187–90
    fetal alcohol syndrome, 233
    general defenses against, 185
    germs causing, 183–85
    and immune system, 185
    noncommunicable, 196–201
    from polluted water, 280
    sexually transmitted infections, 191–95
Distress, 42
Divorce, 57
Doctors, 104, 179
Drowning prevention, *267*
Drugs
    abuse/misuse of, 239, 240
    alcohol, 230–33
    alternatives to using, 248
    definition of, 230
    help for abusers' families, 249
    illegal, 240–45

medicines, 234–39
    and reaching goals, 252–53
    reasons for avoiding, 246
    in schools, 264
    violent acts caused by, *74,* 75

E

Early adulthood, 173
Earplugs, *98*
Ears, 97–99
Earthquakes, 271
Eating. *See* Nutrition
Eating disorders, 131–32
Ecstasy, 243
Egg cells, 171
Electrical safety, 262
Emergencies
    first aid for, 272–77
    weather, 270, 271
Emotional abuse, 58
Emotional fatigue, 43
Emotional health. *See* Mental/emotional health
Emotional neglect, 58
Emotions, 36–40
    during adolescence, 167
    conflict and, *70*
    expressing, 38
    handling strong emotions, 46–47
    physical responses to, *37*
Empathy, 62
Emphysema, *214*
Endocrine system, 152, 165–66
Endurance, 134
Energy, redirection of, 44
Environmental diseases, *196*
Environmental protection, 278–83
Enzymes, 163
Epidermis, 89, 92
Esophagus, *163*

Index

Index

Index

Health Resources

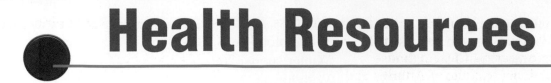

Action on Smoking and Health
2013 H Street NW
Washington, DC 20006

Alcoholics Anonymous
Central Office
15 E. 26th Street
New York, NY 10010-1501

Al-Anon/Alateen Family
Group Headquarters
1600 Corporate Landing Parkway
Virginia Beach, VA 23454-5617

American Academy of Pediatrics
National Headquarters
141 Northwest Point Road
Elk Grove Village, IL 60007-1098

American Automobile Association,
Foundation for Traffic Safety
Administrative Office
1440 New York Avenue NW
Suite 201
Washington, DC 20005

American Cancer Society
National Headquarters
1599 Clifton Road NE
Atlanta, GA 30329

American Counseling Association
5999 Stevenson Avenue
Alexandria, VA 22304

American Dental Association
211 East Chicago Avenue
Chicago, IL 60611

American Heart Association
National Center
7272 Greenville Avenue
Dallas, TX 75231-4596

American Institute of Nutrition
9650 Rockville Pike
Suite 4500
Bethesda, MD 20814

American Insurance Association, Engineering
and Safety Service
85 John Street
New York, NY 10038

American Lung Association
1740 Broadway
New York, NY 10019

American Medical Association
515 North State Street
Chicago, IL 60610

American Optometric Association
243 North Lindbergh Boulevard
St. Louis, MO 63141

American Society of Safety Engineers
1800 East Oakton Street
Des Plaines, IL 60018-2187

Asthma and Allergy Foundation of America
(AAFA)
1233 20th Street, NW
Suite 402
Washington, DC 20036

Centers for Disease Control and Prevention
(CDC)
1600 Clifton Road
Atlanta, GA 30333

Council on Environmental Quality
722 Jackson Place NW
Washington, DC 20503

Department of Health and Human Services
National Clearinghouse for Alcohol and Drug
Information (a service of the Substance
Abuse and Mental Health Services
Administration)
Information Specialist
P.O. Box 2345
Rockville, MD 20847-2345

Juvenile Diabetes Research Foundation
International
120 Wall Street
New York, NY 10005-4001

March of Dimes Birth Defects Foundation
1275 Mamaroneck Avenue
White Plains, NY 10605

National Institute of Arthritis and Musculoskeletal and Skin Diseases Information Clearinghouse
National Institute of Arthritis and Musculoskeletal and Skin Diseases (NIAMS)
National Institutes of Health
1 AMS Circle
Bethesda, MD 20892-3675

National Association of Sports for Cerebral Palsy
66 East 34th Street
New York, NY 10016

National Cancer Institute (NCI)— General Cancer Information
Office of Cancer Communications
31 Center Drive
Building 31, Room 10A07
Bethesda, MD 20892

National Center for Health Statistics
Centers for Disease Control and Prevention
6525 Belcrest Road
Hyattsville, MD 20782

National Council on Alcoholism and Drug Dependence
20 Exchange Place
Suite 2902
New York, NY 10005

National Dairy Council
10255 West Higgins Road
Suite 900
Rosemont, IL 60018-5606

National Fire Protection Association (NFPA)
1 Batterymarch Park
Quincy, MA 02269-9101

National Health Information Center (NHIC)
Referral Specialist
P.O. Box 1133
Washington, DC 20013-1133

The National Institute of Allergy and Infectious Diseases
NIAID Office of Communications and Public Liaison
Building 31, Room 7A-50
31 Center Drive MSC 2520
Bethesda, MD 20892-2520

National Institute of Mental Health (NIMH)
Public Inquiries
6001 Executive Boulevard
Room 8184, MSC 9663
Bethesda, MD 20892-9663

National Mental Health Association
1021 Prince Street
Alexandria, VA 22314-2971

National Parents-Teachers Association
Drug and Alcohol Abuse Prevention Project
330 North Wabash Ave., Suite 2100
Chicago, IL 60611-3690

National Safety Council
1121 Spring Lake Drive
Itasca, IL 60143-3201

National Wildlife Federation
8925 Leesburg Pike
Vienna, VA 22180

Office on Smoking and Health
Centers for Disease Control and Prevention
Publications
Mail Stop K-50
4770 Buford Highway, NE
Atlanta, GA 30341-3717

Students Against Destructive Decisions
255 Main Street
P.O. Box 800
Marlboro, MA 01752

United Cerebral Palsy, Inc.
1660 L Street, NW
Suite 700
Washington, DC 20036

USDA Food and Nutrition Information and Education Resources Center
National Agricultural Library,
U.S. Department of Agriculture
10301 Baltimore Avenue, Room 304
Beltsville, MD 20705

U.S. Food and Drug Administration
Office of Consumer Affairs
5600 Fishers Lane
Rockville, MD 20857-001

Credits

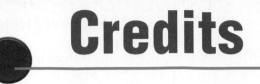

Photographs

Kevin Birch: pages 10, 19, 20 (left), 47, 61 (all), 71, 76, 132, 134 (left), 144–145, 191, 202, 224, 260.

CORBIS: Paul Barton, page 3; Ed Bohon, page 239; Jim Cummings, page 134 (center); Duomo, page 154; C. Hammell, page 164; Lawrence Manning, page 225; Tom & Dee McCarthy, page 224; Kevin R. Morris, page 216; 95 Mugshots, page 169; F. Rossotto, page 280 (top); George Schiavone, page 158; Ariel Skelley, page 224; Joseph Sohm, Visions of America, page 69; Tom Stewart, page 234.

Bob Daemmrich Photography, Inc.: pages 7, 36, 45, 105, 235, 241; Joel Salcido Photography/Bob Daemmrich Associates, page 35.

Mary Kate Denny: pages 91, 94, 110, 128, 186.

Getty Images: Bruce Ayres/Tony Stone, page 170; Chris Baker/Tony Stone, page 242; Kindra Clineff/Tony Stone, page 173; Bill Hickey/Image Bank, page 134 (right); David Madison/Tony Stone, page 161; James Randkley/Tony Stone, page 225; Ian Shaw/Tony Stone, page 165; Zubin Shroff/Tony Stone, page 225; Maria Taglienti/The Image Bank, pages 222–223; Tony Stone, pages 58, 222 (center).

Richard Hutchings: pages 5 (bottom, right), 6, 8, 14, 38, 40, 48, 62, 100.

The Image Works: page 133; L. Kolvoord, page 43; Larry Mulvehill, page 88; N. Richmond, pages 176–177; Skjold, page 269 (right).

International Stock: Kirk Anderson, page 269 (left); Scott Barrow, pages 210–211; Vincent Graziani, page 280 (bottom); Victor Ramos, page 52.

Ken Karp: pages xvi–1, 5 (left), 11, 13, 23, 24, 32, 41, 44, 46, 54 (all), 56, 59, 60, 63, 64, 68, 73 (all), 75, 78, 79 (left), 87, 90, 92, 108 (all), 109 (all), 121, 122 (all), 123 (all), 125, 127, 129, 131, 136, 142, 180–181, 189 (all), 208–209, 212, 220, 228–229, 230, 244, 245, 249, 252, 261, 264, 270, 272 (all), 275 (all), 284, 286.

Ken Lax: page 61 (center).

David Mager: pages 104, 187, 222 (left), 282.

Jordan Miller: pages 16, 118, 194.

PhotoEdit: Robert Brenner, page 20 (right); Myrleen Ferguson, pages 223 (left), 114–115, 266; Tony Freeman, pages 12, 217; Richard Hutchings, pages 148–149, 256–257, 281; Felicia Martinez, page 223 (right); Michael Newman, page 222 (right); Jonathan Nourok, pages 223 (center), 271; David Young-Wolff, pages 93, 240.

Photo Researchers Inc.: Michael Abbey, page 183 (top right); A. Glauberman/Science Source, page 219; Stevie Grand/Science Photo Library, page 276 (left); Dr. P. Marazzi/Science Photo Library, pages 198, 276 (bottom, right); Oliver Meckes/Ottawa, page 183 (bottom right); David M. Phillips, page 183 (bottom left); Tek Image/Science Photo Library, page 182; Jon Wilson/Science Photo Library, page 183 (top left).

PictureQuest: Michael Newman/PhotoEdit, page 126; Frank Siteman/Stock Boston, page 265 (background).

Michael Provost: pages 84–85, 250, 251.

Skjold Photographs: page 27.

Stock Boston: Mark C. Burnett, page 280 (middle); Bob Daemmrich, pages 137, 243; John Lei, page 201.

SuperStock: pages 4, 278, 279; Florian Franke, page 30; Kwame Zikomo, pages 82–83.

Terry Sutherland: pages 99, 120, 130, 141.

Unicorn Stock Photos: Aneal Vohra, page 265 (foreground).

The Terry Wild Studio: pages 22, 26, 34, 79 (right).

Illustrations

Ron Boisvert: pages 157, 214–215.

Max Crandall: page 38.

Robert A. Deverell: pages 49, 98, 101, 102, 103, 135, 139, 143, 144, 177, 185, 193, 196, 197, 204, 205, 218, 232, 246, 283, 285.

Jerry Gonzalez: pages 70, 213, 262.

Jim Higgins/The Mazer Corporation: page 15.

David Kelley Design: pages 89, 95, 97, 153, 156, 166, 171, 200.

Catherine Leery/Martha Productions: pages 33, 55, 138, 174–175, 184, 258–259.

Andy Levine: pages 65, 116–117, 203.

Alvalyn Lundgren: pages 87, 268, 273.

Erin Mauterer/Bluewater: pages 286–287.

Hilda Muinos: pages 86, 150–151, 155 (left), 159, 162, 163.

Network Graphics: pages 42, 93, 96, 160, 167, 231, 233, 236, 267, 274.

Parrot Graphics: pages 119, 237, 238.

Mary Power: page 124.

Precision Graphics: page 155 (right).

Jerry Zimmerman: pages 21, 37, 66, 74, 110–111, 168, 221, 247, 263.